Edited by
Roger Narayan and Paul Calvert

Computer Aided Biomanufacturing

Related Titles

Kumar, C. S. S. R. (ed.)

Tissue, Cell and Organ Engineering

2006
ISBN: 978-3-527-31389-1

Noorani, R. I.

Rapid Prototyping
Principles and Applications

2005
ISBN: 978-0-471-73001-9

Minuth, W. W., Strehl, R., Schumacher, K.

Tissue Engineering
Essentials for Daily Laboratory Work

2005
ISBN: 978-3-527-31186-6

Baltes, H., Brand, O., Fedder, G. K., Hierold, C., Korvink, J. G., Tabata, O. (eds.)

Enabling Technologies for MEMS and Nanodevices
Advanced Micro and Nanosystems

2004
ISBN: 978-3-527-30746-3

Edited by
Roger Narayan and Paul Calvert

Computer Aided Biomanufacturing

WILEY-VCH Verlag GmbH & Co. KGaA

The Editors

Prof. Roger J. Narayan
North Carolina State Univers.
Dept. of Biomed. Engineering
2147 Burlington Labs
Raleigh, NC 27695-7115
USA

Prof. Paul Calvert
Dept. of Textile Sc. Rm 218
Univ. of Massachusetts
285 Old Westport Rd.
Dartmouth, MA 02747
USA

■ All books published by **Wiley-VCH** are carefully produced. Nevertheless, authors, editors, and publisher do not warrant the information contained in these books, including this book, to be free of errors. Readers are advised to keep in mind that statements, data, illustrations, procedural details or other items may inadvertently be inaccurate.

Library of Congress Card No.: applied for

British Library Cataloguing-in-Publication Data
A catalogue record for this book is available from the British Library.

Bibliographic information published by the Deutsche Nationalbibliothek
The Deutsche Nationalbibliothek lists this publication in the Deutsche Nationalbibliografie; detailed bibliographic data are available on the Internet at http://dnb.d-nb.de.

© 2011 Wiley-VCH Verlag & Co. KGaA, Boschstr. 12, 69469 Weinheim, Germany

All rights reserved (including those of translation into other languages). No part of this book may be reproduced in any form – by photoprinting, microfilm, or any other means – nor transmitted or translated into a machine language without written permission from the publishers. Registered names, trademarks, etc. used in this book, even when not specifically marked as such, are not to be considered unprotected by law.

Composition   Thomson Digital, Noida, India
Printing and Binding   Fabulous Printers Pte Ltd
Cover Design   Grafik-Design Schulz, Fußgönheim

Printed in Singapore
Printed on acid-free paper

Print ISBN: 978-3-527-40906-8

Contents

Computer-Aided Biomanufacturing: Introduction *1*
Roger Narayan

1 **Towards a Multi-scale Computerized Bone Diagnostic System: 2D Micro-scale Finite Element Analysis** *8*
Lev Podshivalov, Yaron Holdstein, Anath Fischer, and Pinhas Bar-Yoseph
Update *26*

2 **Hierarchical Starch-Based Fibrous Scaffold for Bone Tissue Engineering Applications** *32*
Albino Martins, Sangwon Chung, Adriano J. Pedro, Sofia G. Caridade, João F. Mano, Rui A. Sousa, Alexandra P. Marques, Rui L. Reis, and Nuno M. Neves
Update *39*

3 **Bacterial and *Candida albicans* Adhesion of Rapid Prototyping-Produced 3D-Scaffolds Manufactured as Bone Replacement Materials** *54*
Ali Al-Ahmad, Margit Wiedmann-Al-Ahmad, Carlos Carvalho, and Elmar Hellwig
Update *66*

4 **Electric Field Driven Jetting: An Emerging Approach for Processing Living Cells** *72*
Suwan N. Jayasinghe, Peter A.M. Eagles and Amer N. Qureshi

5 **Inkjet Printing of Bioadhesives** *82*
Anand Doraiswamy, Timothy M. Dunaway, Jonathan J. Wilker, Roger J. Narayan

6 **Laser Microfabrication of Hydroxyapatite-Osteoblast-Like Cell Composites** *92*
A. Doraiswamy, R. J. Narayan, M. L. Harris, S. B. Qadri, R. Modi, D. B. Chrisey

7   Two Photon Polymerization of Polymer–Ceramic Hybrid
    Materials for Transdermal Drug Delivery   102
    A. Ovsianikov and B. Chichkov, P. Mente, N. A. Monteiro-Riviere,
    A. Doraiswamy, R. J. Narayan

8   Simultaneous Immobilization of Bioactives During 3D Powder
    Printing of Bioceramic Drug-Release Matrices   112
    By Elke Vorndran, Uwe Klammert, Andrea Ewald, Jake E. Barralet,
    and Uwe Gbureck

9   Structural and Mechanical Evaluations of a Topology Optimized Titanium
    Interbody Fusion Cage Fabricated by Selective Laser Melting Process   120
    Chia-Ying Lin, Tobias Wirtz, Frank LaMarca, Scott J. Hollister

10 Monitoring Muscle Growth and Tissue Changes Induced
    by Electrical Stimulation of Denervated Degenerated Muscles
    with CT and Stereolithographic 3D Modeling   130
    Thordur Helgason, Paolo Gargiulo, Sigrun Knutsdottir,
    Vilborg Gudmundsdottir, Helmut Kern, Ugo Carraro,
    Stefan Yngvason, and Pall Ingvarsson
    Update   135

11 CAD-CAM Construction of a Provisional Nasal Prosthesis After
    Ablative Tumour Surgery of the Nose: A Pilot Case Report   148
    Leonardo Ciocca, Massimiliano Fantini, Francesca De Crescenzio,
    and Roberto Scotti
    Update   154

12 Individually Prefabricated Prosthesis for Maxilla
    Reconstruction   162
    Sekou Singare, Yaxiong Liu, Dichen Li, Bingheng Lu, Jue Wang, and Sanhu He
    Update   169

13 The Use of Rapid Prototyping Didactic Models
    in the Study of Fetal Malformations   176
    H. Werner, J.R. Lopes dos Santos, R. Fontes, E.L. Gasparetto,
    P.A. Daltro, Y. Kuroki, and R.C. Domingues
    Update   179

14 Non-invasive Archaeology of Skeletal Material by CT Scanning
    and Three-Dimensional Reconstruction   184
    Niels Lynnerup
    Update   189

    Index   191

Computer-Aided Biomanufacturing: Introduction

Roger Narayan

Computer-aided biomanufacturing, also known as rapid prototyping, layer manufacturing, or solid freeform fabrication, is a technology involving additive layer-by-layer fabrication of a three-dimensional, biologically relevant structure through selective joining of material; fabrication of the structure is guided by a computer-aided design (CAD) model [1–3]. Computer-aided biomanufacturing methods were independently developed in the late twentieth century by investigators working with several groups, including 3D Systems Inc., Stratsys Inc., the Massachusetts Institute of Technology, and the University of Texas at Austin [2].

In computer-aided biomanufacturing, the surface of the computer-aided design model is converted to a series of polygons (in a process known as tessellation) and sliced into collections of cross-sectional layers. The structure is subsequently fabricated in a layer-by-layer manner along the Z-direction; the layers extend in the X- and Y- directions [3]. Direct computer-aided biomanufacturing methods involve addition of material in solid, liquid, or powder form according to the design of the model. Indirect computer-aided biomanufacturing methods may also be used, which involve processing of structures using computer-aided biomanufacturing-fabricated molds or patterns [2]. For example, computer-aided biomanufacturing methods can be used to create structures for subsequent use in investment casting, sand casting, or injection molding [3]. One advantage of indirect methods over direct methods is that the chemical, corrosion, biological, and mechanical properties of the material used to create the final structure may be conserved since this material does not undergo the computer-aided biomanufacturing process.

This book describes recent efforts to fabricate a variety of medical devices, including patient-specific prostheses, microstructured medical devices, and artificial tissues, using computer-aided biomanufacturing techniques. For example, data obtained from computed tomography, magnetic resonance imaging, or other noninvasive imaging techniques may be employed in order to create prostheses or artificial tissues with patient-specific geometries or other patient-specific features [4–8]. One possible application of computer-aided biomanufacturing is the development of cell-seeded scaffolds for replacement of various tissues, including blood vessel, bone, cartilage, liver, nerve, and skin [5, 8]. The demand to replace

Computer Aided Biomanufacturing, Edited by Roger Narayan and Paul Calvert
© 2011 WILEY-VCH Verlag GmbH & Co. KGaA. Published 2011 by WILEY-VCH Verlag GmbH & Co. KGaA.

damaged or diseased tissues has led to the development of tissue engineering, which involves creating artificial tissues by placing living cells within three-dimensional scaffolds created out of resorbable polymers (poly(lactic acid)), hydrogels (poly(vinyl alcohol)), or naturally derived materials (collagen). The scaffold serves as a synthetic extracellular matrix, providing mechanical support and guiding cell development [4–7]. Many primary organ cells are believed to require a scaffold material for attachment and growth [6]. The use of extracellular matrix components and other biologically active materials as scaffold materials has been considered due to the fact that these materials possess protein and polysaccharide molecules, which are believed to promote cell adhesion [8]. The cell-seeded scaffold is then transferred to a bioreactor, which provides nutrients that enable cells to multiply within the scaffold. The cell-seeded scaffold is subsequently implanted in the body, where the artificial tissue assumes the function of its natural counterpart. Many scaffold materials undergo degradation after implantation within the body.

Cells or biological molecules may be incorporated within scaffold structures during the computer-aided biomanufacturing process. For example, growth factors or proteins may be placed at specific locations within hierarchical scaffold structures in order to modulate cell attachment and differentiation [4–6]. Surface features may be incorporated into scaffold structures in order to promote cell–prosthesis interactions; for example, interconnected pores with dimensions between 100 and 300 μm (depending on cell type) and vascular structures may be incorporated within scaffolds in order to allow cell ingrowth, diffusion of nutrients to cells, and diffusion of waste matter from cells [4]. Unlike conventional methods, computer-aided biomanufacturing methods enable the development of scaffolds containing pores with well-defined chemistries, sizes, densities, and orientations [6]. In addition, small-scale surface features may be used to increase cell attachment and/or guide cell growth [4].

Computer-aided biomanufacturing methods may be used to create prostheses (e. g., dental crowns and cranial prostheses) that match patient anatomy for clinical use; patient-specific prostheses may lead to both reduced postoperative complications and improved aesthesis [9, 10]. These methods have also been used to fabricate models for visualizing the anatomical features of a patient in order to facilitate surgical planning; anatomical models may serve to improve diagnosis accuracy and reduce operating time [9]. Finally, computer-aided biomanufacturing methods may also be used to create prototypes of medical devices or prostheses for evaluation, optimization, and iteration purposes [11].

Several computer-aided biomanufacturing techniques, including fused deposition modeling, stereolithography apparatus (SLA), selective laser sintering (SLS), laser direct writing, microcontact printing, and inkjet printing, have been used to prepare medical devices, prostheses, and scaffolds for tissue engineering. The advantages and disadvantages of several computer-aided biomanufacturing techniques are described in Table 1 [1]. Many of these processes (e.g., microsyringe-based systems) allow for computer-aided biomanufacturing of materials at low temperatures. It is important to note that many computer-aided biomanufacturing technologies can be placed in conventional clinical environments (e.g., clinical medicine facilities) that do not contain specialized equipment (e.g., cleanroom facilities). Unlike conventional

Table 1 Comparison of rapid prototyping technologies used in medical devices and tissue engineering.

Rapid Prototyping Technique	Resolution (μm)	Strengths	Weaknesses
3D Bioplotter	250	Compatible with many materials; biomolecules may be incorporated	Completed part may exhibit low mechanical strength; smooth surfaces required; low accuracy; slow processing times
3D Printing™	200	Microscale porosity may be introduced; compatible with many materials; water may be used as binder; no support structure needed; rapid processing times	Material must be in powder form; completed part may exhibit low mechanical strength; powdery surface finish; trapped powder may be present in completed part; may require postprocessing steps
3D inkjet printer	180	Compatible with many materials; control of external and internal morphology	Multiple steps involved
3D Fiber deposition technique	250	Input material in pellet form	High temperature; difficult to prepare structures with microscale porosity
Fused deposition modeling (FDM)	250	Good mechanical strength; control of external and internal morphology	High temperature; need to produce filament material; difficult to prepare structures with microscale porosity
Multinozzle deposition manufacturing (MDM)	400	Compatible with many materials; biomolecules may be incorporated; low-temperature process	Use of solvent required; freeze drying required
Precision extruding deposition (PED)	250	Input material in pellet form	High temperature; difficult to prepare structures with microscale porosity
Precise extrusion manufacturing (PEM)	200–500	Input material in pellet form	High temperature; difficult to prepare structures with microscale porosity
Pressure-assisted microsyringe (PAM)	10–600	Compatible with many materials; biomolecules may be incorporated	Use of solvent required; small nozzle size inhibits incorporation of particles; narrow range of printable viscosities

(*Continued*)

Table .1 (*Continued*)

Rapid Prototyping Technique	Resolution (μm)	Strengths	Weaknesses
Rapid prototyping robotic dispensing system (RPBOD)	400–1000	Compatible with many materials; biomolecules may be incorporated	Precise control of material and medium properties; freeze drying required
Robocasting	100–1000	Compatible with many materials	Precise control of ink properties necessary
Selective laser sintering	500	Microporosity induced in the part; compatible with many materials; no support structure needed; rapid processing times	Material must be in powder form; high temperatures are required; powdery surface finish; trapped powder may be present in finished part
Stereolithography apparatus	250	Compatible with many materials; no support structure needed; rapid processing times	Material must be photocross-linkable and cytocompatible; involves the use of ultraviolet light
TheriForm™	300	Microporosity induced in the part; compatible with many materials; nonorganic binders may be used; no support structures needed; rapid processing times	Material must be in powder form; powdery surface finish; trapped powder may be present in finished part
Two photon polymerization	<1	Control of external and internal morphology; involves the use of infrared light	Material must be photocross-linkable and cytocompatible

Source: Reproduced from Ref. [1] with permission of ASM International®.

machining-based processes, structures with complex internal geometries (e.g., catheters with interlocking tips or organs with complex internal structures) may be generated using computer-aided biomanufacturing processes [3–5, 8, 10, 11]. Most importantly, computer-aided biomanufacturing processes can produce structures more rapidly and with fewer steps than conventional machining-based processes; according to Hou *et al.*, the product development cycle may be decreased to between 10% and 20% of traditional methods [4, 12].

Solid-based computer-aided biomanufacturing techniques involve the joining or fusing of extruded material [13, 14]. In fused deposition modeling, material is melted and subsequently extruded into thin filaments on a mobile platform, which can operate along X-, Y-, and Z- planes. The filaments solidify and cold weld with previously deposited material [3, 13]. Structures containing several thermoplastic polymers, including polyethylene, poly (ε-caprolactone), and polypropylene, have been obtained using this method [8]. Critical processing parameters include the laser spot size and the powder size [6]. One of the disadvantages of fused deposition modeling is the high operating temperature; processing of many biological materials is precluded [14]. In addition, materials prepared using this process exhibit very high porosities and poor mechanical properties. Several variants of the fused deposition modeling process were developed to overcome these limitations, including precision extrusion manufacturing, low-temperature deposition manufacturing, and rapid prototyping robotic dispensing. For example, a technique known as three-dimensional printing has been used to prepare porous scaffolds at room temperature; in this technique, a binder material is used to selectively attach powder located on a powder bed [14].

Liquid-based techniques involve selective solidification of material in the liquid phase [12]. In stereolithography, a liquid resin containing monomers is selectively solidified upon exposure to radiation from an ultraviolet laser (e.g., an argon ion laser or a helium–cadmium laser). In this technique, movement of a Z-height stage controls exposure of the laser to a liquid resin reservoir. X- and Y-stage movements may be used to pattern the material in the Z-plane. The laser polymerizes the photocurable liquid resin layer to generate a layer of solidified material. The table is then lowered and another layer is selectively cured. This layer-by-layer buildup process is repeated until the desired three-dimensional structure is obtained. The structure is then removed from the liquid reservoir, baked (exposed to light for further polymerization), and cleaned. Photosensitive polymers, including acrylate polymers, have been processed using this method. Several factors, including encoder resolution, table step height, laser spot size, and laser performance determine the resolution of structures prepared using stereolithography. The biological, chemical, and mechanical properties of the resins, breakdown products, diluents, and dispersants used in stereolithography may not be suitable for many medical and biological applications [15, 16].

Powder-based computer-aided biomanufacturing techniques involve selective melting of powders or granules in a powder bed using a high-power carbon dioxide laser. In selective laser sintering, the powder is annealed to a temperature close to its transition melting point prior to laser exposure; only a small increase in temperature is required to cause localized melting. A three-dimensional structure is formed by lowering the height-adjustable table containing the powder bed after processing of each layer. This technique has been utilized to fabricate complex porous ceramic structures that are suitable for implantation in a bone defect [17]. Many other materials, including nylon, polystyrene, polyurethane, polystyrene, and titanium, may also be processed using selective laser sintering [2]. The technique has the capability to process three-dimensional structures with complex features, including overhangs and undercuts. In fused deposition modeling, the critical processing parameter is the nozzle diameter [6]. Materials processed using selective laser sintering generally exhibit high porosities and high surface roughness values; this fact may preclude the use of fused deposition modeling in many medical applications. It should be noted that molten metal can be infiltrated within as-prepared structures in order to create dense structures [3]. Thermal distortion of selective laser sintering-fabricated structures is also possible [3].

We anticipate that computer-aided biomanufacturing will play a growing role in medical care in the coming decades. Research activities are needed to overcome limitations associated with present computer-aided biomanufacturing technologies. A reduction in the minimum feature size from the micrometer (10^{-6} m) regime to the nanometer (10^{-9} m) regime would enable more complex cell–material interactions and would expand the number of potential medical applications. The use of computer-aided biomanufacturing processes with a wider variety of materials, including materials with low shrinkage rates and materials that do not require high-temperature processing, would also be of benefit [4]. In addition, the development of computer-aided biomanufacturing-compatible materials with improved biological, chemical, corrosion, mechanical, and tribological properties would be useful. Finally, the capital equipment costs associated with purchasing and operating computer-aided biomanufacturing equipment must fall in line with those of conventional machining equipment. If these obstacles can be overcome, computer-aided biomanufacturing will play a leading role in fabrication of structures for biological and medical applications.

References

1 Boland, T., Chickov, B.N., Chua, C.K., Doraiswamy, A., Leong, K.F., Narayan, R.J., Ovsianikov, A., and Yeong, W.Y. (2007) Rapid prototyping of artificial tissues and medical devices. *Adv. Mater. Proc.*, **4**, 51–53.

2 Groover, M.P. (2007) *Fundamentals of Modern Manufacturing: Materials, Processing, and Systems*, 3rd edn, John Wiley & Sons Ltd., New York.

3 Pham, D.T. and Gault, R.S. (1998) A comparison of rapid prototyping technologies. *Int. J. Mach. Tool Manufact.*, **38**, 1257–1287.

4 Peltola, S.M., Melchels, F.P.W., Grijpma, D.W., and Kelloma, M. (2008) A review of rapid prototyping techniques for tissue engineering purposes. *Ann. Med.*, **40**, 268–280.

5 Sun, W. and Lal, P. (2002) Recent development on computer aided tissue engineering: a review. *Comp. Methods Programs Biomed.*, **67**, 85–103.

6 Yang, S., Leong, K.F., Du, Z., and Chua, C.K. (2002) The design of scaffolds for use

in tissue engineering. Part II. Rapid prototyping techniques. *Tissue Eng.*, **8**, 1–12.
7 Yeong, W., Chua, C., Leong, K., and Chandrasekaran, M. (2004) Rapid prototyping in tissue engineering: challenges and potential. *Trends Biotechnol.*, **22**, 643–652.
8 Sun, W., Darling, A., Starly, B., and Nam, J. (2004) Computer-aided tissue engineering: overview, scope, and challenges. *Biotechnol. Appl. Biochem.*, **39**, 29–47.
9 Webb, P.A. (2000) A review of rapid prototyping (RP) techniques in the medical and biomedical sector. *J. Med. Eng. Technol.*, **24**, 149–153.
10 Azari, A. and Nikzad, S. (2002) The evolution of rapid prototyping in dentistry: a review. *Inform. Software Technol.*, **44**, 579–592.
11 Yan, X. and Gu, P. (1996) A review of rapid prototyping technologies and systems. *Comput. Aided. Des.*, **28**, 307–318.
12 Hou, Y.L., Zhao, T.T., Li, C.H., and Ding, Y.C. (2010) The manufacturing of rapid tooling by stereo lithography. *Adv. Mater. Res.*, **102–104**, 578–582.
13 Kai, C.C., Fai, L.F., and Chu-Sing, L. (2003) *Rapid Prototyping: Principles and Applications*, 2nd edn, World Scientific Publishing, Singapore.
14 Hutmacher, D.W., Sittinger, M., and Risbud, M.V. (2004) Scaffold-based tissue engineering: rationale for computer-aided design and solid free-form fabrication systems. *Trends Biotechnol.*, **22**, 354–362.
15 Despa, F., Orgill, D.P., Neuwalder, J., and Lee, R.C. (2005) The relative thermal stability of tissue macromolecules and cellular structure in burn injury. *Burns*, **31**, 568–577.
16 Nishigori, C. (2006) Cellular aspects of photocarcinogenesis. *Photochem. Photobiol. Sci.*, **5**, 208–214.
17 Vail, N.K., Swain, L.D., Fox, W.C., Aufdlemorte, G., Lee, G., and Barlow, J.W. (1999) Materials for biomedical applications. *Mater. Des.*, **20**, 123–132.

1
Towards a Multi-scale Computerized Bone Diagnostic System: 2D Micro-scale Finite Element Analysis

Towards a multi-scale computerized bone diagnostic system: 2D micro-scale finite element analysis

L. Podshivalov*,†, Y. Holdstein, A. Fischer and P. Z. Bar-Yoseph

Faculty of Mechanical Engineering, Technion—Israel Institute of Technology, Haifa 32000, Israel

SUMMARY

Currently, there is major interest within the biomedical community in developing accurate non-invasive means for analyzing bone micro-structure. This paper presents a new approach for a multi-scale finite element (FE) analysis of a trabecular structure. Two domain decomposition approaches are investigated as a basis for computational analysis at the micro-scale level, which is then applied for solving a 2D elasticity FE problem. In addition, a homogenization procedure from micro- to macro-scale level is presented. The proposed new multi-scale FE method has the potential to provide new insights into bone structure and behavior. Moreover, it is expected that the outcomes of this research will develop into a computerized virtual biopsy system. Copyright © 2008 John Wiley & Sons, Ltd.

Received 31 March 2008; Revised 8 August 2008; Accepted 21 November 2008

KEY WORDS: bone diagnostic system; bone micro-structure; multi-scale finite elements analysis; micro-CT/MRI

1. OVERVIEW

Metabolic bone diseases are at the forefront of scientific and biomedical research worldwide. The United Nations, the World Health Organization (WHO) and more than 60 countries have proclaimed the period 2000–2010 as the Bone and Joint Decade [1]. Bone is composed of hierarchical bio-composite materials with complex multi-scale structural geometry and complex behavior. Metabolic bone diseases such as osteoporosis are characterized by micro-architectural deterioration of bone tissue, leading to micro fractures; therefore, early diagnosis is a key to intervention. Currently, bone disease is diagnosed at the macro-scale of bone structure by decreased bone mineral density

---

*Correspondence to: L. Podshivalov, Faculty of Mechanical Engineering, Technion—Israel Institute of Technology, Haifa 32000, Israel.
†E-mail: slpod@tx.technion.ac.il

Contract/grant sponsor: Technion—Israel Institute of Technology
Contract/grant sponsor: Medical-Engineering Collaboration 2007
Contract/grant sponsor: Irwin and Joan Jacobs Fellowship 2008

Copyright © 2008 John Wiley & Sons, Ltd.
Computer Aided Biomanufacturing, Edited by Roger Narayan and Paul Calvert
© 2011 WILEY-VCH Verlag GmbH & Co. KGaA. Published 2011 by WILEY-VCH Verlag GmbH & Co. KGaA.

(BMD) and/or by characteristic osteoporotic fractures. These techniques provide 2D scalar results at the bone macro-scale level, and thus cannot accurately assess the 3D micro-scale level of the bone. Emerging medical imaging technology provides the means for high resolution *in vivo* and *in vitro* scanning of bone models at the micro-scale level. However, no reliable and complete diagnostic method that incorporates these technical abilities has been proposed to date.

The first step in 3D analysis of scanned tissue is the reconstruction of the 3D model from the medical images. 3D model reconstruction can be divided into two main categories: surface reconstruction [2, 3] and volumetric reconstruction [4]. Subsequently, even if the visualization quality of the reconstructed geometric model is high, it is not sufficient for finite element (FE) analyses. Therefore, optimization and remeshing are required to enable such analyses.

Micro-scale models are analyzed using the micro FE method developed a decade ago. This method has the following disadvantages: (a) the micro FE method can solve only a small bone volume due to computational limits; (b) transition from macro-scale to micro-scale models requires recomputing the entire micro-scale model; and (c) transition from micro-scale to macro-scale models requires homogenizing the micro-scale model, thus disregarding micro-scale characteristics of bone architecture. These disadvantages stem from the fact that the geometrical and computational models of the macro- and micro-scale levels are separate. Therefore, a new multi-scale FE method is needed for robust multi-scale analysis of bone architecture.

The paper is organized as follows. Section 2 describes the bone hierarchical structure and Section 3 presents current macro-scale BMD scanning techniques. Section 4 discusses issues of 3D model reconstruction from micro computed tomography/micro magnetic resonance imaging (μCT/μMRI) images. Sections 5 and 6 are dedicated to an overview of the micro-scale FEA and multi-scale FE methods, respectively. In Section 7 we present our new approach to multi-scale FE analysis. In Section 8 we provide preliminary results of our research for FE analysis at the micro-scale level and the homogenization technique for transition from micro- to macro-scale levels. Finally, Section 9 summarizes this paper and describes future work.

2. BONE HIERARCHICAL STRUCTURE

Bones are composed of hierarchical bio-composite materials characterized by complex multi-scale structural geometry and complex behavior. Bone tissue structure can be classified into five structural levels [5, 6] ranging from macro-scale to nano components:

- Macro-structure (mm–μm): trabecular and cortical bone.
- Micro-structure (10–500 μm): osteons and trabeculae.
- Sub-micro-structure (1–10 μm): lamellae and single trabecula.
- Nano-structure (100 nm–1 μm): fibrillar collagen and embedded mineral.
- Sub-nano-structure (<100 nm): molecular structure of mineral, collagen and non-collagenous organic proteins.

Depending upon the anatomical site, bone architecture differs significantly at the micro-structural level with respect to shape, thickness, element direction and size. For example, the rod-like structures at the vertebra differ significantly from the plate-like structure at the femoral head, as shown in Figure 1. Bone architecture can also vary at different locations on the same site as a result of functionality and locally applied forces characterized by magnitude and direction. Thus,

MULTI-SCALE COMPUTERIZED BONE DIAGNOSTIC SYSTEM

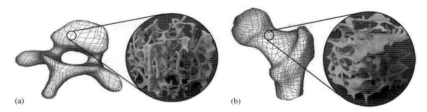

Figure 1. Characteristic bone micro-structure: (a) rod-like structure of the lumbar spine vertebrae and (b) plate-like structure of femoral head bone.

each patient's bone structure is unique and is influenced by gender, age, life style and physical condition. These characteristics are crucial for diagnosis of bone metabolic disease.

3. MACRO-SCALE BONE ANALYSIS

The WHO has chosen BMD measurements for diagnosing osteoporosis [7]. The most widely used techniques for assessing BMD are: (a) dual-energy X-ray absorptiometry (DEXA); (b) dual photon absorptiometry (DPA); (c) ultrasound; and (d) quantitative computerized tomography (QCT), the only technique capable of providing 3D results. BMD results are reported as a scalar representing a statistical value (T-score). Following is a brief description of these techniques:

- DEXA uses two different X-ray beams to estimate real BMD and is widely used in vertebrae and hip bones. It is fast and uses very low doses of radiation. Smaller and less expensive units for assessing the peripheral skeleton, such as the distal forearm and the middle phalanx of the non-dominant upper limb, are also available. These units can be used for monitoring therapy and for comparison with original measurements taken at the hip or vertebrae. A typical image obtained using this method is shown in Figure 2(a).
- DPA uses low doses of a radioactive substance to produce radiation, but has a slower scan time than the other methods.
- Ultrasound is a rapid and painless technique that does not use potentially harmful radiation such as X-rays.
- QCT is the most sensitive method, but involves substantially greater radiation exposure than DEXA. Modern QCT machines can provide spatial resolution of up to 150 µm and thus offer an initial glance at the 3D structure of the bone. A typical image obtained using this method shown in Figure 2(b).

BMD values are compared with a characteristic gender and age-dependent statistical distribution graph, and based on this comparison are used to classify patients into three categories: (a) normal; (b) osteopenic; and (c) osteoporotic. Patients with normal BMD values need no further therapy. Osteopenic patients should be counseled and treated with preventive therapy. Osteoporotic patients should receive active therapy aimed at increasing bone density and decreasing fracture risk. This approach is applicable to the normal and osteopenic BMD groups only in the absence of osteoporotic

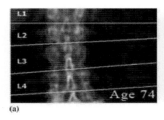
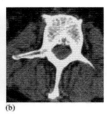

Figure 2. Typical images obtained using: (a) dual-energy X-ray absorptiometry and (b) quantitative CT.

fractures. Although BMD testing is commonly used, it presents a number of limitations:

- The BMD result does not describe the complex 3D bone micro-structure. It only offers an indication with a single scalar value.
- BMD is not applied on 3D micro-architecture.
- BMD assesses bone strength with only 70% reliability.
- BMD is difficult to measure accurately.
- No uniform threshold exists for all instruments and sites.

As a result, the BMD method occasionally fails to diagnose risk of osteoporotic fractures [8], leading to unreliable diagnosis and incorrect treatment.

The necessity for diagnosis of micro-structures has lead to the development of 3D micro-scale scanning methods. 3D models can be constructed from these scans using surface and volumetric reconstruction methods, and then adapted to bone micro-structure analysis. However, these analysis techniques cannot fully incorporate the advantages of high-resolution models.

4. RECONSTRUCTION OF 3D MODELS FROM μCT/μMRI IMAGES

Mesh reconstruction from μCT/μMRI images produced by commercial software often results in a highly distorted triangulation that is not suitable for FE mechanical analysis, and therefore requires remeshing and mesh optimization. These operations are time consuming and sometimes demand manual user interventions. We examined the quality of a 3D mesh model (84 K triangles) created from μCT images by a typical commercial scanning system. For evaluation we used three characteristic parameters [9, 10] commonly used in the professional literature and commercial software: (a) minimum angle that in an ideal mesh equals $60°$; (b) in radius to circumradius ratio; and (c) shortest edge length to circumradius ratio in an ideal mesh; these ratios are equal to 2 and 0.5, respectively. We applied the following two remeshing methods on the original mesh and compared the resulting mesh quality with this set of parameters:

- Neural network (NN)-based method [11].
- Remeshing tool of hypermesh software [12].

We chose the NN-based method because it is characterized as a learning process that uses simplified mathematical models. During the learning process, the mesh is adaptively fitted to the unknown given shape.

The growing neural gas (GNG) method developed by Fritzke [13] approximates a network consisting only of neurons and edges to the cloud of sampled points. The meshing growing neural gas neural network (MGNG) method, described by Holdstein and Fischer [3] extracts surfaces from the NN, thus creating a high-quality triangular mesh. The NN-based remeshing method [11] is an extension of the MGNG method.

In our case, the cloud of sampled points is derived from a low-quality mesh and then remeshed. The mesh quality analyses are presented in Table I. The analyses were classified into two groups, 'poor/average' and 'good/excellent', for each parameter as follows:

- Quality values of all elements were scaled to fit a range (0, 1].
- The scale was classified as 'poor/average', (0, 0.5] or 'good/excellent' (0.5, 1].

Based on the conducted analysis, the following conclusions can be drawn:

- The original mesh is not suitable for FE analysis due to the high percentage of skewed triangles (~40%) as shown in Figure 3.
- The remeshed meshes are of significantly higher quality than the original mesh. The mesh quality improved by an average of 20–30% on all used criteria, thus creating a mesh suitable for FE analysis.
- The number of elements in the high-quality meshes increased threefold using the NN-based remeshing method and almost tenfold with hypermesh. Hence, the number of degrees of freedom (DOFs) of these meshes is increased as well. Micro-structures that are initially characterized by a large number of elements, increasing the number of elements is not desired. This consequence will slow down the solution process and requires additional computer resources.
- The mesh of the highest quality, generated by the hypermesh tool, still includes several hundred (250–500) low-quality triangles. These triangles need to be treated manually before further analysis. Such treatment may involve additional optimization.

Figure 3 shows the original low-quality mesh and the two resulting meshes after applying the above described remeshing methods. In the first mesh, depicted in Figure 3(a), 47% of triangles failed the minimum/maximum angles test. The second mesh (Figure 3(b)) was remeshed using the NN-based method and its quality improved to only 22% failure in the same test. The last mesh

Table I. Mesh quality numerical analysis for three meshes: (a) minimal angle; (b) inradius to circumradius ratio; and (c) shortest edge length to circumradius ratio.

	Mesh					
	Original mesh		NN Remesher		Hypermesh	
Criterion	Poor/Avr. (%)	Good/Exc. (%)	Poor/Avr. (%)	Good/Exc. (%)	Poor/Avr. (%)	Good/Exc. (%)
Minimal angle	39	61	18	82	2	98
Inradius to circumradius ratio	21	79	5	95	1	99
Shortest edge length to circumradius ratio	27	73	9	91	2	98
Number of elements	3K		10K		25K	

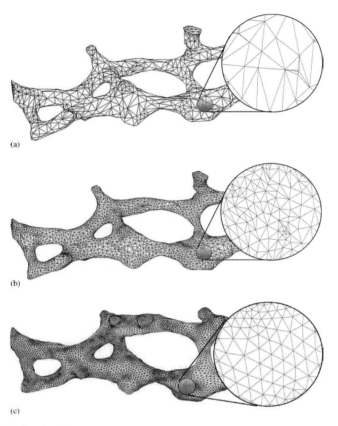

Figure 3. Quality of original and remeshed meshes: (a) original mesh; (b) remeshed with NN-based method; and (c) remeshed with hypermesh remeshing tool.

(Figure 3(c)), remeshed using the hypermesh, tool provides best mesh quality with only a 6% failure rate.

5. MICRO FE ANALYSIS

The growth in the computational resources and in the availability of parallel computing has created two trends in the area of computational mechanics: (a) an increase in the number of elements in analyzed models and (b) a decrease in the size of these elements, leading to an increase in the overall number of DOF. The combination of these two trends led to the development of micro FE analysis techniques [15].

These techniques provide a versatile tool for mechanical evaluation of bone tissue at the microstructural level [16–18]. Many researchers have begun utilizing these techniques for analyzing bone micro-structure These analyses provide better insight into the structural adaptation of bones to internal and external physical loads and better diagnosis of osteoporosis [19].

Existing 3D meshing methods for micro-structure generate brick elements that lack geometrical continuity and precision. Hexahedral elements have become popular due to efficient computational strategies for solution of large FE applications [20]. These strategies are based on direct conversion of a voxel into a 'brick' hexahedral element, thus avoiding time-consuming computations of a stiffness matrix and a force vector for each element.

State-of-the-art micro-FE methods today are based on parallel computing of large high-resolution specimens of human bone reconstructed from μCT/μMRI images, as demonstrated by Arbenz et al. [16] in 2006. More than 1100 AMD processors were used for analyzing the distal part (20% of the length) of the radius of a human forearm with 30 μm spatial resolution. Despite the above achievements, the μFE method has the following disadvantages:

- The accuracy of FE analysis is reduced by the discretization of the structure into brick elements.
- Achieving high precision of the computational model requires a large number of hexahedral elements, thus increasing the computational complexity.
- Uncertainties in choosing boundary conditions at the load patterns result in inaccurate solutions.
- Only a small bone volume can be solved using reasonable computational resources.

The above technique does not represent a mechanical multi-scale analysis that is based on a macro–micro model, and is limited in terms of the precision required for medical applications and reliable diagnosis.

6. MULTI-SCALE FE METHODS

The multi-scale approach is used in problems where we wish to take advantage of both the simplicity and the efficiency of the macroscopic models as well as the accuracy of the detailed microscopic model by coupling macroscopic and microscopic models [21]. The multi-scale models facilitate fast transition between the scales without accumulative errors.

From the viewpoint of computational methods, there has already been a long history of using multi-scale concepts in methods such as the multi-grid method and adaptive mesh refinement [22, 23]. Traditional multi-scale methods, such as the multi grid, are actually micro-scale solvers. Their purpose is to resolve the details of the solutions of the large micro-scale model. As a result, their cost is high.

Bone tissue is a hierarchical material whose architecture differs at each level of hierarchy. Moreover, mechanical properties of the bone at the micro-scale level can vary considerably even on the same bone/model due to bone heterogeneity. Thus, a multi-scale approach for mechanical analysis of the bone is imperative.

Although effective models can be obtained with satisfactory accuracy for microscopic processes, as in the case of μFE, they have limitations. Such models provide too much information that may be of little interest, further complicating the process of extracting useful data.

Recently developed multi-scale methods capture the micro-scale behavior of the model at a cost that is much less than the full cost of micro-scale solvers [21] by focusing only on the small volume at the micro-scale level. These multi-scale methods allow only two binary scales: macro- and micro-scale; no intermediate scales can be represented. The known approach is the adaptive modeling method [24]. This method is based on modeling an entire model using a macro-scale homogeneous model, and embedding this model into the *Volume of Interest*. Such embedding can be performed using the local mechanical energy conservation between the mechanical states of the different scales [25] or the mesh superposition method [26]. However, in this method, enlarging the area of interest will consequently increase the computational complexity of the solution and will require additional computational resources.

Analyzing strengths and weaknesses of the most common multi-scale methods showed that no one method has an overwhelming advantage over the others. Methods that allow hierarchical mesh representations and are simple to implement do not include hierarchical physical criteria that are imperative for bone structure [27]. On the other hand, methods that include hierarchical physical criteria are non-trivial to implement, have high time complexity and lack a detailed method description.

In summary, a new method must include a multi-scale representation, a local solution at the micro-structural level and hierarchical physical criteria. The implementation should have a simple geometrical representation and low time complexity. Furthermore, it must allow rapid transition between different scales for convenient usage. Owing to the limitations in current FE techniques, we intend to re-examine the various multi-scale computational strategies with the goal of developing an efficient and robust computational technique that will form the basis for a computerized virtual biopsy system for diagnosing metabolic bone diseases.

7. THE MULTI-SCALE FE APPROACH

Multi-scale FE analysis is essential for efficient and reliable mechanical analysis of bone structure. Our approach for multi-scale FE analysis will enable physicians to use a 'digital magnifying glass' that provides continuous transition between macro- and micro-scales, as depicted in Figure 4. Our

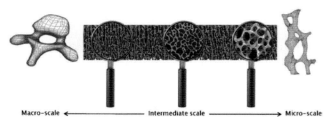

Figure 4. Continuous multi-scale approach.

MULTI-SCALE COMPUTERIZED BONE DIAGNOSTIC SYSTEM

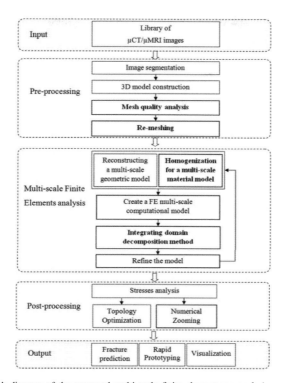

Figure 5. Block diagram of the proposed multi-scale finite element approach (components marked in bold are discussed in this paper).

method uses commonly available computational resources provided by a few PCs or a workstation. In the proposed approach, the amount of computational resources needed for solution of the large-scale problem can be preserved by limiting the total number of DOF in the model. This consideration is of great importance in developing a diagnostic tool to be used by physicians on commonly available workstations rather than on super-computers or grid-based systems. The algorithm of the proposed approach is shown in Figure 5. A brief description the algorithm's main stages follows.

7.1. Acquisition of µCT/µMRI images

Medical imaging technology allows high resolution *in vivo* (up to 50 µm) and *in vitro* (up to 5 µm) scanning of large specimens or even whole bone models. These imaging methods include: (a) peripheral quantitative computed tomography; (b) µCT; and (c) µMRI. All these methods are based on robust CT and MRI technologies.

7.2. Pre-processing

The first step in 3D analysis of scanned tissue is to reconstruct the 3D model from the medical data. 3D model reconstruction can be divided into two main categories: volumetric reconstruction and surface reconstruction. Subsequently, even if the geometry of the reconstructed model has high visualization quality, its quality may be insufficient for FE analysis. The mesh quality enhancement can be handled through optimization and remeshing to enable further analyses, such as FE analysis. This subject is discussed in detail in Section 4.

7.3. Multi-scale FE analysis

Realization of the proposed approach requires synergy between the development of a multi-resolution geometric model for representing each intermediate scale and the assignment of proper mechanical properties of bone tissue for each scale. This process creates a computational FE model for the analyzed scale that requires an efficient solution scheme.

7.3.1. Geometric modeling. A hierarchical geometric multi-resolution model should allow continuous transition from a smooth macro-scale model to a cancellous micro-scale model, in effect a transition from low to high topology models. The intermediate scales, which can be defined as meso-scales of the bone tissue, represent zooming from a dense trabecular structure to a detailed group of trabeculae, and finally to a single trabecula.

7.3.2. Material compliance matrix. Mechanical properties of bone tissue vary at each intermediate scale, from homogeneous material at the macro-scale level to highly heterogeneous material at the micro-scale level that causes discontinuity of the stresses. This variance requires recalculation of material properties, such as Young's and Shear Modulii, at each scale level. Several homogenization approaches are discussed in the literature:

- The *asymptotic analysis* approach is the most frequently mentioned method in the literature [28]. This method assumes periodic material structure and computes material properties for the characteristic cells. However, this approach cannot be applied for trabecular bone structures, since it lacks a periodical pattern structure.
- The *Representative Volume Element* (RVE) approach samples the material properties at a finite number of test-windows and averages the results [29]. The apparent material properties can be extrapolated from these computations. This approach has recently been applied for homogenization of non-periodic masonry structures with a similar irregular structure [30]. This approach will be used as the basis for our algorithm. Preliminary results are presented in Section 8.

7.3.3. Domain decomposition (DD) using parallel computing. It is technically impossible to solve an entire large-scale problem on a single processor due to the high computational complexity and the high memory demands. Thus, parallel computation is imperative at this stage. A natural way to perform parallel computations is by domain decomposition (DD) methods [31]. The solution domain is subdivided into subdomains on which the elasticity problem is computed in parallel.

In this paper, a DD approach is described as the basic technique of the multi-scale FE method. Several DD methods are further discussed in Section 8.

7.4. Post-processing

The outcome of the multi-scale FE analysis can be used for topological optimization of bone micro-structure. Topological optimization methods are used for efficient designing with respect to strength [32]. The topological optimized trabecular bone structure can be compared with the original one to get an indication with respect to topologically optimal structures.

8. PRELIMINARY RESULTS

The preliminary stages of the research included development of a computational method for solving 2D elasticity problems in genus-n domain at the micro-scale level. As previously mentioned, the DD technique served as a major research tool. For the analyses, we used typical trabecular geometry adapted from a 2D image of trabecular bone, as shown in Figure 6. Without loss of generality, the number of holes in the computational model is demonstrated on a grid with at most one single hole per domain (Section 8.1). A general and more complex model, with

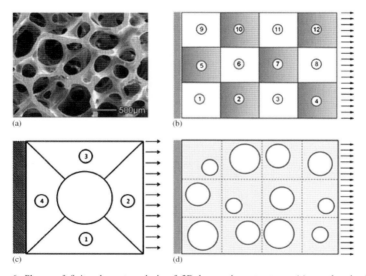

Figure 6. Phases of finite element analysis of 2D bone micro-structures: (a) a trabecular bone structure; (b) domain decomposition of plate subjected to uniform tension; (c) Kirsch-like problem; and (d) 2D simplified trabecular structure.

several holes per cell and partial-holes per cell, is described in Section 8.2. In reality, these holes are cavities filled with bone marrow, whose contribution to material stiffness can be overlooked. In Section 8.3 we present our approach for continuous homogenization from micro- to macro-scales.

8.1. DD technique for the 2D micro-structures

For the 2D elasticity DD problem, we chose a rectangular plate subjected to uniform tension on one boundary and fixed on the opposite boundary The two remaining boundaries had stress-free boundary conditions (Figure 6(b)). This domain's geometry was chosen due to its resemblance to the vertical cross-section of the actual bone biopsy. We divided the plate into 12 equally sized square domains. The number of domains was chosen to create inner domains without global boundary conditions (domains 6 and 7). According to the DD scheme of non-overlapping domains [14, 33], we assigned a black or white 'color' to each domain based on checkerboard rules.

One of the important aspects of DD is data transmission over the interfaces of adjoining domains. In our case, two physical variables were transmitted: tractions (T) and displacement field (u). Since each domain must be well defined as an independent problem, at least one boundary must be assigned displacement boundary conditions. According to the developed scheme, black domains were assigned the displacement (geometric) boundary condition on the left boundary and stress (mechanical) boundary conditions on the other boundaries as depicted in Figure 7. Displacement boundary conditions are applied with the relaxation parameter θ [14].

The DD solution was compared with the one-piece Ansys solution in terms of total strain energy U. After each iteration, strain energy is estimated in each domain using Equation 1. The total strain energy is computed by summing up the strain energy on each subdomain. Figure 8 presents the ratio of the total strain energy in all subdomains to the strain energy of the Ansys solution [34] as a function of number of iterations.

$$U = \tfrac{1}{2}(\sigma_x \varepsilon_x + \sigma_y \varepsilon_y + \tau_{xy} \gamma_{xy}) \tag{1}$$

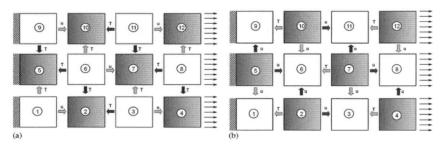

Figure 7. Data transmission scheme for domain decomposition of the rectangular plate: (a) data transmission from white to black domains and (b) data transmission from black to white domains.

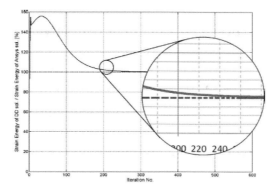

Figure 8. Ratio of total strain energy of domain decomposition solution for rectangular plate to one-piece Ansys solution (domain decomposition solution in solid line, Ansys solution in dashed line).

Based on the conducted analysis, the following conclusions can be drawn:

- The initial jump in strain energy is highly dependent on the quality of the initial guess chosen for the first iteration. The convergence can be influenced by this choice, especially as the number of subdomains increases.
- Convergence occurred only after 240 iterations. Such a result is influenced by the previously mentioned relaxation parameter θ. This parameter decreases as the number of subdomains increases to allow convergence. Thus, a geometrically complex model constructed from a large number of subdomains is in practice unsolvable using this technique.

The main drawback of the above applied DD method is its slow convergence, which makes it impractical for analysis of real micro-scale bone model.

8.2. DD applying finite element tearing and interconnecting (FETI) method for micro-structures

A more practical DD approach is the finite element tearing and interconnecting (FETI) method developed by Farhat and Roux [35] in 1991. Since then, many extensions off this method have been developed; the best known and most widely used are the FETI-DP (dual primal) [36] and the balancing domain decomposition by constraints methods [37].

The basic idea behind the FETI method is based on coupling the adjoining domains using Lagrange multipliers λ that represent the interaction forces between these two subdomains. For implementation issues, see [35] or [38].

The FETI method allows scalability in terms of number of subdomains and is adjusted to parallel computation, as each subdomain at the tearing phase can be solved independently on a separate processor. The interconnecting phase of the algorithm can be resolved using a direct approach for a small number of interface nodes or iteratively otherwise.

The advantages of the FETI over the method utilized in the previous section are:

- The FETI method allows more flexibility in terms of parallel computations, since there is no requirement for solving one domain prior to another.
- The FETI method does not require initial guess to be applied on the domain's boundaries; therefore, the outcome does not depend on the quality of the initial guess.
- A direct solver can be applied for solving the model.

FE code using a Visual C++ application was written to solve 2D plane stress elasticity using the FETI method assuming a homogeneous isotropic material model. The example depicted in Figure 9 illustrates the solution of a 32-domain 2D bone-like structure using the FETI method. A rectangular domain was divided into 32 geometrically equal subdomains, where each subdomain included approximately 2250 DOF, resulting in a total of 72 000 DOF. This time, the domain was subjected to uniform pressure on the right boundary and fixed on the opposite boundary.

The outcomes of the performed analysis are as follows:

- The FETI method can be used for a geometrically complex model, a result that was not possible using the previously utilized method.
- Convergence of each subdomain was not influenced by the total number of subdomains, thus showing the scalability of the method.

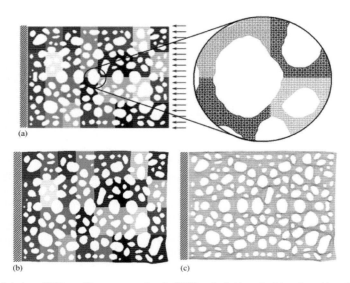

Figure 9. Solution of 2D bone-like structure using the FETI method: (a) meshed domain and its subdomains; (b) solution depicting each subdomains; and (c) von-Mises stress analysis.

Copyright © 2008 John Wiley & Sons, Ltd.   *Commun. Numer. Meth. Engng* (2008)
DOI: 10.1002/cnm

Computer Aided Biomanufacturing, Edited by Roger Narayan and Paul Calvert
© 2011 WILEY-VCH Verlag GmbH & Co. KGaA. Published 2011 by WILEY-VCH Verlag GmbH & Co. KGaA.

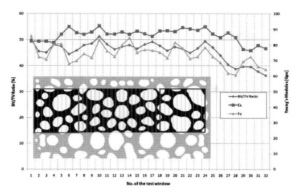

Figure 10. Analysis of material properties as a function of test-window location.

According to the above, the FETI method can be used as a major tool for developing a multi-scale FE method for analysis of macro and micro bone structure. Current work is focused on parallelization of our code for solution on computer clusters. Within the scope of this work, we will discuss the issues of load balancing and optimal domain subdivision.

8.3. Homogenization for micro-structures

We adapted the approach based on RVE. A number of simulations were carried out to analyze the apparent material properties as a function of test-window size and location. In this simulation the dependency between test-window location and the material fraction was analyzed. To this end, 32 overlapping test-windows were used, with an overlap of 96%. Figure 10 depicts the results of one of the applied simulations. The diamond markers illustrate changes in the material fraction in each of test-windows, and square and triangle markers represent Young's moduli in the x- and y-axis accordingly. The results showed that even for a considerable test-window overlap of 96%, material properties at the micro-scale level can change significantly. The change in some of the cases was in the range of 25–30%. Thus, interpolation and extrapolation are very difficult to perform. The results will be further analyzed to determine the optimal test-window size and number of samples required for accurate homogenization.

9. SUMMARY AND FUTURE WORK

In this paper we have presented a new approach to a multi-scale FE analysis of a trabecular structure. Two DD approaches were applied for solving a 2D elasticity FE problem of bone microstructure. We presented the first phase of a transition from the micro- to macro-scale material models based on the RVE homogenization technique.

The proposed method will enable continuous transition between macro- and micro-scales. It is expected that the outcomes of this research will develop into a computerized virtual biopsy system that will include: (a) multi-scale analysis for macro–micro architectures and (b) bone fracture prediction.

Future research will focus on extending this technique to general 3D bone architecture and developing a multi-resolution geometrical model.

ACKNOWLEDGEMENTS

This study was partially supported by the Samuel and Anne Tolkowsky chair at the Technion—Israel Institute of Technology by the Technion Fund for Medical-Engineering collaboration 2007 and by the Irwin and Joan Jacobs Fellowship 2008.

REFERENCES

1. www.boneandjointdecade.org, 2008.
2. Azernikov S, Miropolsky A, Fischer A. Surface reconstruction of freeform objects from 3D camera data based on multiresolution volumetric method. *ASME Transactions, Journal of Computing and Information Science in Engineering (JCISE)* 2003; **3**(4):334–338.
3. Holdstein Y, Fischer A. Reconstruction of volumetric freeform objects using neural networks. *The Visual Computer Journal* 2008; **24**(4):295–302.
4. Azernikov S, Fischer A. A new approach to reverse engineering based on volume warping. *ASME Transactions, Journal of Computing and Information Science in Engineering (JCISE)* 2006; **6**(4):355–363.
5. Weiner S, Wagner HD. The material bone: structure-mechanical function relations. *Annual Review of Materials Science* 1998; **28**:271–298.
6. Rho JY, Kuhn-Spearing L, Zioupos P. Mechanical properties and the hierarchical structure of bone. *Medical Engineering and Physics* 1998; **20**:92–102.
7. NIH Consensus Development Panel. Osteoporosis prevention, diagnosis, and therapy. *Journal of the American Medical Association* 2001; **285**(6):785–795.
8. Schuit SC, van der Klift M, Weel AE, de Laet CE, Burger H, Seeman E, Hofman A, Uitterlinden AG, van Leeuwen JP, Pols HA. Fracture incidence and association with bone mineral density in elderly men and women: the Rotterdam study. *Bone* 2004; **34**(1):195–202.
9. Ho-Le K. Finite element mesh generation methods: a review and classification. *Computer-Aided Design* 1988; **20**(1):27–38.
10. Bar-Yoseph PZ, Mereu S, Chippada S, Kalro VJ. Automatic monitoring of element shape quality in 2D and 3D computational mesh dynamics. *Computational Mechanics* 2001; **27**:378–395.
11. Holdstein Y, Podshivalov L, Fischer A, Bar-Yoseph PZ. A neural network technique for re-meshing of bone micro-structure. *Advanced Research in Virtual and Rapid Prototyping*. Taylor & Francis Group: Leiria, 2008; 237–241.
12. www.altairhyperworks.com, 2008.
13. Fritzke B. A growing neural gas network learns topologies. *Advances in Neural Information Processing Systems 7*. MIT Press: Cambridge, MA, 1995; 625–632.
14. Quarteroni A. Domain decomposition and parallel processing for the numerical solution of partial differential equations. *Surveys on Mathematics for Industry* 1991; **1**:75–118.
15. van-Rietbergen B. Micro-FE analyses of bone: state of the art. *Advances in Experimental Medicine and Biology* 2001; **496**:21–30.
16. Arbenz P, van Lenthe GH, Mennel U, Muller R, Sala M. Multi-level μ-finite element analysis for human bone structure. *Workshop on State-of-the-art in Scientific and Parallel Computing*, Umeå, Sweden, 18–21 June 2006.
17. Müller R, Ruegsegger P. Three-dimensional finite element modeling of non-invasively trabecular bone structure. *Medical Engineering and Physics* 1995; **17**(2):126–133.
18. Niebur GL, Feldstein MJ, Yuen JC, Chen TJ, Keaveny TM. High-resolution FE models with tissue strength asymmetry accurately predict failure of trabecular bone. *Journal of Biomechanics* 2000; **33**:1575–1583.
19. Ruimerman R, Hilbers P, van Rietbergen B, Huiskes R. A theoretical framework for strain-related trabecular bone maintenance and adaptation. *Journal of Biomechanics* 2005; **38**:931–941.

20. van Rietbergen B, Weinans H, Huiskes R, Polman BJW. Computational strategies for iterative solutions of large FEM applications employing voxel data. *International Journal for Numerical Methods in Engineering* 1996; **39**:2743–2767.
21. Weinan E, Engquist B, Li X, Weiqing R, Vanden-Eijnden E. The heterogeneous multiscale method: a review. *Communications in Computational Physics* 2007; **2**(3):367–450.
22. Brandt A. Multiscale scientific computation: review 2001. In *Multiscale and Multiresolution Methods: Theory and Applications*, Barth TJ *et al.* (eds), *Proceedings of the Yosemite Educational Symposium Conference*, 2000. Lecture Notes in Computer Science and Engineering, vol. 20. Springer: Berlin, 2002; 3–96.
23. Fischer A, Bar-Yoseph PZ. Adaptive mesh generation based on Multiresolution Quadtree representation. *International Journal for Numerical Methods in Engineering* 2000; **48**:1571–1582.
24. Liu WK, Park HS, Qian D, Karpov EG, Kadowaki H, Wagner GJ. Bridging scale methods for nanomechanics and materials. *Computer Methods in Applied Mechanics and Engineering* 2006; **195**(13):1407–1421.
25. Ben Dhia H, Rateau G. The Arlequin method as a flexible engineering design tool. *International Journal for Numerical Methods in Engineering* 2005; **52**:1442–1462.
26. Kawagai M, Sando A, Takano N. Image-based multi-scale modelling strategy for complex and heterogeneous porous microstructures by mesh superposition method. *Modelling and Simulation in Materials Science and Engineering* 2006; **13**:53–69.
27. Mitra S, Parashar M, Browne JC. Distributed adaptive grid hierarchy. *User's Guide*, Department of Computer Sciences, University of Texas at Austin, 2001.
28. Zienkiewicz OC, Taylor RL. *The FEM for Solid and Structural Mechanics* (6th edn). Elsevier: Amsterdam, 2005; 547–587.
29. Aboudi J. *Mechanics of Composite Materials*. Studies in Applied Mechanics, vol. 29. Elsevier: Amsterdam, 1991; 1–10.
30. Cluni F, Gusella V. Homogenization of non-periodic masonry structures. *International Journal of Solids and Structures* 2004; **41**:1911–1923.
31. Magoulès F, Rixen D (eds). Domain decomposition methods: recent advances and new challenges in engineering. *Special Issue in the Computer Methods in Applied Mechanics and Engineering* 2007; **196**(8):1345–1346.
32. Bendsøe M, Sigmund O. *Topology Optimization: Theory, Methods and Applications* (2nd edn). Springer: Berlin, Heidelberg, 2003.
33. Marini LD, Quarteroni A. A relaxation procedure for domain decomposition methods using finite elements. *Numerische Mathematik* 1989; **55**:575–598.
34. www.ansys.com, 2008.
35. Farhat C, Roux FX. A method of finite element tearing and interconnecting and its parallel solution algorithm. *International Journal for Numerical Methods in Engineering* 1991; **32**:1205–1227.
36. Farhat C, Lesoinne M, LeTallec P, Pierson K, Rixen D. FETI-DP: a dual-primal unified FETI method—Part I: a faster alternative to the two-level FETI method. *International Journal for Numerical Methods in Engineering* 2001; **50**:1523–1544.
37. Mandel J, Dohrmann CR. Convergence of a balancing domain decomposition by constraints and energy minimization. *Numerical Linear Algebra with Applications* 2003; **10**(63):639–659.
38. Kamath C. *The FETI Level 1 Method: Theory and Implementation*. Lawrence Livermore National Laboratory, U.S. Department of Energy, 2000.

Update

Toward a Multiscale Computerized Bone Diagnostic System: 2D Microscale Finite Element Analysis

Lev Podshivalov, Yaron Holdstein, Anath Fischer, and Pinhas Bar-Yoseph

1
Overview

Bone is composed of hierarchical biocomposite materials that are characterized by complex multiscale structural geometry and heterogeneous material properties. Bone tissue structure may be classified into five structural levels [1, 2], ranging from macro- to nanoscales. Each patient's bone structure is unique and is influenced by gender, age, lifestyle, and physical condition. Depending on the anatomical site, bone architecture differs significantly at the microstructural level with respect to shape, thickness, directionality, and size. It may also vary at different locations of the same site, as a result of functionality and locally applied forces characterized by magnitude and direction. These characteristics are crucial for diagnosis of bone metabolic diseases.

Metabolic bone diseases are characterized by microarchitectural deterioration of bone tissue, leading to microfractures; therefore, early diagnosis is a key to intervention. The most widely used technique for assessing bone quality is bone mineral density (BMD) assessment. BMD data are represented as scalar of a statistical value (T-score). Although BMD testing is used regularly, it has a major limitation. It does not describe the complex 3D bone microstructure, but rather provides an indication using a single scalar value. As a result, the BMD method occasionally fails to diagnose risk of osteoporotic fractures [3], leading to unreliable diagnosis and incorrect treatment.

The need for diagnosis of microstructures has led to the development of emerging 3D microscale scanning methods such as µCT and µMRI, which offer high-resolution *in vivo* and *in vitro* scanning of bone structures. To date, however, no complete diagnostic method incorporating these technical abilities has been proposed.

Computer Aided Biomanufacturing, Edited by Roger Narayan and Paul Calvert
© 2011 WILEY-VCH Verlag GmbH & Co. KGaA. Published 2011 by WILEY-VCH Verlag GmbH & Co. KGaA.

Surface reconstruction and volumetric modeling of the 3D bone structure from medical images constitute the first stages for analysis. Mesh reconstruction from μCT/μMRI images produced by commercial software often results in a highly distorted triangulation that is not suitable for finite element (FE) mechanical analysis, and therefore requires remeshing and mesh optimization [4]. These operations are time consuming and often require manual user interventions. Moreover, a multiresolution volumetric representation should be created [5–7] in order to analyze microscale models using the microfinite element method. The major limitation of current methods [8] is their inability to handle large bone volumes using commonly available computational resources. Therefore, a multiscale approach is required.

State-of-the-art multiscale FE methods currently utilize parallel computing on large, high-resolution models of human bone reconstructed from μCT/μMRI images [9]. However, these multiscale methods include only two binary scales: macro- and microscales; no intermediate scales can be represented. An adaptive approach has recently been proposed [10]. This method is based on modeling an entire model using a macroscale homogeneous model and embedding this model into the volume of interest (VOI). Nevertheless, this method does not provide the complete multiscale method needed for robust multiscale analysis of bone architecture.

The required multiscale analysis approach should take advantage of both the simplicity and efficiency of the macroscopic models and the accuracy of the detailed microscopic model, by coupling macro- and microscopic models [11, 12]. A new multiscale method must include a multiresolution geometric representation and predefined hierarchical physical criteria capable of computing the microstructural level locally. The multiscale models should facilitate fast geometric and material transition between the scales, without accumulative errors. Thus, a multiscale approach for mechanical analysis of bone is imperative. Our main goal is to develop an efficient and robust computational technique that will form the basis of a computerized virtual biopsy system for diagnosing metabolic bone diseases.

2
The Multiscale Finite Element Approach

Our approach to multiscale finite element analysis is based on a "digital magnifying glass" that provides continuous transition between macro- and microscales. In the proposed approach, the computational method for the large-scale high-resolution problem is adaptive, so that the computational resources may be used efficiently. This is essential because a diagnostic tool for physicians must be able to use commonly available workstations rather than supercomputers or clusters. A detailed description of the algorithm is presented in our full paper [13]. The main stages of the algorithm are as follows: (a) acquisition of μCT/μMRI images; (b) 3D reconstruction of a multiresolution volumetric representation; (c) multiscale finite element analysis, and (d) visualization. The multiscale finite element analysis stage is the key module of the proposed approach. It consists of following components:

a) **Geometric, domain-based, multiresolution model**: The multiresolution model enables continuous bidirectional transition between the microscale and macroscale geometric representations of the bone models. The algorithm for generating the progressive multiresolution meshes is based on the edge collapse technique, which is applied to the DCEL boundary representation [13, 14].

b) **Multiscale material properties**: Mechanical properties of bone tissue vary at each intermediate scale due to the discontinuity of the stresses, ranging from homogeneous material at the macroscale level to highly heterogeneous material at the microscale level. This variance requires recalculation of the material compliance matrix at each scale level, as further discussed in the next section.

c) **Multiscale computational method**: Handling large-scale high-resolution bone model on a single processor is technically difficult due to computational complexity and memory demands. Thus, parallel computation is imperative. Domain decomposition methods are natural in parallel computing [15]. The model domain is subdivided into subdomains, and the mechanical problem is computed in parallel on all these subdomains. Several domain decomposition methods are discussed in our detailed paper [13].

In this update, we focus on the multiscale material compliance matrix that is the core of the mechanical model.

3
Domain-Based Multiscale Material Properties

The main challenge when dealing with multiscale computational models is to preserve the prominent geometric features and mechanical properties at all structural levels. Since the multiresolution modeling alters the geometry at every structural level, the mechanical properties also change. Therefore, the local mechanical properties should be defined for each level. To this end, we applied the *representative volume element* (RVE) *homogenization* approach to each subdomain of the bone model. The main stages in the proposed method are as follows:

a) Calculating the progressive multiresolution meshes from the microscale level to the macroscale level. Each mesh represents the complete geometric model but at a different level of detail (scales).

b) Calculating the material parameters for each scale using the homogenization technique. In this stage, an anisotropy direction of the material is calculated and the tensor is then transformed in this direction. The local material model is assumed to be an isotropic linear model, where the tissue model is assumed to be an orthotropic material model.

c) Defining the behavior of material parameters as a function of model porosity.

d) Calculating the inverse material model that preserves the global material properties for all structural levels. Local material properties for each structural level are then computed from this model. At this stage, the local material model is assumed to be orthotropic to compensate for geometry changes.
e) Verifying the model for all structural levels (scales).

The outcomes of stages (a)–(d) are depicted in Figure 1. In (a)–(c), the first row depicts three meshes at the macro-, meso-, and microscales. The corresponding

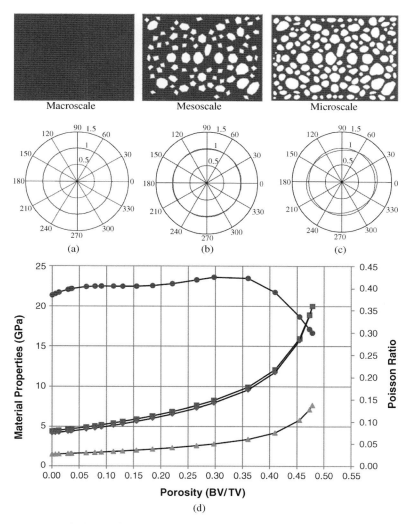

Figure 1 Calculation of the local material properties for the structural levels. Anisotropy and direction for all levels (a–c) and local material (d) as a function of porosity (circles: Poisson ratio; squares and rhombuses: Young's moduli in principal directions; triangles: shear modulus).

anisotropy directions of these meshes are depicted in the second row. The curve on the polar coordinates represents a ratio between Young's moduli for a given orientation. The principal axes of the material directionality can be calculated from this curve. At the microscale, the tissue is anisotropic due to the cancellous geometry. At the macroscale, the tissue material properties are preserved by replacing an isotropic local material with an orthotropic material, as shown in Figure 1d. At this scale, the tissue becomes isotropic without correcting the local material properties. Such adjustment compensates for the changes in geometry and preserves tissue material properties at all scales.

4
Summary and Future Work

This update describes a new approach for a 2D multiscale finite element analysis of a trabecular bone structure. The proposed method includes reconstruction of the geometric multiresolution model, thus facilitating continuous geometric transition from macro- to microscale, and vice versa. In addition, the method includes a bidirectional transition from micro- to macroscale of the material models based on the RVE homogenization approach. Our current research focuses on extending this technique to general 3D bone architecture for a computerized 3D virtual biopsy system.

The proposed method can be used as a stand-alone tool for mechanical analysis of bone tissue and for diagnostic biopsies. Moreover, it can be used as a tool for simulating bone regeneration [16] and bone in-growth into bone microscaffolds. A future extension may include development of new methods at the cell level for fracture healing [17].

Acknowledgments

This study has been partially supported by the Samuel and Anne Tolkowsky chair at the Technion, by the Irwin and Joan Jacobs Fellowship 2008, and by the Phyllis and Joseph Gurwin Fund for Scientific Advancement at the Technion 2009.

References

1 Weiner, S. and Wagner, H.D. (1998) The material bone: structure–mechanical function relations. *Annu. Rev. Mater. Sci.*, **28**, 271–298.

2 Rho, J.Y., Kuhn-Spearing, L., and Zioupos, P. (1998) Mechanical properties and the hierarchical structure of bone. *Med. Eng. Phys.*, **20**, 92–102.

3 Schuit, S.C., van der Klift, M., Weel, A.E., de Laet, C.E., Burger, H., Seeman, E., Hofman, A., Uitterlinden, A.G., van Leeuwen, J.P., and Pols, H.A. (2004) Fracture incidence and association with bone mineral density in elderly men and women: the Rotterdam Study. *Bone*, **34** (1), 195–202.

4 Zaideman, O. and Fischer, A. (2009) Geometrical bone modeling: from macro to micro structures. *J. Comput. Sci. Technol.*, **25** (3), 614–622.
5 Fischer, A. (2002) Multi-level of detail models for reverse engineering in remote CAD systems. *J. Eng. Comput.*, **18** (1), 50–58.
6 Fischer, A. and Bar-Yoseph, P.Z. (2000) Adaptive mesh generation based on multiresolution quadtree representation. *Int. J. Numer. Methods Eng.*, **48** (11), 1571–1582.
7 Azernikov, A. and Fischer, A. (2006) A new approach to reverse engineering based on volume warping. *J. Comput. Inf. Sci. Eng.*, **6** (4), 355–363.
8 Van Rietbergen, B. (2001) Micro-FE analyses of bone: state of the art. *Adv. Exp. Med. Biol.*, **496**, 21–30.
9 Arbenz, P., van Lenthe, G.H., Mennel, U., Muller, R., and Sala, M. (2006) Multi-level u-finite element analysis for human bone structure. Workshop on State-of-the-Art in Scientific and Parallel Computing, Sweden.
10 Yu, Q. (2001) Computational homogenization for the advanced materials and structures with multiple spatial and temporal scales. The Scientific Computation Research Center (SCOREC).
11 Weinan, E., Engquist, B., Li, X., Weiqing, R., and Vanden-Eijnden, E. (2007) The heterogeneous multiscale method: a review. *Commun. Comput. Phys.*, **2** (3), 367–450.
12 Brandt, A. (2002) Multiscale scientific computation: review 2001, in *Multiscale and Multiresolution Methods: Theory and Applications, Lecture Notes in Computational Science and Engineering*, vol. 20 (eds T.J. Barth *et al.*), Springer, pp. 3–96.
13 Podshivalov, L., Holdstein, Y., Fischer, A., and Bar-Yoseph, P.Z. (2009) Towards a multi-scale computerized bone diagnostic system: 2D micro-scale finite element analysis. *Commun. Numer. Methods Eng.*, **25** (6), 733–749.
14 Podshivalov, L., Fischer, A., and Bar-Yoseph, P.Z. (2010) 2D multiresolution geometric meshing for multiscale FE analysis of bone microstructures. *Virtual Phys. Prototyping*, **5** (1), 33–43.
15 Magoulès, F. and Rixen, D. (2007) Domain decomposition methods: recent advances and new challenges in engineering. *Comput. Methods Appl. Mech. Eng.*, **196** (8) 1345–1346.
16 Van Oers, R., Ruimerman, R., Tanck, E., Hilbers, P., and Huiskes, R. (2008) A unified theory for osteonal and hemi-osteonal remodeling. *Bone*, **42** (2), 250–259.
17 Ouaknin, G. and Bar-Yoseph, P.Z. (2009) Stochastic collective movement of cells and fingering morphology: no maverick cells. *Biophys. J.*, **97** (7), 1811–1821.

2
Hierarchical Starch-Based Fibrous Scaffold for Bone Tissue Engineering Applications

RESEARCH ARTICLE

Hierarchical starch-based fibrous scaffold for bone tissue engineering applications

Albino Martins[1,2]*, Sangwon Chung[1,2], Adriano J. Pedro[1,2], Rui A. Sousa[1,2,3], Alexandra P. Marques[1,2], Rui L. Reis[1,2,3] and Nuno M. Neves[1,2]

[1]*3B's Research Group – Biomaterials, Biodegradables and Biomimetics, Department of Polymer Engineering, University of Minho, and Headquarters of the European Institute of Excellence on Tissue Engineering and Regenerative Medicine, AvePark, Zona Industrial da Gandra, S. Cláudio do Barco, 4806-909 Caldas das Taipas, Guimarães, Portugal*
[2]*Institute for Biotechnology and Bioengineering (IBB), PT Government Associated Laboratory; Braga, Portugal*
[3]*Stemmatters, Biotechnology and Regenerative Medicine Ltd, AvePark, Zona Industrial da Gandra, S. Cláudio do Barco, Apartado 4152-4805 Caldas das Taipas, Portugal*

Abstract

Fibrous structures mimicking the morphology of the natural extracellular matrix are considered promising scaffolds for tissue engineering. This work aims to develop a novel hierarchical starch-based scaffold. Such scaffolds were obtained by a combination of starch–polycaprolactone micro- and polycaprolactone nano-motifs, respectively produced by rapid prototyping (RP) and electrospinning techniques. Scanning electron microscopy (SEM) and micro-computed tomography analysis showed the successful fabrication of a multilayer scaffold composed of parallel aligned microfibres in a grid-like arrangement, intercalated by a mesh-like structure with randomly distributed nanofibres (NFM). Human osteoblast-like cells were dynamically seeded on the scaffolds, using spinner flasks, and cultured for 7 days under static conditions. SEM analysis showed predominant cell attachment and spreading on the nanofibre meshes, which enhanced cell retention at the bulk of the composed/hierarchical scaffolds. A significant increment in cell proliferation and osteoblastic activity, assessed by alkaline phosphatase quantification, was observed on the hierarchical fibrous scaffolds. These results support our hypothesis that the integration of nanoscale fibres into 3D rapid prototype scaffolds substantially improves their biological performance in bone tissue-engineering strategies. Copyright © 2008 John Wiley & Sons, Ltd.

Received 2 September 2008; Accepted 14 September 2008

Keywords electrospinning; rapid prototyping; starch-based fibres; micro/nano multilayer scaffolds; human osteoblastic cells; bioreactor

1. Introduction

Biodegradable scaffolds are generally recognized as indispensable elements in tissue engineering and regenerative medicine strategies. Scaffolds are used as temporary templates for cell seeding, migration, proliferation and differentiation prior to the regeneration of biologically functional tissue or natural extracellular matrix (ECM) (Lutolf and Hubblell, 2005; Hutmacher et al., 2007). Ideally, to create a tissue-engineered construct capable of regenerating a fully functional tissue, it should mimic both the fibrous form and the complex function of the native ECM (Agrawal and Ray, 2001). Like natural ECM, a range of topographic features at the macro-, micro- and even nano-scale levels must lead cell response (Norman and Desai, 2006). A multi-scale network structure can be developed by integrating microfibrous structures, produced by wet-spinning or rapid prototyping, with electrospun nanofibres (Tuzlakoglu et al., 2005; Santos et al., 2007; Moroni et al., 2008).

Electrospun fibres typically have dimensions varying from the nano- to the micro-scale, although fibre diameters in the sub-micrometer range are mainly

*Correspondence to: Albino Martins, 3Bs Research Group – Biomaterials, Biodegradables and Biomimetics, Department of Polymer Engineering, University of Minho, Portugal. E-mail: amartins@dep.uminho.pt

observed (Huang *et al.*, 2003). These mesh-like scaffold are characterized by high porosity, high surface : volume ratio and, most importantly, they can closely mimic the morphology of the native ECM of many tissues. Such physical cues enhance cell adhesion, proliferation and differentiation, and consequently neo-tissue formation on nanofibrous meshes of both natural and synthetic polymers (Zhang *et al.*, 2005; Martins *et al.*, 2007).

Rapid prototyping has emerged as a powerful polymer-processing technique for the production of scaffolds in the area of tissue engineering (Hutmacher *et al.*, 2004; Leong *et al.*, 2003; Mironov *et al.*, 2003; Peltola *et al.*, 2008; Pfister *et al.*, 2004; Yang *et al.*, 2002; Yeong *et al.*, 2004). The main advantage of this technique is the possibility of creating structures with customized shapes linked with computer-aided design (CAD), thus providing more flexibility, versatility and reproducibility in creating scaffolds (Hutmacher *et al.*, 2004; Moroni *et al.*, 2005; Moroni *et al.*, 2006; Capes *et al.*, 2005). However, the typical pore size of RP scaffold constitutes a limitation in the cell-seeding efficiency (Pfister *et al.*, 2004), once it is relatively large as compared to cell dimensions.

Therefore, the aim of this study was to characterize a novel hierarchical starch-based fibrous scaffold obtained by the combination of starch–polycaprolactone (SPCL) micro- and polycaprolactone (PCL) nano-motifs, respectively produced by rapid prototyping (RP) and electrospinning. The defined strategy aimed at overcoming the high number of cells needed to attain sufficient adherent cells to the RP scaffolds (Moroni *et al.*, 2008), which can be accomplished by alternately integrating electrospun nanofibre meshes every two consecutive layers of plotted microfibres. In this way these nanofibre meshes will act as cell entrapment systems, increasing cell attachment efficiency, cell proliferation and tissue regeneration. Ultimately, this integration will enhance the potential application of such three-dimensional (3D) fibrous structures in bone tissue-engineering strategies. This work reports the results of a set of experiments in which human osteoblast-like cells were dynamically seeded and statically cultured for 7 days on micro-nano fibre polymeric scaffolds designed to validate this hypothesis.

2. Materials and methods

2.1. Scaffold fabrication

Three-dimensional (3D) rapid prototyping scaffolds (6RP) were fabricated using a 3D plotting technique (Bio-plotter, EnvisionTec GmbH, Germany), using a 30 : 70 (wt%) blend of starch and polycaprolactone (SPCL, Novamont, Italy). SPCL polymer powder was placed into a metal barrel and heated at 140 °C through a heated cartridge unit, then plotted through a nozzle by air pressure control. The nozzle comprises a stainless steel needle with internal diameter 0.5 mm and length 6 mm. A metal piston plunger with a Teflon seal was used to apply pressure to the molten polymer. The machine was linked to CAD software (PrimCam, Germany) which required inputs of dispensing and processing parameters (e.g. speed of the head, dispensing pressure and temperature) and the design parameters of the scaffold (e.g. scaffold dimensions, spacing between the polymer strands, and number of layers). The strand spacing was set to 1 mm, without offsets between the consecutive equivalent layers. The orientation was changed by plotting the polymer with 90° angle steps between two successive layers. The production of hierarchical fibrous scaffolds (6RP + 5NFM) was achieved by integrating nanofibre meshes (NFM) every two consecutive layers of plotted microfibres. The nanofibre meshes were previously produced by electrospinning, as described elsewhere (Araujo *et al.*, 2007). Briefly, a polymeric solution of 17% w/v PCL, dissolved in an organic solvent mixture of chloroform : dimethylformamide (7 : 3 ratio), was electrospun by establishing a electric tension of 9.5 kV, a needle tip-to-ground collector distance of 200 mm and a flow rate of 1 ml/h. The scaffolds (6RP and 6RP + 5NFM scaffolds) were all cut into 5 × 5 mm cubical samples from the originally deposited bulk 20 × 20 mm cube (12 layers) and sterilized using ethylene oxide (EtO) before the cell culture assays.

2.2. Scaffold characterization

Scaffold architecture was analysed using micro-computed tomography (μ-CT) with a desktop micro CT scanner (SkyScan 1072, Aartselaar, Belgium). The scanner was set to a voltage of 40 kV and a current of 248 µA, and the samples were scanned at 8.71 µm pixel resolutions by approximately 350 slices covering the sample height of 2.5 mm. For imaging, the sliced 2D tomographic raw images were reconstructed using CT Analyser software, and the threshold levels of the greyscale images were equally adjusted for all the samples to allow the measurement of the volume of pores, providing the data for scaffold porosity. 3D modelling was also used to analyse the scaffold structure in a non-destructive manner, using imaging software. The morphology of the scaffold was also analysed, using scanning electron microscopy (SEM; Leica Cambridge, Model S360, UK). All samples were previously sputter-coated with gold (Sputter Coater, Model SC502, Fisons Instruments, UK).

2.3. Cell seeding and culture

Human osteosarcoma-derived cells [Saos-2 cell line, European Collection of Cell Cultures (ECACC), UK], were maintained in Dulbecco's modified Eagle's medium (DMEM; Sigma-Aldrich; Germany) supplemented with 10% heat-inactivated fetal bovine serum (Biochrom AG, Berlin, Germany) and 1% antibiotic–antimycotic solution (Gibco, UK). Cells were cultured in a humidified incubator at 37 °C in a 5% CO_2 atmosphere and the medium was routinely replaced every 3–4 days.

Confluent osteoblastic-like cells were harvested and dynamically seeded onto the polymeric scaffolds as follows. The combined and the RP (controls) scaffolding structures were placed between stainless steel holding wires in spinner flasks (12 scaffolds/spinner flask) containing a suspension of osteoblast-like cells with a concentration of 0.5×10^6 cells/ml in a total volume of 35 ml. The stirrer was set at 80 r.p.m. and the spinner flasks left on for 72 h to allow the cells to colonize the entire scaffold. After this time period the osteoblasts/scaffold constructs were transferred to 24-well cell culture plates (Costar®, Corning, NY, USA) and statically cultured for 1 and 7 days under the culture conditions previously described for maintenance of the cell line.

2.4. Evaluation of cell adhesion, morphology and distribution

To evaluate the cell morphology, the cells–scaffold constructs were fixed with 2.5% glutaraldehyde (Sigma, USA) in phosphate-buffered saline (PBS; Sigma) solution for 1 h at 4 °C. Then, the samples were dehydrated through a graded series of ethanol and allowed to dry overnight. Finally, they were sputter-coated with gold (Model SC502, Fisons Instruments, UK) and observed in a scanning electron microscope (Model S360, Leica Cambridge, UK).

2.5. Cell viability assay

At each defined time culture period, the cell viability was determined using the CellTiter 96® Aqueous One Solution Cell Proliferation Assay (Promega, USA). This assay is based on the bioreduction of a tetrazolium compound, 3-(4,5-dimethylthiazol-2-yl)-5-(3-carboxymethoxyphenyl)-2-(4-sulphofenyl)-2H-tetrazolium (MTS), into a water-soluble brown formazan product. This conversion is accomplished by NADPH or NADH production by the dehydrogenase enzymes in metabolically active cells. The absorbance, measured at 490 nm in a microplate reader (Bio-Tek, Synergie HT, USA), is related to the quantity of formazan product and directly proportional to the number of living cells in the constructs. Three samples per type of scaffold and per time point were characterized.

2.6. DNA Quantification

Cell proliferation was evaluated by quantifying the total amount of double-stranded DNA throughout the culture time. Quantification was performed using the Quant-iT™ PicoGreen dsDNA Assay Kit (Invitrogen, Molecular Probes, OR, USA), according to the manufacturer's instructions, and after the cells in the construct were lysed by osmotic and thermal shock. The intensity of the fluorescence, proportional to the amount of double-strand DNA, was measured at an excitation wavelength of 485/20 nm and at an emission wavelength of 528/20 nm, in a microplate reader (Bio-Tek, Synergie HT, USA). Triplicates of each sample, allowed for a statistical analysis. The DNA concentration for each sample was calculated using a standard curve relating quantity of DNA and fluorescence intensity.

2.7. Alkaline phosphatase (ALP) quantification

To assess the osteogenic activity of cells seeded into the 3D scaffolds (6RP and 6RP + 5NFM), the expression of ALP was determined for both culture time periods, in the same samples used for DNA quantification. In each well of a 96-well plate (Costar®, Corning, NY, USA), 20 μl of each sample were mixed with 60 μl substrate solution and 0.2% wt/v p-nytrophenyl phosphate (Sigma, USA), in a substrate buffer of 1 M diethanolamine HCl (Merck, Germany) at pH 9.8. The plate was then incubated in the dark for 45 min at 37 °C. After the incubation period, 80 μl stop solution, 2 M NaOH (Panreac; Barcelona, Spain) plus 0.2 mM EDTA (Sigma), was added to each well. Standards were prepared with 10 μM/ml p-nytrophenol (pNP, Sigma, USA) solution, to obtain a standard curve covering the range 0–0.3 μM/ml. Triplicates of each sample and standard were made. Absorbance was read at 405 nm in a microplate reader (Bio-Tek, Synergie HT) and sample concentrations were read off from the standard curve. These ALP concentrations were normalized against the DNA concentrations of the same samples to determine the ALP activity.

2.8. Statistical analysis

Statistical analysis was performed using the SPSS statistic software (release 8.0.0 for Windows). First, a Shapiro–Wilk test was used to ascertain about data normality. Once biological results did not follow a normal distribution, Kruskal–Wallis test was performed to compare the effect of scaffold architecture over cell performance. In the analysis of the results, $p < 0.05$ was considered statistically significant.

3. Results and discussion

A novel hierarchical fibrous scaffold was developed, combining starch–polycaprolactone micro- and polycaprolactone nano-motifs, respectively produced by rapid prototyping (RP) and electrospinning (ES). These scaffolds were characterized by a 3D structure of parallel aligned rapid prototyped microfibres (average fibre diameter, 300 μm), periodically intercalated by randomly distributed electrospun nanofibres (fibre diameters in the range 400 nm–1.4 μm) (Figure 1B). When nanofibre meshes were integrated within the 3D scaffold, no

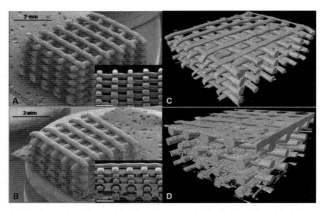

Figure 1. SEM and μ-CT micrographs of the starch-based rapid prototyped, 6RP (A, C) and hierarchical fibrous scaffolds, 6RP + 5NFM (B, D)

delamination between consecutive layers of RP fibres was observed, resulting in a stable scaffold. Additionally, this micro–nano scaffold architecture comprises a high-throughput scaffold process methodology, with regular control over RP-produced structure and nanofibres distribution within the scaffold. The integration of these nano-motifs resulted in a decrease of scaffold porosity of around 11% (from 79.4% on 6RP scaffolds to 68.3% on 6RP + 5NFM scaffolds), as determined by μ-CT analysis (Figure 1C, D). Despite a decrease in porosity, a fully interconnected porous structure was observed, allowing gas, nutrient and waste transport through the 3D structure.

Starch-based scaffolds have been proposed as candidates for bone tissue-engineering strategies in multiple studies (Gomes et al., 2001, 2003, 2006, 2008; Salgado et al., 2004, Salgado et al., 2005, 2007; Tuzlakoglu et al., 2005), supporting the choice of SPCL to develop the structures proposed in this study. Indeed, successful results were demonstrated in terms of cell viability, proliferation and maturation of osteoblastic cells or differentiation of bone marrow stromal cells. Moreover, other starch-based blends (corn starch, dextran and gelatine, 50:30:20 wt%) have already been used to produce different scaffold designs by 3D printing (3DP) (Lam et al., 2002). Although showing suitable physicochemical properties for tissue-engineering applications, the biocompatibility of those 3DP geometric scaffolds, with a highly interconnected porous network, remains to be tested. The hierarchical starch-based fibrous scaffolds developed in the present study were seeded with human osteoblast-like cells to observe how the scaffold architecture affects their behaviour. Cells were initially allowed to attach to the scaffold using a dynamic system; this spinner flask bioreactor allows the cells to efficiently penetrate into the inner regions of the scaffolds, avoiding in a certain extent the preferential colonization of the outer most parts of the scaffolds (Oliveira et al., 2007). Consequently, a homogeneous distribution of cells throughout the entire scaffold was observed. However, SEM micrographs demonstrated that osteoblastic cells preferentially adhered to the nanofibrous meshes (Figure 2B, D, G, H). This phenomenon of cellular preference was previously described by our group and others (Tuzlakoglu et al., 2005, Kwon et al., 2005, Yang et al., 2005), when different cell types (osteoblastic, endothelial and neural stem cells) were seeded in micro- and nano-fibre-based scaffolds. Additionally, the integration of nanofibre meshes into the 3D rapid prototyped scaffolds seemed to act as a cell entrapment system within the RP scaffold. It was reported by others (Pfister et al., 2004) that cells go through the pores of rapid prototyped scaffolds and accumulate at the bottom of the well plate during the seeding process, without attaching the scaffold, and thus reducing the seeding efficiency typically down to values of 25–35%. Thus, the integration of nanofibre meshes constitutes an innovative strategy to enhance cell seeding efficiency into 3D RP scaffolds.

The quantification of cell viability and metabolic activity of human osteoblast-like cells seeded into the combined electrospun nanofiber meshes and RP scaffolds was evaluated by MTS assay (Figure 3). The results revealed a steadily increasing trend, with culture time, although there was no significant difference on the effect of the type of scaffold architectures ($p > 0.05$). From the morphological evaluation of the constructs, it seems that the integrated nanofibre meshes into the 3D rapid prototyped structure also acted as a cell entrapment system within the scaffold. Consequently, a significant increment of cell proliferation and maturation, respectively assessed by DNA and ALP activity quantification, along the culture time, was observed on the hierarchical fibrous scaffolds (Figures 4, 5) in comparison to the rapid prototyped scaffolds ($p <$

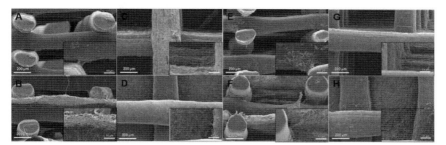

Figure 2. SEM micrographs of rapid prototyped (A, C, E, G) and **hierarchical fibrous** (B, D, F, H) scaffolds cultured with human osteoblast-like cells (Saos-2 cell line) for 1 (A–D) and 7 (E–H) days. Cross-sections (A, B, E, F) and top views (C, D, G, H) of the constructs. Insets, higher magnifications

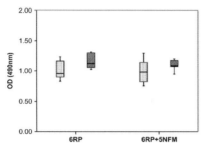

Figure 3. Box plot of cell viability results of human osteoblastic cells cultured on rapid prototyped (6RP) and **hierarchical fibrous** (6RP + 5NFM) scaffolds for 1 and 7 days. Data were analysed by the non-parametric method of a Kruskal–Wallis test ($p < 0.05$)

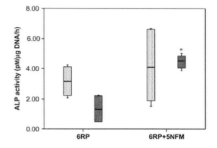

Figure 5. Box plot of ALP activity, normalized against dsDNA amount, from osteoblastic cells (Saos-2 cell line) cultured on rapid prototyped (6RP) and **hierarchical fibrous** (6RP + 5NFM) scaffolds for 1 and 7 days. Data were analysed by the non-parametric method of a Kruskal–Wallis test; *$p < 0.05$

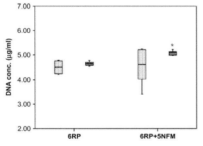

Figure 4. Box plot of DNA content of osteoblast-like cells cultured on rapid prototyped (6RP) and **hierarchical fibrous** (6RP + 5NFM) scaffolds for 1 and 7 days. Data were analysed by the non-parametric method of a Kruskal–Wallis test; *$p < 0.05$

0.05), especially for longer culture periods. However, for the RP scaffolds, the osteoblastic activity was not maintained throughout the experiment, as observed by a decrease in ALP activity from day 1 to day 7 of culture. It was previously reported by Schantz *et al.* (2003) that rabbit calvarial osteoblasts, seeded onto PCL scaffolds fabricated via fused deposition modelling (FDM) and embedded into a fibrin matrix (Tisseel, Baxter Hyland Immuno), showed no significant differences in their ALP activity along time. These results are in accordance with those of our study.

4. Conclusion

A novel hierarchical fibrous scaffold was developed, combining starch-polycaprolactone micro- and polycaprolactone nano-motifs, respectively produced by rapid prototyping and electrospinning. It is evident that the nanofiber meshes supply topological cues at the ECM level, whereas the micro 3D fibrous structure provide the required mechanical stability. We here demonstrated that the integration of these two hierarchial structures lead to improved biological performance. Indeed, human osteoblast-like cells presented significantly higher proliferation and maturation when seeded on these hierarchical starch-based fibrous scaffolds. Overall, the results corroborate our hypothesis that the hierarchical fibrous structure of the scaffolds, mimicking the hierarchical structure of the native ECM, is favourable for bone tissue-engineering strategies.

Acknowledgements

This work was partially supported by the European Integrated Project GENOSTEM (Grant No. LSH-STREP-CT-2003-503161) and the European Network of Excellence EXPERTISSUES (Grant No. NMP3-CT-2004-500283). We also acknowledge the Portuguese Foundation for Science and Technology for the project Naturally Nano (Grant No. POCI/EME/58982/2004) and a PhD grant to A. Martins (Grant No. SFRH/BD/24382/2005).

References

Agrawal CM, Ray RB. 2001; Biodegradable polymeric scaffolds for musculoskeletal tissue engineering. *J Biomed Mater Res* **55**: 141–150.

Araújo JV, Martins A, Leonor IB, *et al.* 2008; Surface controlled biomimetic coating of polycaprolactone nanofibre meshes to be used as bone extracellular matrix analogues. *J Biomater Sci Polym Ed* **19**: 1239–1256.

Capes JS, Ando HY, Cameron RE. 2005; Fabrication of polymeric scaffolds with a controlled distribution of pores. *J Mater Sci Mater Med* **16**: 1069–1075.

Gomes ME, Azevedo HS, Moreira AR, *et al.* 2008; Starch-poly(ε-caprolactone) and starch-poly(lactic acid) fibre-mesh scaffolds for bone tissue engineering applications: structure, mechanical properties and degradation behaviour. *J Tissue Eng Regen Med* **2**: 243–252.

Gomes ME, Holtorf HL, Reis RL, *et al.* 2006; Influence of the porosity of starch-based fibre mesh scaffolds on the proliferation and osteogenic differentiation of bone marrow stromal cells cultured in a flow perfusion bioreactor. *Tissue Eng* **12**: 801–809.

Gomes ME, Reis RL, Cunha AM, *et al.* 2001; Cytocompatibility and response of osteoblastic-like cells to starch-based polymers: effect of several additives and processing conditions. *Biomaterials* **22**: 1911–1917.

Gomes ME, Sikavitsas VI, Behravesh E, *et al.* 2003; Effect of flow perfusion on the osteogenic differentiation of bone marrow stromal cells cultured on starch-based three-dimensional scaffolds. *J Biomed Mater Res A* **67**: 87–95.

Huang ZM, Zhang YZ, Kotaki M, *et al.* 2003; A review on polymer nanofibres by electrospinning and their applications in nanocomposites. *Compos Sci Technol* **63**: 2223–2253.

Hutmacher DW, Schantz JT, Lam CX, *et al.* 2007; State of the art and future directions of scaffold-based bone engineering from a biomaterials perspective. *J Tissue Eng Regen Med* **1**: 245–260.

Hutmacher DW, Sittinger M, Risbud MV. 2004; Scaffold-based tissue engineering: rationale for computer-aided design and solid free-form fabrication systems. *Trends Biotechnol* **22**: 354–362.

Kwon IK, Kidoaki S, Matsuda T. 2005; Electrospun nano- to microfibre fabrics made of biodegradable copolyesters: structural characteristics, mechanical properties and cell adhesion potential. *Biomaterials* **26**: 3929–3939.

Lam CXF, Mo XM, Teoh SH, *et al.* 2002; Scaffold development using 3D printing with a starch-based polymer. *Mater Sci Eng C* **20**: 49–56.

Leong KF, Cheah CM, Chua CK. 2003; Solid freeform fabrication of three-dimensional scaffolds for engineering replacement tissues and organs. *Biomaterials* **24**: 2363–2378.

Lutolf MP, Hubbell JA. 2005; Synthetic biomaterials as instructive extracellular microenvironments for morphogenesis in tissue engineering. *Nature Biotechnol* **23**: 47–55.

Martins A, Araújo JV, Reis RL, *et al.* 2007; Electrospun nanostructured scaffolds for tissue engineering applications. *Nanomedicine* **2**: 929–942.

Mironov V, Boland T, Trusk T, *et al.* 2003; Organ printing: computer-aided jet-based 3D tissue engineering. *Trends Biotechnol* **21**: 157–161.

Moroni L, de Wijn JR, van Blitterswijk CA. 2005; Three-dimensional fibre-deposited PEOT/PBT copolymer scaffolds for tissue engineering: influence of porosity, molecular network mesh size, and swelling in aqueous media on dynamic mechanical properties. *J Biomed Mater Res A* **75**: 957–965.

Moroni L, de Wijn JR, van Blitterswijk CA. 2006; 3D fibre-deposited scaffolds for tissue engineering: influence of pores geometry and architecture on dynamic mechanical properties. *Biomaterials* **27**: 974–985.

Moroni L, Schotel R, Hamann D, *et al.* 2008; 3D fibre-deposited electrospun integrated scaffolds enhance cartilage tissue formation. *Adv Func Mater* **18**: 53–60.

Norman JJ, Desai TA. 2006; Methods for fabrication of nanoscale topography for tissue engineering scaffolds. *Ann Biomed Eng* **34**: 89–101.

Oliveira JT, Crawford A, Mundy JM, *et al.* 2007; A cartilage tissue engineering approach combining starch-polycaprolactone fibre mesh scaffolds with bovine articular chondrocytes. *J Mater Sci Mater Med* **18**: 295–302.

Peltola SM, Melchels FP, Grijpma DW, *et al.* 2008; A review of rapid prototyping techniques for tissue engineering purposes. *Ann Med* **40**: 268–280.

Pfister A, Landers R, Laib A, *et al.* 2004; Biofunctional rapid prototyping for tissue-engineering applications: 3D bioplotting versus 3D printing. *J Polym Sci Part A Polym Chem* **42**: 624–638.

Salgado AJ, Coutinho OP, Reis RL. 2004; Novel starch-based scaffolds for bone tissue engineering: cytotoxicity, cell culture, and protein expression. *Tissue Eng* **10**: 465–474.

Salgado AJ, Coutinho OP, Reis RL, *et al.* 2007; In vivo response to starch-based scaffolds designed for bone tissue engineering applications. *J Biomed Mater Res A* **80**: 983–989.

Salgado AJ, Figueiredo JE, Coutinho OP, *et al.* 2005; Biological response to pre-mineralized starch based scaffolds for bone tissue engineering. *J Mater Sci Mater Med* **16**: 267–275.

Santos MI, Fuchs S, Gomes ME, *et al.* 2007; Response of micro- and macrovascular endothelial cells to starch-based fibre meshes for bone tissue engineering. *Biomaterials* **28**: 240–248.

Schantz JT, Teoh SH, Lim TC, *et al.* 2003; Repair of calvarial defects with customized tissue-engineered bone grafts I. Evaluation of osteogenesis in a three-dimensional culture system. *Tissue Eng* **9**: S113–126.

Tuzlakoglu K, Bolgen N, Salgado AJ, *et al.* 2005; Nano- and microfibre combined scaffolds: a new architecture for bone tissue engineering. *J Mater Sci Mater Med* **16**: 1099–1104.

Yang F, Murugan R, Wang S, *et al.* 2005; Electrospinning of nano/micro scale poly(L-lactic acid) aligned fibres and their potential in neural tissue engineering. *Biomaterials* **26**: 2603–2610.

Yang S, Leong KF, Du Z, *et al.* 2002; The design of scaffolds for use in tissue engineering. Part II. Rapid prototyping techniques. *Tissue Eng* **8**: 1–11.

Yeong WY, Chua CK, Leong KF, *et al.* 2004; Rapid prototyping in tissue engineering: challenges and potential. *Trends Biotechnol* **22**: 643–652.

Zhang YZ, Lim CT, Ramakrishna S, *et al.* 2005; Recent development of polymer nanofibres for biomedical and biotechnological applications. *J Mater Sci Mater Med* **16**: 933–946.

Update

Hierarchical Starch-Based Fibrous Scaffold for Bone Tissue Engineering Applications

Albino Martins, Sangwon Chung, Adriano J. Pedro, Sofia G. Caridade, João F. Mano, Rui A. Sousa, Alexandra P. Marques, Rui L. Reis, and Nuno M. Neves

Abstract

Fibrous structures mimicking the morphology of the natural extracellular matrix are considered promising scaffolds for tissue engineering. This study aims to develop a novel hierarchical starch-based scaffold. Such scaffolds were obtained by a combination of starch-polycaprolactone micromotif and polycaprolactone nanomotif, respectively produced by rapid prototyping and electrospinning techniques. Scanning electron microscopy and microcomputed tomography analysis showed the successful fabrication of a multilayer scaffold composed of parallel aligned microfibers in a grid-like arrangement, intercalated by a mesh-like structure with randomly distributed nanofibers (NFM). The combination of rapid prototyped microfibers with electrospun nanofiber meshes results in a minor decrease in the scaffolds' stiffness, being more significant in wet conditions. Human osteoblast-like cells were dynamically seeded in the scaffolds, using spinner flasks, and cultured for 7 days under static conditions. SEM analysis showed predominant cell attachment and spreading on the nanofiber meshes, which enhanced cell retention at the bulk of the composed/hierarchical scaffolds. A significant increase in cell proliferation and osteoblastic activity, assessed by alkaline phosphatase quantification, was observed on the hierarchical fibrous scaffolds. These results support our hypothesis that the integration of nanoscale fibers into 3D rapid prototype scaffolds substantially improves their biological performance in bone tissue engineering strategies.

1
Introduction

Biodegradable scaffolds are generally recognized as indispensable element in tissue engineering and regenerative medicine strategies. They are used as temporary templates for cell seeding, migration, proliferation, and differentiation prior to the regeneration of biologically functional tissue or natural extracellular matrix (ECM) [1, 2]. Ideally, to create a tissue-engineered construct capable of regenerating a fully functional tissue, it should mimic both the fibrous form and the complex function of the native ECM [3]. Like the natural ECM, a range of topographic features at the macro-, micro-, and even nanoscale levels must lead cell response [4]. The understanding that the natural ECM is a multifunctional nanocomposite motivated researchers to rationally design synthetic ECM-substitute scaffolds. A combination of nanofibers with conventionally designed microfibers may mimic some morphological features of the native ECM [5]. A multiscale network structure can be developed by integrating microfibrous structures, produced by wet spinning or rapid prototyping (RP), with electrospun nanofibers [6–8]. However, most attempts to take advantage of nanofiber structure in mimicking the complexity and hierarchical organization of natural ECM, in the literature, are mostly restricted to the use of nanofibers for coating implants and biomedical devices or are used as processed in random nanofibrous meshes [9].

Electrospun fibers typically have dimensions varying from nano- to microscale, although fiber diameters in the submicrometer range are mainly observed [10]. These mesh-like scaffolds are characterized by high porosity and high surface–volume ratio and, most importantly, they can closely mimic the morphology of native ECM of many tissues. Such physical cues enhance cell adhesion, proliferation, and differentiation, and consequently neotissue formation on nanofibrous meshes of both natural and synthetic polymers [11, 12].

Rapid prototyping has emerged as a powerful polymer processing technique for the production of scaffolds in the area of tissue engineering [13–19]. The main advantage of this technique is the possibility of creating structures with customized shapes linked with computer-aided design (CAD), thus providing more flexibility, versatility, and reproducibility in creating scaffolds [13, 20–22]. However, the typical pore size of RP scaffold constitutes a limitation in cell seeding efficiency [17], once it is relatively large compared to cell dimensions.

Therefore, the aim of this study was to characterize a novel hierarchical starch-based fibrous scaffold obtained by the combination of starch-polycaprolactone (SPCL) micromotif and polycaprolactone (PCL) nanomotif, respectively produced by rapid prototyping and electrospinning (ES). The defined strategy aimed at overcoming the high number of cells needed to attain sufficient adherent cells to the RP scaffolds [8], which can be accomplished by alternately integrating electrospun nanofiber meshes (NFM) every two consecutive layers of plotted microfibers. In this way these nanofiber meshes will act as cell entrapment systems, increasing cell attachment, cell proliferation, and tissue regeneration. Ultimately, this integration will enhance the potential application of such three-dimensional (3D) fibrous structures in bone tissue engineering strategies. This study reports the results of a set of experiments where human osteoblast-like cells were dynamically seeded and statically cultured for 7 days in the micro–nano fiber polymeric scaffolds designed to validate this hypothesis.

2
Materials and Methods

2.1
Scaffold Fabrication

Three-dimensional rapid prototyping scaffolds (6RP) were fabricated by a 3D plotting technique (Bioplotter, EnvisionTec GmbH, Germany), using a 30 : 70 (wt%) blend of starch and polycaprolactone (SPCL; Novamont, Italy). SPCL polymer powder was put into a metal barrel and heated at 140 °C through a heated cartridge unit, and then plotted through a nozzle by air pressure control. The nozzle comprises a stainless steel needle with internal diameter of 0.5 mm and length of 6 mm. A metal piston plunger with a Teflon seal was used to apply pressure to the molten polymer. The machine was linked to a CAD software (PrimCam, Germany) that required inputs of dispensing and processing parameters (e.g., speed of the head, dispensing pressure, and temperature) and the design parameters of the scaffold (e.g., scaffold dimensions, spacing between the polymer strands, and number of layers). The strand spacing was set to 1 mm, without any offset between the consecutive equivalent layers. The orientation was changed by plotting the polymer with 90° angle steps between two successive layers. The production of hierarchical fibrous scaffolds (6RP + 5NFM) was achieved by integrating nanofiber meshes every two consecutive layers of plotted microfibers. The nanofiber meshes were previously produced by electrospinning, as described elsewhere [23–25]. Briefly, a polymeric solution of 17% (w/v) PCL, dissolved in an organic solvent mixture of chloroform/dimethylformamide (7 : 3 ratio), was electrospun by establishing an electric tension of 9.5 kV, a needle tip-to-ground collector distance of 200 mm and a flow rate of 1 ml/h. The scaffolds (6RP and 6RP + 5NFM scaffolds) were all cut into $5 \times 5 \times 5$ mm^3 cubical samples from the originally deposited bulk $20 \times 20 \times 20$ mm^3 cube (12 layers) and sterilized by ethylene oxide (EtO) before the cell culture assays.

2.2
Scaffolds' Structure Characterization

Scaffold architecture was analyzed using microcomputed tomography (μ-CT) with a desktop micro CT scanner (SkyScan 1072, Aartselaar, Belgium). The scanner was set to a voltage of 40 kV and a current of 248 μA, and the samples were scanned at 8.71 μm pixel resolutions by approximately 350 slices covering the sample height of 2.5 mm. For imaging, the sliced 2D tomographic raw images were reconstructed using CT Analyzer software, and the threshold levels of the gray scale images were equally adjusted for all the samples to allow the measurement of the volume of pores providing the data for scaffold porosity. Three-dimensional modeling was also used to analyze the scaffold structure in a nondestructive manner using imaging software.

The morphology of the scaffold was also analyzed using scanning electron microscopy (SEM) (Leica Cambridge, Model S360; UK). All samples were previously sputter-coated with gold (Sputter Coater, Model SC502, Fisons Instruments, UK).

2.3
Dynamic Mechanical Analysis

The viscoelastic measurements were performed using a TRITEC8000B Dynamic mechanical analysis (DMA) from Triton Technology (UK), equipped with the compressive mode. Samples were cut in cubic shapes of 4 mm (dimensions were characterized for each individual sample). Three samples were used for DMA testing that were performed both in wet and dry environment. In the wet condition, scaffolds were previously immersed in a PBS solution for a period of 24 h, their geometry measured, and, then, clamped in the DMA apparatus and immersed in a PBS solution. After reaching equilibrium at 37 °C, the DMA spectra were obtained during a frequency scan between 0.1 and 15 Hz. The experiments were performed under constant strain amplitude (50 µm). A small preload was applied to each sample to ensure that the entire scaffold surface was in contact with the compression plates before testing, and the distance between plates was equal for all scaffolds being tested. The aforementioned measurement conditions were also established for the experiments in the dry state, without the referred immersion periods.

2.4
Cell Seeding and Culture

Human osteosarcoma-derived cells (Saos-2 cell line, European Collection of Cell Cultures (ECACC), UK) were maintained in Dulbecco's modified Eagle's medium (DMEM) (Sigma-Aldrich, Germany) supplemented with 10% heat-inactivated fetal bovine serum (Biochrom AG, Germany) and 1% antibiotic–antimycotic solution (Gibco, UK). Cells were cultured in a humidified incubator at 37 °C in 5% CO_2 atmosphere, and the medium was routinely replaced every 3–4 days.

Confluent osteoblast-like cells were harvested and dynamically seeded into the polymeric scaffolds as follows. The combined and the RP (controls) scaffolding structures were placed between stainless steel holding wires in spinner flasks (12 scaffolds/spinner flask) containing a suspension of osteoblast-like cells with a concentration of 0.5×10^6 cells/ml in a total volume of 35 ml. The stirrer was set at 80 rpm and the spinner flasks left for 72 h to allow the cells to colonize the entire scaffold. After the seeding was completed, the osteoblast/scaffold constructs were transferred to 24-well cell culture plates (Costar®; Corning, NY) and statically cultured at days 1 and 7, under the cultured conditions previously described for maintenance of the cell line.

2.5
Evaluation of Cell Adhesion, Morphology, and Distribution

To evaluate the cell morphology, the cell–scaffold constructs were fixed with 2.5% glutaraldehyde (Sigma, USA) in phosphate-buffered saline (PBS) (Sigma, USA) solution for 1 h at 4 °C. Then, the samples were dehydrated through a graded series of ethanol and let to dry overnight. Finally, they were sputter-coated with gold (Model SC502, Fisons Instruments, UK) and observed in a scanning electron microscope (Model S360, Leica Cambridge, UK).

2.6
Cell Viability Assay

At each defined time culture period, the cell viability was determined using CellTiter 96® aqueous one solution cell proliferation assay (Promega, USA). This assay is based on the bioreduction of a tetrazolium compound, 3-(4,5-dimethylthiazol-2-yl)-5-(3-carboxymethoxyphenyl)-2-(4-sulfofenyl)-2H-tetrazolium (MTS), into a water-soluble brown formazan product. This conversion is accomplished by NADPH or NADH production by the dehydrogenase enzymes in metabolically active cells. The absorbance, measured at 490 nm in a microplate reader (Bio-Tek, Synergie HT, USA), is related to the quantity of formazan product and directly proportional to the number of living cells in the constructs. Three samples per type of scaffold and per time point were characterized.

2.7
DNA Quantification

Cell proliferation was evaluated by quantifying the total amount of double-stranded DNA throughout the culturing time. Quantification was performed using the Quant-iT™ PicoGreen dsDNA assay kit (Invitroge, Molecular Probe, OR), according to the manufacturer's instructions after the cells in the construct were lysed by osmotic and thermal shock. The intensity of fluorescence proportional to the amount of double-stranded DNA was measured at an excitation wavelength of 485/20 nm and at an emission wavelength of 528/20 nm in a microplate reader (Bio-Tek, Synergie HT, USA). Triplicates of each sample allowed a statistical analysis. The DNA concentration for each sample was calculated using a standard curve relating quantity of DNA and fluorescence intensity.

2.8
Alkaline Phosphatase Quantification

To assess the osteogenic activity of cells seeded into the 3D scaffolds (6RP and 6RP + 5NFM), the expression of alkaline phosphatase (ALP) was determined for both culture time periods in the same samples for DNA quantification. In each well of a 96-well plate (Costar; Corning, NY), 20 µl of each sample were mixed with 60 µl substrate solution and 0.2% (w/v) p-nitrophenyl phosphate (Sigma, USA) in a substrate buffer of 1 M diethanolamine HCl (Merck, Germany) at pH 9.8. The plate was then incubated in dark for 45 min at 37 °C. After the incubation period, 80 µl stop solution, 2 M NaOH (Panreac, Barcelona, Spain) and 0.2 mM EDTA (Sigma, USA), was added to each well. Standards were prepared with 10 µmol/ml p-nitrophenol (p-NP) (Sigma, USA) solution to obtain a standard curve ranging from 0 to 0.3 µmol/ml. Triplicates of each sample and standard were made. Absorbance was read at 405 nm in a microplate reader (Bio-Tek, Synergie HT, USA) and sample concentrations were read off from the standard curve. These ALP concentrations were normalized against the DNA concentrations of the same samples to determine the ALP activity.

2.9
Statistical Analysis

Statistical analysis was performed using the SPSS statistic software (Release 8.0.0 for Windows). First, a Shapiro–Wilk test was used to ascertain the data normality. Once the biological results did not follow a normal distribution, Mann–Whitney U test was performed to compare the effect of scaffold architecture over cell performance. In the analysis of the results, $p < 0.05$ was considered statistically significant.

3
Results and Discussion

A novel hierarchical fibrous scaffold was developed, combining starch-polycaprolactone micromotif and polycaprolactone nanomotif, respectively produced by rapid prototyping and electrospinning. These scaffolds were characterized by a 3D structure of parallel-aligned rapid prototyped microfibers (average fiber diameter, 300 μm), periodically intercalated by randomly distributed electrospun nanofibers (fiber diameters in the range of 400 nm–1.4 μm) (Figure 1b). When nanofiber meshes were integrated within the 3D scaffold, no delamination between consecutive layers of RP fibers was observed, resulting in a stable scaffold. In addition, this micro–nano scaffold architecture comprises a high-throughput scaffold process methodology, with regular control over RP-produced structure and nanofibers distribution within the scaffold. The integration of these nano motifs results in a decrease of scaffold porosity of around 11% (from 79.4% on 6RP scaffolds to 68.3% on 6RP + 5NFM scaffolds), as determined by μ-CT analysis (Figure 1c and d). Despite a decrease in porosity, a fully interconnected porous structure was observed, allowing gas, nutrient, and waste transport through the 3D structure.

DMA is an adequate tool to characterize the mechanical/viscoelastic properties of polymeric materials. The storage (elastic) modulus E' and the loss factor tan δ can be measured using a DMA apparatus. E' is related with the stiffness of the material and the loss factor is the ratio of the amount of energy dissipated by viscous mechanisms to the energy stored in the elastic component providing information about the damping properties of the material. Figure 2a presents the viscoelastic behavior of the two kinds of scaffolds. The storage modulus (E') of all scaffolds tends to increase with increasing frequency. For the 6RP scaffolds, E' increases from 17.8 to 25 MPa, while for the 6RP + 5NFM scaffolds, E' increases from 15.2 to 18.9 MPa. Mechanical data indicate that the 6RP scaffolds are stiffer than the 6RP + 5NFM scaffolds. Such differences were expected and attributed to the processing of such structures, as already reported by Kim et al. [26]. Figure 2a also presents the variation of the loss factor tan δ with increasing frequency. We observe that both type of scaffolds present similar behaviors of tan δ, although the values for the 6RP scaffolds are higher than the 6RP + 5NFM scaffolds. The decreasing of tan δ indicates that both scaffolds are becoming viscous with the increasing frequency.

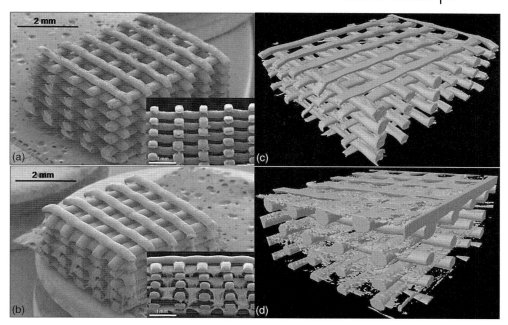

Figure 1 SEM and μ-CT micrographs of the starch-based rapid prototyped, 6RP (a and c) and hierarchical fibrous scaffolds 6RP + 5NFM (b and d).

It has been reported that polymeric materials present different behaviors depending on the testing environment [27–29]. In order to probe how scaffolds behave in physiological conditions, DMA experiments were also performed in a hydrated environment at 37 °C. The variations of the viscoelastic properties with the frequency

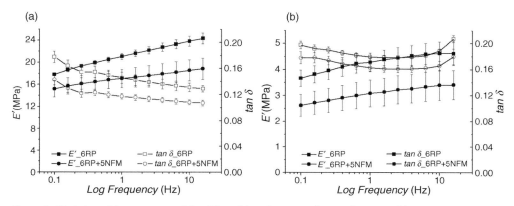

Figure 2 Variation of the storage modulus (E') and loss factor (tan δ), as a function of the frequency, for starch-based rapid prototyped (6RP) and hierarchical fibrous scaffolds (6RP + 5NFM), under dry (a) and wet conditions (b).

are present in Figure 2b. The trend of the mechanical behavior observed in dry state was also verified in the wet conditions. The strong difference in wet conditions is that E' is much lower than that in dry conditions. As observed in Figure 2b, E' increases from 3.7 to 4.6 MPa for the 6RP scaffolds, while for the 6RP + 5NFM scaffolds, E' increases from 2.6 to 3.4 MPa. This decrease in the E' values is due to the plasticization effect of water, which has a profound impact on the scaffolds' viscoelastic properties at physiological conditions [30, 31]. Again, for both scaffold architectures, tan δ slightly decreases with the increasing frequency, indicating that the scaffolds become more elastic and less viscous.

Starch-based scaffolds have been proposed as candidates for bone tissue engineering strategies in multiple studies [6, 32–38], supporting the choice of SPCL to develop the structures proposed in this study. Indeed, successful results were demonstrated in terms of cell viability, proliferation, and maturation of osteoblastic cells or differentiation of bone marrow stromal cells. Moreover, other starch-based blends (corn starch, dextran, and gelatin, 50 : 30 : 20 wt%) have already been used to produce different scaffold designs by 3D printing (3DP) [39]. Although showing suitable physicochemical properties for tissue engineering applications, the biocompatibility of these 3DP geometric scaffolds, with a highly interconnected porous network, remains to be tested. The hierarchical starch-based fibrous scaffolds developed in this study were seeded with human osteoblast-like cells to observe how the scaffold architecture affects their behavior. Cells were initially allowed to attach to the scaffold using a dynamic system; this spinner flask bioreactor allows the cells to efficiently penetrate into the inner regions of the scaffolds, avoiding to a certain extent the preferential colonization of the outermost parts of the scaffolds [40]. Consequently, a homogeneous distribution of cells throughout the entire scaffold was observed. However, SEM micrographs demonstrated that osteoblastic cells preferentially adhered to the nanofibrous meshes (Figure 3b, d, g, and h). This phenomenon of cellular preference was previously described by our group and others [6, 41, 42], when different cell types (osteoblastic, endothelial, and neural stem cells) were seeded into micro- and nanofiber-based scaffolds. In addition, the integration of nanofiber meshes into the 3D rapid prototyped scaffolds seemed to act as a cell entrapment system within the RP scaffold. It was reported by others [17] that cells go through the pores of rapid prototyped scaffolds and accumulate at the bottom of the well plate during the seeding process, without attaching the scaffold, and thus reduces the seeding efficiency typically down to values of 25–35%. Thus, the integration of nanofiber meshes constitutes an innovative strategy to enhance cell seeding efficiency into 3D RP scaffolds.

The quantification of cell viability and metabolic activity of human osteoblast-like cells seeded into the combined electrospun fiber meshes and RP scaffolds was evaluated by MTS assay (Figure 4). The results revealed a steadily increasing trend, with culture time, although there was no significant difference in the effect of the type of scaffold architectures ($p > 0.05$). From the morphological evaluation of the constructs, it seems that the integrated nanofiber meshes into the 3D rapid prototyped structure also acted as a cell entrapment system within the scaffold. Consequently, a significant increase in cell proliferation and maturation, respectively

3 Results and Discussion

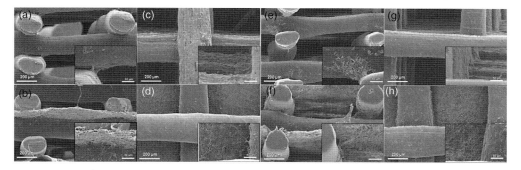

Figure 3 SEM micrographs of rapid prototyped (a, c, e, and g) and hierarchical fibrous (b, d, f, and h) scaffolds cultured with human osteoblast-like cells (Saos-2 cell line) at day 1 (a–d) and day 7 (e–h). Cross sections (a, b, e, and f) and top view (c, d, g, and h) of the constructs. Higher magnifications enclosed.

assessed by DNA and ALP activity quantification, along the culture time, was observed in the hierarchical fibrous scaffolds (Figures 5 and 6) in comparison to the rapid prototyped scaffolds ($p < 0.05$), especially for longer culture periods. However, for the RP scaffolds, the osteoblastic activity was not maintained throughout the experiment, as observed by a decrease in ALP activity from day 1 to day 7 of culture. It was already reported by Schantz et al. [43] that rabbit calvarial osteoblasts, seeded into PCL scaffolds fabricated via fused deposition modeling (FDM) and embedded into a fibrin matrix (Tisseel, Baxter Hyland Immuno, Glendale, CA),

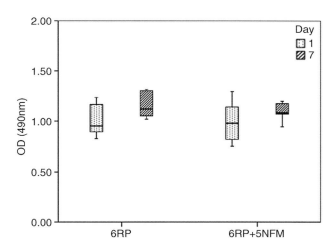

Figure 4 Box plot of cell viability results of human osteoblastic cells cultured in rapid prototyped (6RP) and hierarchical fibrous (6RP + 5NFM) scaffolds, at day 1 and day 7. Data were analyzed by nonparametric way of a Mann–Whitney U test ($p < 0.05$).

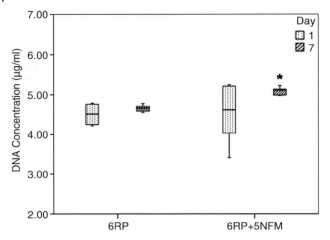

Figure 5 Box plot of DNA content of osteoblast-like cells cultured in rapid prototyped (6RP) and hierarchical fibrous (6RP + 5NFM) scaffolds, at day 1 and day 7. Data were analyzed by nonparametric way of a Mann–Whitney U test ($^*p < 0.05$).

showed no significant differences in their ALP activity along time. These results are in accordance with those of our study.

Similar strategies were already described in the literature [8, 26, 44], describing a hybrid fabrication process of integrated/hierarchical scaffolds. Briefly, PCL or PCL/collagen nanofiber meshes were directly electrospun (i.e., by 3D plotting or by direct

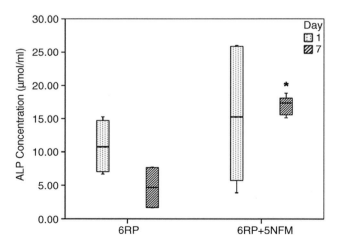

Figure 6 Box plot of ALP activity, normalized against dsDNA amount, from osteoblastic cells (Saos-2 cell line) cultured in rapid prototyped (6RP) and hierarchical fibrous (6RP + 5NFM) scaffolds, at day 1 and day 7. Data were analyzed by nonparametric way of a Mann–Whitney U test ($^*p < 0.05$).

polymer melt deposition) over rapid prototyped microfibers, during shorter deposition periods. These micro–nanofibrous structures were biologically tested envisioning cartilage tissue engineering strategies. Cell culture data demonstrated the preferential adhesion of bovine or porcine primary chondrocytes to the electrospun nanofiber matrices, as well as a statistically significant increase in cell proliferation on the hybrid processed scaffolds. Integrating these observations with our data, it could be speculated that the cell behavior is directly related with the topographical cues provided by the electrospun nanofibers. In addition, the integration of nanofibrous structure into 3D fibrous scaffolds could enhance serum protein adsorption, due to the high specific surface area of the nanofibers, mediating an efficient adhesion of the cells at the surface of these structures [45].

4
Conclusions

A novel hierarchical fibrous scaffold was developed, combining starch-polycaprolactone micromotif and polycaprolactone nanomotif, respectively produced by rapid prototyping and electrospinning. It is evident that the nanofiber meshes supply topological cues at the ECM level, whereas the micro 3D fibrous structure provides the required mechanical stability. The combination of rapid prototyped microfibers with electrospun nanofiber meshes results in a minor decrease in the scaffolds' stiffness, being more significant in wet conditions. The mechanical properties of these structures follow the general trend to decrease the compression modulus in wet conditions. We here demonstrated that the integration of these two hierarchical structures lead to improved biological performance. Indeed, human osteoblast-like cells presented significantly higher proliferation and maturation when seeded in these hierarchical starch-based fibrous scaffolds. Overall, the results corroborate our hypothesis that the hierarchical structure of the scaffolds, mimicking the hierarchical structure of the native ECM, is favorable for bone tissue engineering strategies.

5
Future Perspectives

The application of hierarchical fibrous scaffolds could be an outstanding starting point for the *in vitro* generation of hierarchically structured tissues, namely, vascularized and highly organized 3D tissues like bone and skin, involving more than one cell communities. The functional complexity of the hierarchical fibrous scaffolds could also be improved by incorporating the bioactive molecules into nanofibers. It is also very important to evaluate the performance of these complex structures *in vivo*, for specific applications, taking advantage of the enhanced opportunities to deliver communities of cells and to also release locally specific bioactive molecules.

Acknowledgments

This work was partially supported by the European Integrated Project GENOSTEM (LSH-STREP-CT-2003-503161) and the European Network of Excellence EXPERTISSUES (NMP3-CT-2004-500283). It was also funded by the Portuguese Foundation for Science and Technology for the project Naturally Nano (POCI/EME/58982/2004) and the PhD grant to A. Martins (SFRH/BD/24382/2005).

References

1 Lutolf, M.P. and Hubbell, J.A. (2005) Synthetic biomaterials as instructive extracellular microenvironments for morphogenesis in tissue engineering. *Nat. Biotechnol.*, **23**, 47–55.

2 Hutmacher, D.W., Schantz, J.T., Lam, C.X., Tan, K.C., and Lim, T.C. (2007) State of the art and future directions of scaffold-based bone engineering from a biomaterials perspective. *J. Tissue Eng. Regen. Med.*, **1**, 245–260.

3 Agrawal, C.M. and Ray, R.B. (2001) Biodegradable polymeric scaffolds for musculoskeletal tissue engineering. *J. Biomed. Mater. Res.*, **55**, 141–150.

4 Norman, J.J. and Desai, T.A. (2006) Methods for fabrication of nanoscale topography for tissue engineering scaffolds. *Ann. Biomed. Eng.*, **34**, 89–101.

5 Dzenis, Y.A. (1996) Hierarchical nano-/micromaterials based on electrospun polymer fibers: predictive models for thermomechanical behavior. *J. Comput. Aid. Mater. Des.*, **3**, 403–408.

6 Tuzlakoglu, K., Bolgen, N., Salgado, A.J., Gomes, M.E., Piskin, E., and Reis, R.L. (2005) Nano- and micro-fiber combined scaffolds: a new architecture for bone tissue engineering. *J. Mater. Sci. Mater. Med.*, **16**, 1099–1104.

7 Santos, M.I., Fuchs, S., Gomes, M.E., Unger, R.E., Reis, R.L., and Kirkpatrick, C.J. (2007) Response of micro- and macrovascular endothelial cells to starch-based fiber meshes for bone tissue engineering. *Biomaterials*, **28**, 240–248.

8 Moroni, L., Schotel, R., Hamann, D., de Wijn, J.R., and van Blitterswijk, C.A. (2008) 3D fiber-deposited electrospun integrated scaffolds enhance cartilage tissue formation. *Adv. Funct. Mater.*, **18**, 53–60.

9 Teo, W.E. and Ramakrishna, S. (2009) Electrospun nanofibers as a platform for multifunctional, hierarchically organized nanocomposite. *Compos. Sci. Technol.*, **69**, 1804–1817.

10 Huang, Z.M., Zhang, Y.Z., Kotaki, M., and Ramakrishna, S. (2003) A review on polymer nanofibers by electrospinning and their applications in nanocomposites. *Compos. Sci. Technol.*, **63**, 2223–2253.

11 Zhang, Y.Z., Lim, C.T., Ramakrishna, S., and Huang, Z.M. (2005) Recent development of polymer nanofibers for biomedical and biotechnological applications. *J. Mater. Sci. Mater. Med.*, **16**, 933–946.

12 Martins, A., Araujo, J.V., Reis, R.L., and Neves, N.M. (2007) Electrospun nanostructured scaffolds for tissue engineering applications. *Nanomedicine*, **2**, 929–942.

13 Hutmacher, D.W., Sittinger, M., and Risbud, M.V. (2004) Scaffold-based tissue engineering: rationale for computer-aided design and solid free-form fabrication systems. *Trends Biotechnol.*, **22**, 354–362.

14 Leong, K.F., Cheah, C.M., and Chua, C.K. (2003) Solid freeform fabrication of three-dimensional scaffolds for engineering replacement tissues and organs. *Biomaterials*, **24**, 2363–2378.

15 Mironov, V., Boland, T., Trusk, T., Forgacs, G., and Markwald, R.R. (2003) Organ printing: computer-aided jet-based 3D tissue engineering. *Trends Biotechnol.*, **21**, 157–161.

16 Peltola, S.M., Melchels, F.P., Grijpma, D.W., and Kellomaki, M.

(2008) A review of rapid prototyping techniques for tissue engineering purposes. *Ann. Med.*, **40**, 268–280.

17 Pfister, A., Landers, R., Laib, A., Hubner, U., Schmelzeisen, R., and Mulhaupt, R. (2004) Biofunctional rapid prototyping for tissue-engineering applications: 3D bioplotting versus 3D printing. *J. Polym. Sci. Polym. Chem.*, **42**, 624–638.

18 Yang, S., Leong, K.F., Du, Z., and Chua, C.K. (2002) The design of scaffolds for use in tissue engineering. Part II. Rapid prototyping techniques. *Tissue Eng.*, **8**, 1–11.

19 Yeong, W.Y., Chua, C.K., Leong, K.F., and Chandrasekaran, M. (2004) Rapid prototyping in tissue engineering: challenges and potential. *Trends Biotechnol.*, **22**, 643–652.

20 Moroni, L., De Wijn, J.R., and van Blitterswijk, C.A. (2005) Three-dimensional fiber-deposited PEOT/PBT copolymer scaffolds for tissue engineering: influence of porosity, molecular network mesh size, and swelling in aqueous media on dynamic mechanical properties. *J. Biomed. Mater. Res.*, **75**, 957–965.

21 Moroni, L., De Wijn, J.R., and Van Blitterswijk, C.A. (2006) 3D fiber-deposited scaffolds for tissue engineering: influence of pores geometry and architecture on dynamic mechanical properties. *Biomaterials*, **27**, 974–985.

22 Capes, J.S., Ando, H.Y., and Cameron, R.E. (2005) Fabrication of polymeric scaffolds with a controlled distribution of pores. *J. Mater. Sci. Mater. Med.*, **16**, 1069–1075.

23 Araujo, J.V., Martins, A., Leonor, I.B., Pinho, E.D., Reis, R.L., and Neves, N.M. (2008) Surface controlled biomimetic coating of polycaprolactone nanofiber meshes to be used as bone extracellular matrix analogues. *J. Biomater. Sci. Polym. Ed.*, **19**, 1261–1278.

24 da Silva, M.A., Crawford, A., Mundy, J., Martins, A., Araujo, J.V., Hatton, P.V., Reis, R.L., and Neves, N.M. (2009) Evaluation of extracellular matrix formation in polycaprolactone and starch-compounded polycaprolactone nanofiber meshes when seeded with bovine articular chondrocytes. *Tissue Eng.*, **15**, 377–385.

25 Martins, A., Pinho, E.D., Faria, S., Pashkuleva, I., Marques, A.P., Reis, R.L., and Neves, N.M. (2009) Surface modification of electrospun polycaprolactone nanofiber meshes by plasma treatment to enhance biological performance. *Small*, **5**, 1195–1206.

26 Kim, G., Son, J., Park, S., and Kim, W. (2008) Hybrid process for fabricating 3D hierarchical scaffolds combining rapid prototyping and electrospinning. *Macromol. Rapid Commun.*, **29**, 1577–1581.

27 Mano, J.F., Neves, N.M., and Reis, R.L. (2005) Mechanical characterization of biomaterials, in *Biodegradable Systems in Tissue Engineering and Regenerative Medicine* (eds R.L. Reis and J.S. Román), CRC Press.

28 Mano, J.F. (2008) Viscoelastic properties of chitosan with different hydration degrees as studied by dynamic mechanical analysis. *Macromol. Biosci.*, **8**, 67–76.

29 Mano, J.F., Reis, R.L., and Cunha, A.M. (2002) Dynamic mechanical analysis in polymers for medical applications, in *Polymer Based Systems on Tissue Engineering, Replacement and Regeneration* (eds R.L. Reis and D. Cohn), Kluwer Academic Publishers, The Netherlands.

30 Caridade, S.G., da Silva, R.M.P., Reis, R.L., and Mono, J.F. (2009) Effect of solvent-dependent viscoelastic properties of chitosan membranes on the permeation of 2-phenylethanol. *Carbohydr. Polym.*, **75**, 651–659.

31 Bras, A.R., Viciosa, M.T., Dionisio, M., and Mano, J.F. (2007) Water effect in the thermal and molecular dynamics behavior of poly(L-lactic acid). *J. Therm. Anal. Calorim.*, **88**, 425–429.

32 Gomes, M.E., Holtorf, H.L., Reis, R.L., and Mikos, A.G. (2006) Influence of the porosity of starch-based fiber mesh scaffolds on the proliferation and osteogenic differentiation of bone marrow stromal cells cultured in a flow perfusion bioreactor. *Tissue Eng.*, **12**, 801–809.

33 Gomes, M.E., Reis, R.L., Cunha, A.M., Blitterswijk, C.A., and de Bruijn, J.D. (2001) Cytocompatibility and response of osteoblastic-like cells to starch-based polymers: effect of several additives and processing conditions. *Biomaterials*, **22**, 1911–1917.

34 Gomes, M.E., Sikavitsas, V.I., Behravesh, E., Reis, R.L., and Mikos, A.G. (2003) Effect of flow perfusion on the osteogenic differentiation of bone marrow stromal cells cultured on starch-based three-dimensional scaffolds. *J. Biomed. Mater. Res.*, **67**, 87–95.

35 Salgado, A.J., Coutinho, O.P., and Reis, R.L. (2004) Novel starch-based scaffolds for bone tissue engineering: cytotoxicity, cell culture, and protein expression. *Tissue Eng.*, **10**, 465–474.

36 Salgado, A.J., Coutinho, O.P., Reis, R.L., and Davies, J.E. (2007) *In vivo* response to starch-based scaffolds designed for bone tissue engineering applications. *J. Biomed. Mater. Res.*, **80**, 983–989.

37 Salgado, A.J., Figueiredo, J.E., Coutinho, O.P., and Reis, R.L. (2005) Biological response to pre-mineralized starch based scaffolds for bone tissue engineering. *J. Mater. Sci. Mater. Med.*, **16**, 267–275.

38 Gomes, M.E., Azevedo, H.S., Moreira, A.R., Ella, V., Kellomaki, M., and Reis, R.L. (2008) Starch-poly(epsilon-caprolactone) and starch-poly(lactic acid) fibre-mesh scaffolds for bone tissue engineering applications: structure, mechanical properties and degradation behaviour. *J. Tissue Eng. Regen. Med.*, **2**, 243–252.

39 Lam, C.X.F., Mo, X.M., Teoh, S.H., and Hutmacher, D.W. (2002) Scaffold development using 3D printing with a starch-based polymer. *Mater. Sci. Eng. C*, **20**, 49–56.

40 Oliveira, J.T., Crawford, A., Mundy, J.M., Moreira, A.R., Gomes, M.E., Hatton, P.V., and Reis, R.L. (2007) A cartilage tissue engineering approach combining starch-polycaprolactone fibre mesh scaffolds with bovine articular chondrocytes. *J. Mater. Sci. Mater. Med.*, **18**, 295–302.

41 Kwon, I.K., Kidoaki, S., and Matsuda, T. (2005) Electrospun nano- to microfiber fabrics made of biodegradable copolyesters: structural characteristics, mechanical properties and cell adhesion potential. *Biomaterials*, **26**, 3929–3939.

42 Yang, F., Murugan, R., Wang, S., and Ramakrishna, S. (2005) Electrospinning of nano/micro scale poly(L-lactic acid) aligned fibers and their potential in neural tissue engineering. *Biomaterials*, **26**, 2603–2610.

43 Schantz, J.T., Teoh, S.H., Lim, T.C., Endres, M., Lam, C.X., and Hutmacher, D.W. (2003) Repair of calvarial defects with customized tissue-engineered bone grafts I. Evaluation of osteogenesis in a three-dimensional culture system. *Tissue Eng.*, **9** (Suppl. 1), S113–S126.

44 Park, S.H., Kim, T.G., Kim, H.C., Yang, D.Y., and Park, T.G. (2008) Development of dual scale scaffolds via direct polymer melt deposition and electrospinning for applications in tissue regeneration. *Acta Biomater.*, **4**, 1198–1207.

45 Woo, K.M., Chen, V.J., and Ma, P.X. (2003) Nano-fibrous scaffolding architecture selectively enhances protein adsorption contributing to cell attachment. *J. Biomed. Mater. Res. A*, **67**, 531–537.

3
Bacterial and *Candida albicans* Adhesion on Rapid Prototyping-Produced 3D-Scaffolds Manufactured as Bone Replacement Materials

Bacterial and *Candida albicans* adhesion on rapid prototyping-produced 3D-scaffolds manufactured as bone replacement materials

A. Al-Ahmad,[1] M. Wiedmann-Al-Ahmad,[2] C. Carvalho,[3] M. Lang,[1] M. Follo,[4]
G. Braun,[1] A. Wittmer,[5] R. Mülhaupt,[3] E. Hellwig[1]

[1]Department of Operative Dentistry and Periodontology, Albert Ludwigs University, Freiburg, Germany
[2]Department of Oral and Maxillofacial Surgery, Albert Ludwigs University, Freiburg, Germany
[3]Freiburg Material Research Center and Institute for Macromolecular Chemistry, Albert Ludwigs University, Freiburg, Germany
[4]Department of Hematology and Oncology, Albert-Ludwigs-University, Freiburg, Germany
[5]Institute for Medical Microbiology and Hygiene, Albert Ludwigs University, Freiburg, Germany

Received 15 June 2007; revised 2 October 2007; accepted 18 October 2007
Published online 28 January 2008 in Wiley InterScience (www.interscience.wiley.com). DOI: 10.1002/jbm.a.31832

Abstract: Rapid prototyping (RP)-produced scaffolds are gaining increasing importance in scaffold-guided tissue engineering. Microbial adhesion on the surface of replacement materials has a strong influence on healing and long-term outcome. Consequently, it is important to examine the adherence of microorganisms on RP-produced scaffolds. This research focussed on manufacturing of scaffolds by 3D-bioplotting and examination of their microbial adhesion characteristics. Tricalciumphosphate (TCP), calcium/sodium alginate, and poly(lactide-*co*-glycolic acid) (PLGA) constructs were produced and used to study the adhesion of dental pathogens. Six oral bacterial strains, one *Candida* strain and human saliva were used for the adhesion studies. The number of colony forming units (CFU) were determined and scanning electron microscopy (SEM) and confocal laser scanning microscopy (CLSM) were performed. Microorganisms adhered to all scaffolds. All strains, except for *Streptococcus oralis*, adhered best to PLGA scaffolds. *Streptococcus oralis* adhered to each of the biomaterials equally. *Streptococcus mutans* and *Enterococcus faecalis* adhered best to PLGA scaffolds, followed by alginate and TCP. *Prevotella nigrescens*, *Porphyromonas gingivalis*, *Streptococcus sanguis*, and *Candida albicans* showed the highest adherence to PLGA, followed by TCP and alginate. In contrast, the microorganisms of saliva adhered significantly better to TCP, followed by PLGA and alginate. SEM observations correlated with the results of the CFU determinations. CLSM detected bacteria within deeper sheets of alginate. In conclusion, because of the high adherence rate of oral pathogens to the scaffolds, the application of these biomaterials for bone replacement in oral surgery could result in biomaterial-related infections. Strategies to decrease microbial adherence and to prevent infections due to oral pathogens are discussed. © 2008 Wiley Periodicals, Inc. J Biomed Mater Res 87A: 933–943, 2008

Key words: rapid prototyping; tissue engineering; bacterial colonization; dental pathogens; saliva

INTRODUCTION

The field of scaffold-guided tissue or bone engineering has rapidly developed in recent years. This method offers a promising new approach in reconstructive surgery. The loss of bone due to congenital or acquired pathology, such as trauma, tumor, or infection can be reconstructed by the use of vitalised biomaterials (cell/scaffold constructs). The scaffolds have to be biocompatible, biodegradable, and should also have good bone replacement properties. Additionally, the scaffold material should enhance cell attachment, proliferation, and the expression of the native phenotype. However, at the same time it should reduce the extent and the kinetics of bacterial adhesion.[1,2] This is of primary importance because during surgical procedures the RP-produced scaffolds which should be applied in patients could be exposed to bacteria from saliva or dental plaque. Thus, the scaffolds should have surfaces with properties which are antimicrobial or which limit bacterial adhesion. Bacterial adhesion and colonization on scaffold surfaces can lead to foreign body infections or directly to the degradation of the scaffold by proteolytic bacterial enzymes and consequently to the failure of the replacement material.[3] Hung et al.[4]

Correspondence to: A. Al-Ahmad; e-mail: ali.al-ahmad@uniklinik-freiburg.de

© 2008 Wiley Periodicals, Inc.
Computer Aided Biomanufacturing, Edited by Roger Narayan and Paul Calvert
© 2011 WILEY-VCH Verlag GmbH & Co. KGaA. Published 2011 by WILEY-VCH Verlag GmbH & Co. KGaA.

reported the microbial colonization of barrier materials used in guided tissue regeneration and described the negative influence of *Streptococcus mutans* and *Actinobacillus actinomycetemcomitans* on the attachment of periodontal ligament fibroblasts onto these membranes and consequently on the healing process. Different mechanisms for the bacteria and biomaterial surface interactions have been reported. Among these are molecular mechanisms such as electrostatic and hydrophobic forces, van der Waals forces and adhesins, for example lectins.[5,6] Bacterial adhesion is an essential step for bacteria to colonize biomaterial surfaces, forming biofilms which can cause different infections. Bacterial proliferation on biomaterials varies with the material and microorganism. The scaffold composition, especially surface modifications by coupling different end groups (-OH, -NH$_2$, -SO$_3$) and the scaffold structure, play a major role in bacterial adhesion.[6] There have been many studies done on the colonization of bacteria on the surface of conventionally produced 2D-biomaterials for example collagen membranes, polytetra-fluoroethylene, polyurethane, or hydroxyapatite and about medical adhesion on medical devices such as intravenous catheters and sutures.[3,4,6–9] Sela et al.[3] examined the adherence of periodontal bacteria (*Porphyromonas gingivalis*, *Treponema denticola*, and *Actinobacillus actinomycetemcomitans*) to different commercially available collagen membranes and demonstrated the degradation of these membranes by bacterial enzymes.

Reproducibility and precision are required to the manufacturing of scaffolds for use in tissue or bone engineering. In the past few years, a wide range of rapid prototyping (RP) techniques have been developed for the construction of 3D-scaffolds and for their application in the field of tissue engineering. These are capable of overcoming many of the limitations encountered with conventional manual-based fabrication processes (salt or particulate leaching) such as limited thickness, irregular pore sizes, and no reproducibility.[1,10–13] The most widely reported RP-techniques for the manufacturing of scaffolds for tissue engineering include 3D-printing, fused deposition modeling, stereolithography, selective laser sintering, and inkjet printing.[11] In 2000 a new RP technology, 3D-bioplotting, was developed at the Freiburg Materials Research Center. It enables the 3D dispensing of liquids and pastes into liquid media to construct objects layer by layer with predefined macro- and microstructures.[14] Recent studies from our own group have shown the potential for 3D-bioplotting in the field of bone engineering: Human osteoblast-like cells and ovine osteoblast-like cells showed good potential for use on RP-produced scaffolds because of their proliferation, adhesion, and morphology.[15]

To our knowledge there has been no study to date about bacterial adherence on RP-produced scaffolds manufactured as potential bone replacement material. Our research focused on the manufacturing of scaffolds through the use of 3D-bioplotting and on microbial adhesion to these 3D-matrices. Three different scaffolds, hydroxyapatite (TCP), alginate, and poly(lactide-*co*-glycolic acid) (PLGA), were produced and then used to study the adhesion of dental pathogens and other microorganisms. The aim of this study was to examine whether there are any significant differences in microbial adherence to 3D-plotted materials, to discuss the potential risk of biomaterial-associated infections on such 3D-plotted scaffolds and also to determine whether there is a need for scaffold surface modification to prevent bacterial adhesion.

MATERIALS AND METHODS

Biomaterials

The copolymer PLGA, which has a composition of 85:15, was purchased as a granulate from Boehringer Ingelheim, Germany (PLGA Resomer 824) and was kept melted at 180°C in a glass syringe in the dispenser of the 3D bioplotter throughout the process. The movement of the dispenser was controlled by the PrimCAM software (Primus Data, Einsiedeln, Switzerland) to create scaffolds of 25 mm × 25 mm × 1 mm, using a xy-velocity of 300 mm per min and a z-velocity of 200 mm per min. A needle with an inner diameter of 0.25 mm was chosen, with which a strand thickness of 300 μm was achieved. The interval between strands was 700 μm for each layer. The slower cooling and hardening process gave the strands of the PLGA scaffolds a slightly ellipsoid shape. By changing the direction of each layer by 90°, a fine mesh of four layers high was fabricated with an interval of 250 μm between parallel layers. The porosity of the PLGA scaffolds was 0.45–0.52. The Young's modulus of the PLGA scaffolds acquired in compressive strength tests averaged around 92.66 MPa.

The ceramic scaffolds were created from a fine tricalcium phosphate powder (TCP), purchased from cfb Budenheim, Budenheim, Germany, sieved to particle sizes ranging between 1 and 10 μm. To create a plottable paste, a 10% solution of polyvinyl alcohol (PVA) was first made by dissolving this polymer in boiling water. Next, 37.5 g of TCP were mixed with 62.5 g of PVA and stirred steadily for 20 min, which created a white paste. This was then pressed through a 100-μm sieve to remove larger aggregates. The TCP-PVA paste was inserted into a PE syringe for the plotting process. Scaffolds with 25 mm × 25 mm × 1 mm were fabricated, using a xy-velocity of 1000 mm per min and a z-velocity of 800 mm per min onto a cooled surface. A PE needle with an inner diameter of 0.25 mm was chosen, which produced strands with a thickness of 250 μm. The interval between layers was 750 μm. After plotting, the scaffolds were kept frozen at −15°C for 12 h and then freeze-dried (LYOVAC GT 2, Finn-Aqua Santasalo-Sohlberg GmbH, Essen, Germany) for 24 h using 3.6×10^2 Pa and −40°C. The dried scaffolds were placed in an oven (Nabertherm, Lilienthal, Germany—Model HT04/17), which was slowly heated to 250°C at a heating rate of 25 K/h. This temperature was maintained for 5 h and then raised to 1150°C using a heating rate of 100 K/h, at which point the scaffolds were sintered for 12 h. This removed the PVA from the scaffold and melted the TCP particles together to create a solid porous ceramic scaffold. The oven was then cooled down slowly at a rate of 50 K/h to room temperature, to avoid the creation of cracks.

The calcium/sodium alginate scaffolds were fabricated from a 5% solution of sodium alginate, purchased from Fluka, Buchs, Switzerland, and were made using boiling phosphate buffered saline (PBS) (PAA Laboratories GmbH, Pasching, Germany). The solution was cooled down to 40°C and inserted into a glass syringe, which was kept at that temperature during the plotting process. Scaffolds with 25 mm × 25 mm × 1 mm were fabricated onto a cooled petri dish, using a xy-velocity of 400 mm per min and a z-velocity of 300 mm per min. A needle with an inner diameter of 0.25 mm was chosen, with which a strand thickness of 300 μm was achieved, with an interval of 700 μm between each layer. After the plotting process, PBS with 5% calcium chloride (Sigma, Steinheim, Germany) was carefully added to the petri dish and the scaffold was kept at room temperature for at least one hour to fully solidify the strands.

The PLGA- and TCP scaffolds were plasma sterilized, whereas alginate scaffolds were sterilized by incubation in a 1% calcium chloride dihydrate solution in 70% ethanol (Merck, Darmstadt, Germany).

Strains and culture conditions

The following strains were used for the adhesion experiments: *Streptococcus mutans* ATCC 25175, *Streptococcus oralis* DSM 20068, *Streptococcus sanguis* ATCC 35037, *Porphyromonas gingivalis* W 381, *Prevotella nigrescens* NCTC 9336 and additionally, the eukaryotic strain *Candida albicans* ATCC 90028 were kindly provided by the Institute of Medical Microbiology and Hygiene, University of Freiburg, Germany. The strain *Enterococcus faecalis* T 9 described by Maekawa et al.[16] was obtained by Prof. Dr. J. Hübner, Department of Medical Infectiology, University Freiburg, Germany. In addition, unstimulated human saliva from a healthy 40-year-old volunteer who did not use antibacterial mouthrinses or antibiotics for 6 months prior to the start of the experiment was investigated for the adhesion studies on the RP-produced scaffolds. Table I shows an overview of the tested microorganisms and their occurrence.

All *Streptococcus* strains, *Enterococcus faecalis* and saliva were cultivated on Columbia blood (CoBl; Difco 0793-17-2, Germany) agar plates at 37°C, for the overnight cultures and the inoculation in brain heart infusion (BHI) bouillon (Oxoid, Basingstoke, Hampshire, England). *Porphyromonas gingivalis* and the *Prevotella* strains were cultivated under anaerobic conditions (anaerobic jars, Anaerocult A, Merck,

TABLE I
Overview of the Oral Microorganisms Investigated and Their Occurrence to Examine the Adhesion on 3D-Scaffolds Manufactured by Rapid Prototyping

Microorganism	Occurrence
Streptococcus mutans	supragingivale plaque
Streptococcus oralis	supragingivale plaque
Streptococcus sanguis	supragingivale plaque
Porphyromonas gingivalis	supragingivale plaque
Prevotella nigrescens	subgingival plaque
Enterococcus faecalis	endodontic infections
Candida albicans	oral infections in immunesupressed patients
Saliva	oral flora

Darmstadt, Germany) on yeast-cysteine blood agar (HCB) plates and in GC-HP bouillon for the overnight cultures and the inoculation, respectively.[7] *Candida albicans* was cultivated in Sabouraud Dextrose agar and bouillon.

Inoculation and colonization

Logarithmic-phase cells were used for the adhesion studies. Eight-milliliter cell suspensions of each organism were centrifuged at 4000g for 10 min (Hettich, Tuttlingen, Germany). The supernatants were removed, the pellets were washed in PBS (Biochrom AG, Berlin, Germany), and the centrifugation step was repeated. After removing the supernatant, 8 mL PBS was added. Except for the adhesion experiments using alginate scaffolds, the pellets were washed and resuspended in 1% calcium chloride dihydrate solution (Merck, Darmstadt, Germany). One hundred microliter of each organism were streaked onto CoBl, HCB, and Sabouraud Dextrose agar plates, respectively, to determine the number of colony forming units (CFU's) present. The optical densities of the bacterial and *Candida* solutions were measured at 595 nm (Bio-Rad, Life Science Group, Hercules) against PBS as a blank.

Four samples (cut from the original scaffolds, each now 4 mm × 4 mm × 1 mm in size) of each RP-produced scaffold were placed into wells of multiwell plates (24-well plate, Greiner bio-one, Frickenhausen, Germany). Then 2 mL of the bacterial and *Candida* suspensions were added to each well and the samples were incubated at 37°C for 2 h with constant swirling. After the incubation period the probes were rinsed two times with PBS to remove the nonadherent microorganisms. For scanning electron microscopy (SEM) one scaffold with adherent microorganisms was fixed in 8% formaldehyde. The other three probes for determining the CFU's were treated by sonication in 1 mL PBS on ice to elute the microorganisms from the surface of the scaffold. Dilutions were then streaked onto the appropriate media (CoBl, HCB, Sabouraud Dextrose, respectively).

Scanning electron microscopy

For examination by scanning electron microscope, the scaffolds inoculated with bacteria were fixed in 8% formal-

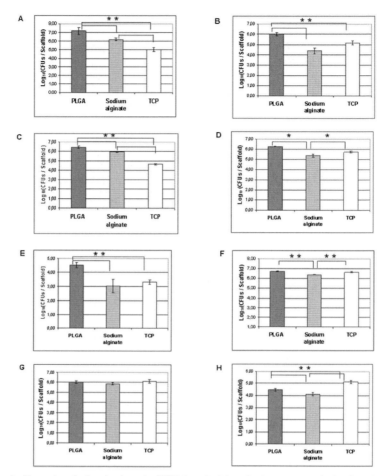

Figure 1. The number of colony forming units (CFUs) determined for each microorganism and saliva for each scaffold. *Streptococcus mutans* (A), *Streptococcus sanguis* (B), *Enterococcus faecalis* (C), *Candida albicans* (D), *Prevotella nigrescens* (E), *Porphyromonas gingivalis* (F), *Streptococcus oralis* (G), saliva (H). **represent highly significant differences, *represent significant differences.

dehyde for 3 days at 4°C and dehydrated in graded alcohol (30, 50, 70, 80, 90, one time each and two times in 99.8% for 1 h). After critical point drying (Critical Point Dryer CPD 030, Bal-Tec, Wallruf, Germany) using liquid carbon dioxide according to standard procedure, the samples were sputtered with gold in a SCD 050 coater (Bal-Tec, Wallruf, Germany). The samples were examined via a Zeiss Leo 435 VP scanning electron microscope (Leo Electron Microscopy Ltd Cooperation Zeiss Leica, Cambridge, England) at 10 kV.

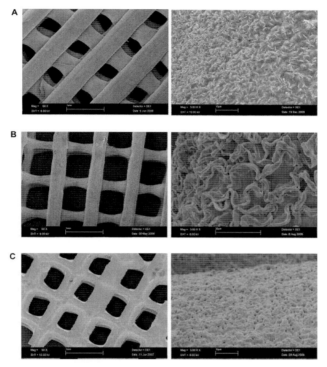

Figure 2. Scanning electron micrographs of the surface of the scaffolds prior to microbial colonization. PLGA (A), calcium/sodium alginate (B), and TCP (C). Each scaffold is shown in lower (50×) and higher (3000×) magnification.

Confocal laser scanning microscopy

To examine the location of adherent bacteria in the lamellar surface of alginate, CLSM was used. The samples were stained using 4′,6-diamino-2-phenylindole (DAPI, Merck, Darmstadt, Germany) solution (1 μg/mL distilled water) for 10 min in the dark. The scaffolds were then washed in distilled water. Immediately after staining a drop of saline buffer was placed onto a chambered coverslip (μ-Slide 8 well, ibidi GmbH, Munich, Germany). The scaffolds with the adherent bacteria were inverted into the saline buffer drops. Confocal images were obtained using a CLSM inverted microscope (Leica TCS SP2 AOBS, Mannheim, Germany) and a 63× water immersion objective (HCX PLAPO ibd.BL). Standard images were made with a zoom setting of 1× and 630× magnification. The area of each section was transformed into a digital image containing 1024 × 1024 pixels.

Statistical analysis

One way ANOVA (PROC GLM, SAS 8.2) and the Tukey test were used to detect significant differences for the different microorganism adhesion targets with respect to the CFU values. In addition to calculating global significance-values (p-values), the biomaterials were analyzed pairwise using the Tukey test to deliver detailed significant differences between the different CFU values for each strain and saliva. Bonferroni's corrections as a post-test were not necessary.

RESULTS

In total, six oral bacterial strains, one *Candida* strain, and human saliva were used for the adhesion studies on three different 3D-RP-produced scaffolds.

Figure 1 shows the number of CFU's determined for each microorganism and saliva on each scaffold. The adherence activities differed from strain to strain and all type strains except for *Streptococcus oralis* [Fig. 1(G)] adhered best to PLGA scaffolds.

Streptococcus oralis adhered equally well to each of the investigated biomaterials, with no significant difference ($p = 0.157$) in adhesion detected. In contrast, the microorganisms of human saliva [Fig. 1(H)] adhered significantly better to TCP, followed by the PLGA scaffold and alginate ($p = 0.0002$). *Streptococcus mutans* [Fig. 1(A)] and *Enterococcus faecalis* [Fig. 1(C)] adhered best to the PLGA scaffolds, followed by alginate and TCP ($p = 0.0007$ and $p = 0001$, respectively). The strains *Prevotella nigrescens* [Fig. 1(E)], *Porphyromonas gingivalis* [Fig. 1(F)], *Streptococcus sanguis* [Fig. 1(B)], and *Candida albicans* [Fig. 1(D)] showed the highest adherence to PLGA followed by TCP (*Prevotella nigrescens* $p = 0.0004$, *Porphyromonas gingivalis* $p = 0.0007$, *Streptococcus sanguis* $p = 0.0003$, *Candida albicans* $p = 0.0014$) and alginate.

The three RP-produced biomaterials were examined both with and without microbial colonization by SEM. Figure 2 shows the surface of all scaffolds without any microbial colonization. In the lower resolution image the interconnecting grid structures of all three materials can be observed. At higher resolution the surface topography of PLGA [Fig. 2(A)], alginate [Fig. 2(B)], and TCP [Fig. 2(C)] shows smooth, wavy surface, which leads to an increase in surface area. The wavy surface of alginate is markedly stronger than either TCP or PLGA. Scanning micrographs (Figs. 3–5) give an example of bacterial and *Candida* adherence for each material. Figure 3 shows the adhesion of *Streptococcus sanguis*, one of the predominant organisms in dental plaque, on PLGA [Fig. 3(A)], alginate [Fig. 3(B)], and TCP [Fig. 3(C)]. *Streptococcus sanguis* is only sporadically visible on alginate. In contrast, on PLGA and on TCP the typical pairwise or chain grouping can be observed. Figure 4 shows the adhesion of *Candida albicans* on PLGA [Fig. 4(A)], alginate [Fig. 4(B)], and TCP [Fig. 4(C)]. *Candida albicans* can only sporadically be observed on alginate, whereas on PLGA and TCP a significant increase in adhesion is visible. Many round to oval shaped cells adhered to the surfaces. Figure 5 shows the adhesion of saliva, which contains a complex mixture of different microorganisms, on PLGA [Fig. 5(A)], alginate [Fig. 5(B)], and TCP [Fig. 5(C)]. The microorganisms of saliva showed a significantly higher affinity to TCP, followed by PLGA and alginate ($p = 0.0002$). Cocci and rods were visible. In general, the results of the scanning electron microscope observations correlated with the measurements of the CFUs (Fig. 1).

The use of confocal laser scanning microscopy (CLSM) revealed an adherence of the bacteria to the surface of alginate (Fig. 6). Single optical sections containing DAPI stained *Enterococcus faecalis* were obtained at a depth of 10–20 μm, whereas DAPI stained bacteria were found only on the surface of PLGA and TCP.

DISCUSSION

The purpose of our study was to evaluate the *in vitro* adherence of different microorganisms on RP-

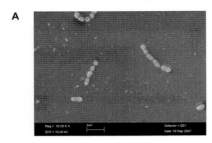
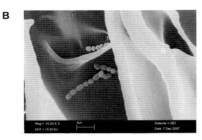
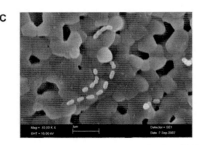

Figure 3. Scanning electron micrographs of each scaffold type colonized with *Streptococcus sanguis*. PLGA (A), calcium/sodium alginate (B), and TCP (C). Magnification 10000×.

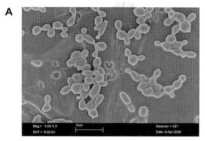
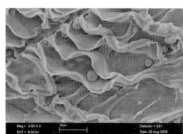
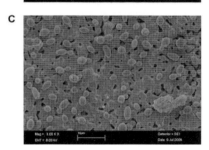

Figure 4. Scanning electron micrographs of each scaffold type colonized with *Candida albicans*. PLGA (A), calcium/sodium alginate (B), and TCP (C). Magnification 3000×.

cause degradation and subsequent failure of the replacement material.[3] For these reasons it is important to examine the adherence of microorganisms on RP-produced scaffolds. These have been gaining importance in the area of scaffold-guided tissue engineering, because this technique shows more advantages and less limitations compared to conventional manual-based fabrication techniques. Some of these advantages include reproducibility, precision, and the ability to manufacture complex biomaterials with

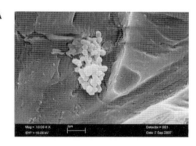
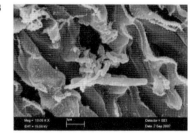
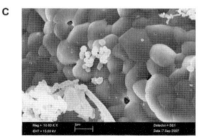

Figure 5. Scanning electron micrographs of each scaffold type colonized with the microorganisms of saliva. PLGA (A), calcium/sodium alginate (B), and TCP (C). Magnification 10000×.

produced (3D-bioplotting) scaffolds.[14] The microorganisms investigated populate the oral cavity, with examples chosen to represent bacteria from gram-negative as well as gram-positive cell wall types. Microbial adhesion on the surface of replacement materials has a strong influence on healing and long-term outcome. These microorganisms can lead to a higher risk of infection, especially in the case of tissue or bone engineering to regenerate specific and functional human tissues or bone. Such infections can

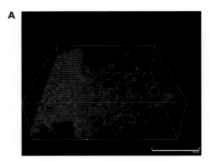

Figure 6. Confocal laser scanning micrographs of adherent and DAPI stained *Enterococcus faecalis* on calcium/sodium alginate (A) and single optical section at a z-depth of 15 μm (B). The bar marker length in panel A is 80 μm.

predefined macro- and microstructures.[14,17] To our knowledge, no study to date has examined the adherence of selected microorganisms to RP-produced scaffolds. All three RP-manufactured scaffolds are materials typically used for bone engineering.[18–25]

The investigated oral bacteria strains, *Candida albicans* and bacteria from saliva adhered to each of the 3D-scaffolds examined. *In vitro* and *in vivo* studies confirmed the important role of oral streptococci, particularly in early formed dental plaque biofilm, which is the trigger for most dental diseases such as gingivitis, caries, and periodontitis.[26–28] In an *in vivo* study we isolated *Enterococcus faecalis* from endodontic infections and compared these results with a number of other epidemiological studies.[29] *Prevotella nigrescens* and *Porphyromonas gingivalis* are associated with periodontitis.[30,31] *Candida albicans* is associated with candidosis in the elderly and in patients undergoing immunosuppression therapy.[32,33] In general, the highest adhesion amount for the type strains which were investigated was found on PLGA scaffolds, except for *Streptococcus oralis*. *Streptococcus oralis* adhered to all of the biomaterials equally with no significant differences detected. Interestingly, the complex microorganisms of saliva adhered significantly better to tricalcium phosphate (TCP) compared to PLGA. The results of the CFU determinations were in accordance with the morphological observations obtained by SEM. PLGA scaffolds possess a smooth, directional fibrous sheet-like structure. PLGA has recently been described as a material with good biocompatibility which promotes vascular ingrowth, guaranteeing adequate engraftment within the host tissue.[32,33] However, because of the high adherence rate of the investigated oral pathogens to PLGA, the application of this scaffold for bone replacement in oral surgery could result in biomaterial-related infections. Acute bone infections can be treated parenterally by antibiotic therapy, however, this can be associated with nephrotoxic, ototoxic, and allergic complications.[34] Taking these disadvantages into consideration, Yenice et al.[34] described the advantages of antibiotic-loaded polymer material. Makinen et al.[35] reported on the efficacy of a bioabsorbable ciprofloxacin containing bone screw (Ab-PLGA) against *Staphylococcus aureus* infection. This local antimicrobial prophylaxis was effective in the prevention of biomaterial-related infections caused by *S. aureus in vivo*. Garvin and Feschuk[36] have already described the use of polymers or copolymers of antibiotic-impregnated polylactide acid and polyglycolic acid as absorbable systems for antibiotic delivery to treat infected bone in dogs and rabbits. The application of PLGA as a replacement material in oral surgery could consequently be loaded prophylactically with antibiotics to prevent infections due to oral pathogens.

Another strategy is the modification of the surface to decrease bacterial adhesion.[37–39] Balazs et al.[37] reported on chemical modifications by radio-frequency-oxygen glow discharge, sodium hydroxide, and silver nitrate solutions. These modifications, which incorporate silver ions, very effectively reduced bacterial adhesion and colonization. Wilson and Harvey[39] studied the effect of polysaccharide coatings on adhesion to dentures. They showed that coating acrylic with a polysaccharide drastically reduced bacterial adhesion. They reported that sodium alginate was found to be one of the most effective in reducing the adhesion of *Streptococcus salivarius*. These results are in accordance with our results: both the determination of CFU's as well as SEM showed that the adhesion of *Streptococcus sanguis*, which also belongs to the so-called viridans group of streptococci, was significantly lower on calcium/sodium alginate compared to the other two RP-produced scaffolds which were investigated.[40] Wilson and Harvey[39] explained this decrease in the number of adherent bacteria as an effect of the high proportion of negatively charged groups.

On TCP and alginate the adhesion rate of the type strains was in general significantly lower compared to that of PLGA. Scanning electron microscopic examinations showed that all three scaffolds have a smooth surface and yet the increase in surface area of TCP and alginate is bigger compared to PLGA. However, this seeming contradiction can be explained because the surfaces of TCP and alginate are not smooth, unlike the surface of PLGA. Previous studies reported that oral bacteria attach better to rough surfaces than to smooth ones.[41] The increase in surface area would lead one to expect more adherent bacteria. Because of this, we examined the adherence of microorganisms to the biomaterial with the largest increase in surface area, alginate, by CLSM to gain knowledge about whether or not bacteria adhere in deeper sheets. Indeed, the results of CLSM showed that bacteria in deeper lamellar parts of the alginate scaffold were found. Thus the question arises about the efficacy of detaching the adherent bacteria using sonication. We would suggest the use of additional methods to directly quantify adherent bacteria, in addition to the determination of CFUs. Since chemical modification of material surfaces was shown to have a big influence on bacterial adhesion, the chemical constitution of PLGA could be the main reason for the high bacterial adhesion seen in this study.

There are different interactions occurring at the biomaterial surface which could affect bacterial adhesion. Among them are electrostatic forces, van der Waals forces, and hydrophobic interactions.[42] Previous studies reported that the adhesion should be higher on hydrophobic than on hydrophilic surfaces.[43,44] The strength of the chemical interactions during the initial contact of microorganisms with the biomaterial influences colonization and biofilm formation.[43] The strength of the chemical interaction depends not only on the biomaterial but also on the microorganism surface structure itself, which explains differences in the adherence rate of different microorganisms to the same biomaterial. Moreover, surface roughness plays an important role in bacterial adhesion. The roughened surface provides more favorable sites for colonization.[42]

Further studies have to be performed to examine the influence of human plasma on the adherence of dental bacteria on the biomaterials investigated in this study. During surgical procedures the biomaterials come into contact with components of the blood, which triggers different reaction. These reactions could lead to thrombus formation and infections. Some evidence suggests a possible association between thrombosis and infection, in that adherent bacteria may provide a nidus for thrombus formation, or alternatively, that adherent thrombi composed of platelets and fibrin may form sheltered sites for bacterial adhesion.[45] Different studies have described that thrombin activation enhances the formation and polymerisation of fibrin, which increases bacterial adhesion on biomaterials.[6] Carlen et al.[46] examined the adherence of periodontopathogenic bacteria to experimental plasma and saliva pellicles. Their results showed that plasma components mediate the adherence of *Porphyromonas gingivalis*, *Fusobacterium nucleatum*, and *Actinomyces naeslundii*.[46] Taking these results into consideration, and if bacterial adhesion would prove to be enhanced by plasma components on the biomaterials used in this study, additional strategies would need to be developed to prevent thrombosis after the contact of blood with biomaterials for example by coating the biomaterials with anticoagulation drugs.[47]

Bacterial adhesion should also be tested *in situ* in the oral cavity to allow pellicle formation, which serves as a conditioning biofilm. The composition of the salivary pellicle formed *in vitro* was found to be different than that formed *in situ* which means that pellicle formation *in vitro* cannot simulate the *in vivo* situation.[48] In studies from our laboratory, the use of dental splints loaded with bovine enamel samples to study bacterial adhesion and dental plaque formation *in situ* has shown differences in comparison to *in vitro* results.[28] Nevertheless, the results shown in this study have revealed different bacterial adhesive properties for three important kinds of biomaterials manufactured by 3D-ribotyping technology. Our results also call attention to the risk of bacterial contamination during the clinical application of these biomaterials, especially with regards to PLGA.

The authors thank Prof. Jürgen Schulte-Monting, Department of Medical Biometry and Statistics, Albert Ludwigs-University-Freiburg, Germany for the statistical analysis. They also thank Brunhild Saaler for her excellent technical help.

References

1. Tan KH, Chua CK, Leong KF, Cheah CM, Cheang P, Abu Bakar MS, Cha SW. Scaffold development using selective laser sintering of polyetherketone-hydroxyapatite biocomposite blends. Biomaterials 2003;24:3115–3123.
2. Dexter SJ, Pearson RG, Davies MC, Camara M, Shakesheff KM. A comparison of the adhesion of mammalian cells and *Staphylococcus epidermidis* on fibronectin-modified polymer surfaces. J Biomed Mater Res 2001;56:222–227.

3. Sela MN, Kohavi D, Krausz E, Steinberg D, Rosen G. Enzymatic degradation of collagen-guided tissue regeneration membranes by periodontal bacteria. Clin Oral Implants Res 2003;14:263–268.
4. Hung SL, Lin YW, Wang YH, Chen YT, Su CY, Ling LJ. Permeability of Streptococcus mutans and Actinobacillus actinomycetemcomitans through guided tissue regeneration membranes and their effects on attachment of periodontal ligament cells. J Periodontol 2002;73:843–851.
5. Gibbons RJ. Bacterial adhesion to oral tissues: A model for infectious diseases. J Dent Res 1989;68:750–760.
6. Park KD, Kim YS, Han DK, Kim JH, Lee EH, Suh H, Coi KS. Bacterial adhesion on PEG modified polyurethane surfaces. Biomaterials 1998;19:851–859.
7. Otten JE, Wiedmann-Al-Ahmad M, Jahnke H, Pelz K. Bacterial colonization on different suture materials—A potential risk for intraoral dentoalveolar surgery. J Biomed Mater Res Part B: Appl Biomater 2005;74:627–635.
8. Gibbons RJ, Hay DI. Adsorbed salivary acidic proline-rich proteins contribute to the adhesion of Streptococcus mutans JBP to apatitic surfaces. J Dent Res 1989;68:1303–1307.
9. Malaisrie SC, Malekzadeh S, Biedlingmaier JF. In vivo analysis of bacterial biofilm formation on facial plastic bioimplants. Lanyngoscope 1998;108:1733–1738.
10. Ciardelli G, Chiono V, Cristallini C, Barbani N, Ahluwalia A, Vozzi G, Previti A, Tantussi G, Giusti P. Innovative tissue engineering structures through advanced manufacturing technologies. J Mater Sci Mater Med 2004;15:305–310.
11. Tan KH, Chua CK, Leong KF, Naing MW, Cheah CM. Fabrication and characterization of three-dimensional poy(etherether-ketone)/-hydroxyapatite biocomposite scaffolds using laser sintering. Proc Inst Mech Eng [H] 2005;219:183–194.
12. Thomson R, Shung AK, Yaszemski MJ, Mikos AG. Polymer scaffold processing. In: Lanza R, Langer R, Chick W, editors. Principles of Tissue Engineering, 2nd ed. Austin, TX: R. G. Landes; 2000. p 251.
13. Ma PX, Choi J. Biodegradable polymer scaffolds with well-defined interconnected spherical pore network. Tissue Eng 2003;7:23–33.
14. Landers R, Huebner U, Schmelzeisen R, Muelhaupt R. Rapid prototyping of scaffolds derived from thermoreversible hydrogels and tailored for application in tissue engineering. Biomaterials 2002;23:4437–4447.
15. Wagner M, Kiapur N, Wiedmann-Al-Ahmad M, Hübner U, Al-Ahmad A, Schön R, Schmelzeisen R, Mülhaupt R, Gellrich NC. Comparative in vitro study of ovine and human osteoblast-like cells on conventionally and rapid prototyping produced scaffolds tailored for application as potential bone replacement material. J Biomed Mater Res A 2007;83:1154–1164.
16. Maekawa S, Yoshioka M, Kumamoto Y. Proposal of a new scheme for the serological typing of Enterococcus faecalis strains. Microbiol Immunol 1992;36:671–681.
17. Chua CK, Leong KF, Tan KH, Wiria FE, Cheah CM. Development of tissue scaffolds using selective laser sintering of polyvinyl alcohol/hydroxyapatite biocomposite for craniofacial and joint defects. J Mater Sci Mater Med 2004;15:1113–1121.
18. Sanchez-Salcedo S, Izquierdo-Barba I, Arcos D, Vallet-Regi M. In vitro evaluation of potential calcium phosphate scaffolds for tissue engineering. Tissue Eng 2006;12:279–290.
19. Matsuno T, Nakamura T, Kuremoto K, Notazawa S, Nakahara T, Hashimoto Y, Satoh T, Shimizu Y. Development of beta-tricalcium phosphate/collagen sponge for bone regeneration. Dent Mater J 2006;25:138–144.
20. Yuan J, Cui L, Zhang WJ, Liu W, Cao Y. Repair of canine mandibular bone defects with bone marrow stromal cells and porous beta-tricalcium phosphate. Biomaterials 2007;28:1005–1013.
21. Weng Y, Wang M, Liu W, Hu X, Chai G, Yan Q, Zhu L, Cui L, Cao Y. Repair of experimental alveolar bone defects by tissue-engineered bone. Tissue Eng 2006;12:1503–1513.
22. Alsberg E, Kong HJ, Hirano Y, Smith MK, Albeiuti A, Mooney DJ. Regulation bone formation via controlled scaffold degradation. J Dent Res 2003;82:903–908.
23. Cohen SR, Mittermiller PA, Holmes RE, Broder KW. Clinical experience with a new fast-resorbing polymer for bone stabilization in craniofacial surgery. J Craniofac Surg 2006;17:40–43.
24. Landes CA, Ballon A, Roth C. Maxillary and mandibular osteosyntheses with PLGA and P(L/DL)LA implants: A 5-year inpatient biocompatibility and degradation experience. Plast Reconstr Surg 2006;117:2347–2360.
25. Rücker M, Laschke MW, Junker D, Carvalho C, Schramm A, Mülhaupt R, Gellrich NC, Menger MD. Angiogenic and inflammatory response to biodegradable scaffolds in dorsal skinfold chambers of mice. Biomaterials 2006;27:5027–5038.
26. Nyvad B, Kilian M. Comparison of the initial streptococcal microflora on dental enamel in caries-active and in caries-inactive individuals. Caries Res 1990;24:267–272.
27. Foster JS, Kolenbrander PE. Development of a multispecies oral bacterial community in saliva-conditioned flow cell. Appl Environ Microbiol 2004;70:4340–4348.
28. Al-Ahmad A, Wunder A, Auschill TM, Follo M, Braun G, Hellwig E, Arweiler NB. The in vivo dynamics of Streptococcus spp., Actinomyces naeslundii, Fusobacterium nucleatum and Veillonella spp. In dental plaque biofilm as analysed by five colour multiplex-FISH. J Med Microbiol 2007;56:681–687.
29. Schirrmeister JF, Liebenow AL, Braun G, Wittmer A, Hellwig E, Al-Ahmad A. Detection and eradication of microorganisms in root-filled teeth associated with periradicular lesions: An in vivo study. J Endod 2007;33:536–540.
30. Marsh P, Martin MV. Orale Mikrobiologie, 4th ed. Stuttgart New York: Georg Thieme Verlag; 1999. p 15.
31. Beikler T, Schnitzer S, Abdeen G, Ehmke B, Eisenacher M, Flemmig TF. Sampling strategy for intraoral detection of periodontal pathogens before and following periodontal therapy. J Periodontol 2006;77:1323–1332.
32. de Resende MA, de Sousa LV, de Oliveira RC, Koga-Ito CY, Lyon JP. Prevalence and antifungal susceptibility of yeasts obtained from the oral cavity of elderly individuals. Mycopathologia 2006;162:39–44.
33. Golecka M, Oldakowska-Jedynak U, Mierzwinska-Nastalska E, Adamczyk-Sosinska E. Candida-associated denture stomatitis in patients after immunosuppression therapy. Transplant Proc 2006;38:155–156.
34. Yenice I, Calis S, Kas H, Ozalp M, Ekizoglu M, Hincal A. Biodegradable implantable teicoplanin beads for the treatment of bone infections. Int J Pharm 2002;242:271–275.
35. Makinen TJ, Veiranto M, Knuuti J, Jalava J, Tormala P, Aro HT. Efficacy of bioabsorbable containing bone screw in the prevention of biomaterial-related infection due to Staphylococcus aureus. Bone 2005;36:292–299.
36. Garvin K, Feschuke C. Polylactide-polyclycolide antibiotic implants. Clin Orthop Relat Res 2005;473:105–110.
37. Balazs DJ, Triandafillu K, Wood P, Chevolot Y, van Delden C, Harms H, Hollenstein C, Mathieu HJ. Inhibition of bacterial adhesion on PVC endotracheal tubes by RF-oxygen glow discharge, sodium hydroxide and silver nitrate treatments. Biomaterials 2004;25:2139–2151.
38. Triandafillu K, Balazs DJ, Aronsson BO, descout P, Tu Quoc P, van Delden C, Mathieu HJ, Harms H. Adhesion of Pseudomonas aeruginosa strains to untreated and oxygen-plasma treated poly (vinyl chloride) (PVC) from endotracheal intubation devices. Biomaterials 2003;24:1507–1518.
39. Wilson M, Harvey W. Prevention of bacterial adhesion to denture acrylic. J Dent 1989;17:166–170.
40. Teng LJ, Hsueh PR, Tsai JC, Chen PW, Hsu JC, Lai HC, Lee CN, Ho SW. groESL sequence determination, phylogenetic analysis, and species differentiation for viridans group streptococci. J Clin Microbiol 2002;40:3172–3178.

41. Wu-Yuan CD, Eganhouse KJ, Keller JC, Walters KS. Oral bacterial attachment to titanium surfaces: A scanning electron microscopy study. J Oral Implantol 1995;21:207–213.
42. An YH, Friedman RJ. Concise review of mechanisms of bacterial adhesion to biomaterial surfaces. J Biomed Mater Res 1998;43:338–348.
43. Sperenza G, Gottardi G, Pederzolli C, Lunelli L, Canteri R, Pasquardini L, Carli E, Lui A, Maniglio D, Brugnara M, Anderle M. Role of chemical interactions in bacterial adhesion to polymer surfaces. Biomaterials 2004;25:2029–2037.
44. Gottenbos B, van der Mei HC, Busscher HJ. Initial adhesion and surface growth of *Staphylococcus epidermidis* and *Pseudomonas aeruginosa* on biomedical polymers. J Biomed Mater Res 2000;50:208–240.
45. Baumgartner JN, Cooper SL. Bacterial adhesion on polyurethane surfaces conditioned with thrombus components. ASAIO J 1996;42:476–479.
46. Carlen A, Rüdiger SG, Loggner I, Olsson J. Bacteria-binding plasma proteins in pellicles formed on hydroxyapatite in vitro and on teeth in vivo. Oral Microbiol Immunol 2003;18:203–207.
47. Stemberger A, Schmidmaier G, Förster C, Alt E, Kohn J, Calatzis A. New antithrombin agents: Potential for coating biomaterials used in cardiopulmonary bypass. In: Pifarré R, editor. New Anticoagulants for the Cardiovascular Patient. Philadelphia: Hanleys & Belfus Med. Pub; 1997. pp 377–386.
48. Carlen A, Borjesson AC, Nikdel K, Olsson J. Composition of pellicles formed in vivo on tooth surfaces in different parts of the dentition, and in vitro on hydroxyapatite. Caries Res 1998;32:447–455.

Update

Adhesion of Microorganisms on Rapid Prototyping-Produced 3D Scaffolds: A Challenge in Tissue Engineering

Ali Al-Ahmad, Margit Wiedmann-Al-Ahmad, Carlos Carvalho, and Elmar Hellwig

1
Perspective of 3D Scaffold Development

Advanced research on biomaterial manufacturing to treat human skeletal defects has been a major focus in recent years. In addition to conventional scaffold fabrication techniques (e.g., gas foaming, particulate leaching, and freeze drying), novel fabrication techniques (rapid prototyping, electrospinning, and surface-based technologies) have also been developed [1]. Particular areas of recent research have examined the rapid prototyping (RP) technique and the development of 3D scaffolds with defined pore size, interconnectivity, and permeability, as well as studying their load-bearing characteristics, transport properties, degradation rate, and chemical and surface characteristics [2]. These scaffold characteristics have influences both on cell proliferation and differentiation and on bacterial attachment. One of the advantages of the RP technique is that it can process a large number of natural and synthetic polymers. To date, many biomaterials with different mechanical properties have been examined for their usefulness in RP fabrication. These include materials such as alginate, gelatin, hydroxyapatite (HA), polyurethane, polycaprolactone (PCL), PCL-HA, and polylactideglycolic acid (PLGA) [1, 3, 4]. Some RP scaffolds have also been used in clinical trials [5, 6]. As Moroni *et al.* [1] have reported, each novel fabrication technology used for the manufacture of 3D scaffolds has disadvantages, and it is difficult to manufacture scaffolds that satisfy all the requirements desirable for tissue or bone engineering using only a single technology. Consequently, in the future the strategy of manufacturing 3D scaffolds with optimal characteristics will be to use a combination of both conventional and novel technologies [7, 8].

Because of microbial contamination during, for example, the insertion of implants, and the very real risk of biomaterial-associated infections, one of the surface-finish requirements of 3D scaffolds is to reduce bacterial adhesion in order to decrease infection while at the same time increase integration into the tissue [9].

Computer Aided Biomanufacturing, Edited by Roger Narayan and Paul Calvert
© 2011 WILEY-VCH Verlag GmbH & Co. KGaA. Published 2011 by WILEY-VCH Verlag GmbH & Co. KGaA.

Many studies have looked at the influence of surface topography with regard to cell and bacterial adhesion, but interestingly their results have varied. Some publications showed a correlation of a decrease in adhesion with an increase in surface roughness, while others have shown an increase in adhesion with roughness, presumably dependent both on the type of cells examined or bacteria used and on the physicochemical characteristics of the materials investigated [10]. Decuzzi and Ferrari [10] reported that not only the surface topography but also the surface energy (gamma) of materials can have an influence on cellular and bacterial adhesion. For materials with small gamma, any increase in roughness is detrimental to adhesion; for large gamma, there is an optimal roughness that maximizes adhesion; for intermediate gamma, surface roughness has only a minor effect on adhesion. The authors concluded that nanotopography and surface biofunctionalization of biomaterials could be modulated in such a way that there is an increase in the level of cell adhesion, while simultaneously bacterial adhesion is decreased or even prevented. This would be a step further in the development of optimal biomaterials for the field of tissue engineering. Ploux *et al.* [11] studied cellular (human osteoprogenitor cells) and bacterial (*Escherichia coli* K12) responses to surface chemistry and surface topography at the nanoscale level. Interestingly, the behavior of bacteria was opposite to that of eukaryotic cells in response to surface chemistry and surface topography with regard to proliferation and orientation.

The adhesion of bacteria to implants fabricated through RP processes will gain in importance in the future as the technology matures and grows into a larger market in modern medical surgery. There are three different strategies that could be undertaken to limit bacterial adhesion. The first strategy uses the knowledge gained in coating conventional, non-RP implants either with drug release systems using antibiotics [12, 13] or permanent silver coatings [14, 15]. The second strategy would involve research done on the surface finish of the created implants, which could be changed either physically (roughness, porosity) or chemically (hydrophobicity, charge) [16, 17]. Both the first and the second strategies, while being based on the already existing research, have the disadvantage of trying to improve on the bacterial adhesion properties of complex, highly porous implants. Coatings and surface finishing would have to be done on a layer-by-layer basis to ensure complete surface modification. Furthermore, cell adhesion on the modified surfaces of these implants could be compromised, and the osteoinductive effects of ceramic implants greatly reduced.

The third strategy, which takes advantage of the material flexibility of the 3D Bioplotter, involves the addition of antibiotics to the material itself prior to implant fabrication. It would be possible to achieve controlled drug release both by using the structure of the implant and its porosity and by carefully positioning the different concentrations of antibiotics within the three-dimensional scaffold using multi-material deposition. Rapid prototyping techniques for controlled drug release have been proposed by several research groups [18–20], but have not been used in animal testing or clinical trials. At present, this strategy has the advantage over the better researched ones because it retains the surface of the biomaterials used, including cell adhesion properties and any osteoinductive property that the material may have, while greatly reducing the risk of inflammation.

2
Monitoring of Microbial Adhesion and Infection

During the development of new 3D scaffolds, the *in vitro* or *in vivo* bacterial adhesive characteristics should be monitored using an appropriate method to visualize adherent microorganisms [21]. Because of the different options available for tissue engineering, and in order to avoid false positive or negative results, the choice of study design is the bottleneck in gaining realistic adhesive characteristics of the 3D scaffolds used. When considering the oral cavity as a tissue engineering application area, the salivary pellicle and the contaminating microorganisms should also be taken into account [4, 22].

A number of techniques can be used to visualize and quantify adherent microorganisms on biomaterials. A short review summarizing these techniques is given by Hannig *et al.* [21]. The relative advantages and disadvantages of the various methods need to be considered in order to choose the appropriate combination of methods. High-resolution microscopic techniques include scanning electron microscopy (SEM), environmental scanning electron microscopy (ESEM), transmission electron microscopy (TEM), and atomic force microscopy (AFM). These techniques can deliver detailed insight into the ultrastructure of the bacteria and the surrounding matrix. An easy-to-use staining technique is DAPI (4′,6-diamidino-2-phenylindole) staining, which enables visualization of all adherent microorganisms via epifluorescence microscopy, but it cannot differentiate between live and dead cells. In contrast, live/dead staining techniques, which combine different dyes for vital and avital bacteria, would allow studying the effects of the biomaterials on microorganisms that are already adherent. The suitability of live/dead staining dyes depends on the matrix and the microorganisms themselves, which means that they should be tested before use. For example, the combination of SYTO 9 with propidium iodide appears to be appropriate for oral streptococcal strains [23, 24]. Fluorescein diacetate (FDA) has also been used in combination with ethidium bromide to detect vital and avital bacteria after initial bacterial adhesion *in vivo*. FDA becomes modified by esterase in vital cells resulting in green fluorescent active bacteria, whereas ethidium bromide enters only dead cells leading to orange red fluorescent microorganisms. Other dye combinations are discussed by Hannig *et al.* [21]. Fluorescence *in situ* hybridization (FISH) is required in order to differentiate between bacterial species adherent to biomaterials [25, 26]. This technique is based on oligonucleotide probes labeled with fluorescent dyes that bind specifically to rRNA. It is therefore dependent on the presence of a large number of intact ribosomes, representing the biological activity of the tested cells. This means that primarily vital bacteria are detected by FISH [27]. The determination of colony forming units (CFU) by prior desorption and subsequent plating on agar plates is the traditional method that has been used to estimate the number of viable adherent microorganisms. This classical plating technique is both labor intensive and time consuming and may select specific species when studying multispecies infections [27]. Furthermore, the quantification of semiplanktonic adherent bacteria (e.g., from saliva) is difficult and could result in high scatter since flocks or agglomerates of adherent bacteria can be dispersed during the desorption process [4, 22].

Recently, Sjollema *et al.* [28] summarized the state of the art concerning nondestructive and noninvasive bioluminescence and fluorescent imaging technologies as used in observing the course of biomaterial-associated infections *in vivo* without the necessity of sacrificing the animals at different time points. This allows monitoring of biomaterial infections while simultaneously overcoming the problem of animal-to-animal variations. The authors discussed the advantages and disadvantages of these biooptical techniques and emphasized that, despite their primarily qualitative character, they are an appropriate tool to evaluate the antimicrobial coating of biomaterials *in vivo*.

The use of biomaterials in tissue engineering should not only emphasize biocompatibility with the different cells growing on them but also consider the aspect of microbial adhesion and infection, which should be a main concern in future studies.

References

1 Moroni, L., de Wijn, J.R., and van Blitterswijk, C.A. (2008) Integrating novel technologies to fabricate smart scaffolds. *J. Biomater. Sci. Polym. Ed.*, **19**, 543–572.

2 Guda, T., Appleford, M., Oh, S., and Ong, J.L. (2008) A cellular perspective to bioceramic scaffolds for bone tissue engineering: the state of the art. *Curr. Top. Med. Chem.*, **8**, 290–299.

3 Leong, K.F., Chua, C.K., Sudarmadji, N., and Yeon, W.Y. (2008) Engineering functionally graded tissue engineering scaffolds. *J. Mech. Behav. Biomed. Mater.*, **1**, 140–152.

4 Al-Ahmad, A., Wiedmann-Al-Ahmad, M., Carvalho, C., Lang, M., Follo, M., Braun, G., Wittmer, A., Mülhaupt, R., and Hellwig, E. (2008) Bacterial and *Candida albicans* adhesion on rapid prototyping-produced 3D scaffolds manufactured as bone replacement materials. *J. Biomed. Mater. Res. A*, **87**, 933–943.

5 Moroni, L., Hendriks, J.A., Schotel, R., de Wijn, J.R., and van Blitterswijk, C.A. (2007) Design of biphasic polymeric 3-dimensional fiber deposited scaffolds for cartilage tissue engineering applications. *Tissue Eng.*, **13**, 361–371.

6 Wilson, C.E., Kruyt, M.C., de Bruijn, J.D., van Blitterswijk, J.R., Oner, F.C., Verbout, A.J., and Dhert, W.J. (2006) A new *in vivo* screening model for posterior spinal bone formation: comparison of ten calcium phosphate ceramic material treatments. *Biomaterials*, **27**, 302–314.

7 Tuzlakoglu, K., Bolgen, N., Salgado, A.J., Gomes, M.E., Piskin, E., and Reis, R.L. (2005) Nano- and micro-fiber combined scaffolds: a new architecture for bone tissue engineering. *J. Mater. Sci. Mater. Med.*, **16**, 1099–1104.

8 Williamson, M.R., Black, R., and Kielty, C. (2006) PCL-PU composite vascular scaffold production for vascular tissue engineering: attachment, proliferation and bioactivity of human vascular endothelial cells. *Biomaterials*, **27**, 3608–3616.

9 Kuijer, R., Jansen, E.J., Emans, P.J., Bulstra, S.K., Riesle, J., Pieper, J., Grainger, D.W., and Busscher, H.J. (2007) Assessing infection risk in implanted tissue-engineered devices. *Biomaterials*, **28**, 5148–5154.

10 Decuzzi, P. and Ferrari, M. (2010) Modulating cellular adhesion through nanotopography. *Biomaterials*, **31**, 173–179.

11 Ploux, L., Anselme, K., Dirani, A., Ponche, A., Soppera, O., and Roucoules, V. (2009) Opposite responses of cells and bacteria to micro/nanopatterned surfaces

prepared by pulsed plasma polymerization and UV-irradiation. *Langmuir*, **25**, 8161–8169.
12 Fuchs, T., Schmidmaier, G., Raschke, M.J., and Stange, R. (2008) Bioactive-coated implants in trauma surgery. *Eur. J. Trauma Emerg. Surg.*, **34**, 60–68.
13 Aykut, S., Oztürk, A., Ozkan, Y., Yanik, K., Ilman, A.A., and Ozdemir, R.M. (2010) Evaluation and comparison of the antimicrobial efficacy of teicoplanin- and clindamycin-coated titanium implants: an experimental study. *J. Bone Joint Surg. Br.*, **92**, 159–163.
14 Gosheger, G., Hardes, J., Ahrens, H., Streitburger, A., Buerger, H., Erren, M., Gunsel, A., Kemper, F.H., Winkelmann, W., and Von Eiff, C. (2004) Silver-coated megaendoprostheses in a rabbit model: an analysis of the infection rate and toxicological side effects. *Biomaterials*, **25**, 5547–5556.
15 Hardes, J., Ahrens, H., Gebert, C., Streitbuerger, A., Buerger, H., Erren, M., Gunsel, A., Wedemeyer, C., Saxler, G., Winkelmann, W., and Gosheger, G. (2007) Lack of toxicological side-effects in silver-coated megaprostheses in humans. *Biomaterials.*, **28**, 2869–2875.
16 Katsikogianni, M. and Missirlis, Y.F. (2004) Concise review of mechanisms of bacterial adhesion to biomaterials and of techniques used in estimating bacteria–material interactions. *Eur. Cell Mater.*, **8**, 37–57.
17 Vasilev, K., Cook, J., and Griesser, H.J. (2009) Antibacterial surfaces for biomedical devices. *Expert Rev. Med. Devices*, **6**, 553–567.
18 Wu, B.M., Borland, S.W., Giordano, R.A., Cima, L.G., Sachs, E.M., and Cima, M.J. (1996) Solid free-form fabrication of drug delivery devices. *J. Control Release*, **40**, 77–87.
19 Lu, Y. and Chen, S.C. (2004) Micro and nano-fabrication of biodegradable polymers for drug delivery. *Adv. Drug Deliv. Rev.*, **56**, 1621–1633.
20 Ryu, W.H., Vyakarnam, M., Greco, R.S., Prinz, F.B., and Fasching, R.J. (2007) Fabrication of multi-layered biodegradable drug delivery device based on micro-structuring of PLGA polymers. *Biomed. Microdevices.*, **9**, 845–853.
21 Hannig, C., Follo, M., Hellwig, E., and Al-Ahmad, A. (2010) Visualization of adherent micro-organisms using different techniques. *J. Med. Microbiol.*, **59**, 1–7.
22 Hannig, C. and Hannig, M. (2009) The oral cavity: a key system to understand substratum-dependent bioadhesion on solid surface in man. *Clin. Oral Invest.*, **13**, 123–139.
23 Weiger, R., Decker, E.M., Krastl, G., and Brecx, M. (1999) Deposition and retention of vital and dead *Streptococcus sanguinis* cells on glass surfaces in a flow-chamber system. *Arch. Oral Biol.*, **44**, 621–628.
24 Decker, E.M. (2001) The ability of direct fluorescence-based, two-colour assays to detect different physiological states of oral streptococci. *Lett. Appl. Microbiol.*, **33**, 188–192.
25 Amann, R.I., Binder, B.J., Olson, R.J., Chisholm, S.W., Devereux, R., and Stahl, D.A. (1990) Combination of 16S rRNA-targeted oligonucleotide probes with flow cytometry for analyzing mixed microbial populations. *Appl. Environ. Microbiol.*, **56**, 1919–1925.
26 Paster, B.J., Bartoszyk, I., and Dewhirst, F.E. (1998) Identification of oral streptococci using PCR-based, reverse-capture, checkerboard hybridization. *Methods Cell Sci.*, **20**, 223–231.
27 Amann, R.I., Ludwig, W., and Schleifer, K.H. (1995) Phylogenetic identification and *in situ* detection of individual microbial cells without cultivation. *Microbiol. Rev.*, **59**, 143–169.
28 Sjollema, J., Sharma, P.K., Dijkstra, R.J., van Dam, G.M., van der Mei, H.C., Engelsman, A.F., and Busscher, H.J. (2010) The potential for bio-optical imaging of biomaterial-associated infection *in vivo*. *Biomaterials*, **31** (8), 1984–1995.

4
Electric Field Driven Jetting: An Emerging Approach for Processing Living Cells

Regular Article

Electric field driven jetting:
an emerging approach for processing living cells

Suwan N. Jayasinghe[1]*, Peter A.M. Eagles[2] and Amer N. Qureshi[2]

[1] BioPhysics Group, Department of Mechanical Engineering, University College London, Torrington Place, London WC1E 7JE, United Kingdom
[2] Randall Division of Cell and Molecular Biophysics, Kings College London, United Kingdom

This paper reports for the first time the ability to process living cellular materials by means of electrified jets at electric field strengths of up to 2 kV/mm. Bio-suspensions containing living human Jurkat cells at different concentrations were processed via this jetting approach. The jetting process was carried out at an electric field strength between 0.67 kV/mm and 2 kV/mm, corresponding to an applied voltage of 10–30 kV between two electrodes ~15 mm apart. The Jurkat cells were jetted under sterile conditions, collected in petri dishes and incubated for 24 and 48 hours. During and after incubation, cells were assessed for survival and structural damage; cells were found to be unharmed and to retain their integrity under all electric field strengths examined. At all field strengths jetting took place in the unstable mode. Good correlation was observed between droplet distribution plots generated by way of laser spectroscopy and estimated values from measurements of droplet relics.

Received 11 October 2005
Revised 24 November 2005
Accepted 25 November 2005

Keywords: Advanced electrified bio-jets · Bioengineering · Bioprocessing · Living human jurkat cells · Biofabrication

1 Introduction

The processing of suspensions containing living cellular materials is an emerging field of research that is rapidly and constantly evolving. The demand for such technology is centre-stage in the nano- and micro-biotechnology industry for the production of bio-chips, biosensors, tissue engineering as well as for gene manipulation and extends into a whole host of widespread technological applications [1–13].

Currently there are several widely used routes for processing cell-suspensions. These range from non-jetting processes such as soft lithography, laser-directed cell writing, photolithography techniques, dip-pen lithography to jet-based processes like ink-jet printing. In soft lithography, microcontact and microfluidic patterning predominate, and of the two the former is the most popular. This technique uses an elastomeric stamp to create patterns on surfaces; several different organic biomolecules have been assembled via this technique [14]. When a nonplannar surface has been stamped, the resulting pattern is used as an absorbing surface for biological molecules such as proteins. These proteins then promote molecular interactions with cells. The primary benefit of this technique is that it can tether cell processes and single cells because it has a resolution ranging from 500 μm down to 2 μm [15, 16].

Another approach is the use of laser-directed cell writing to place single living cells onto substrates by physically guiding them through hollow fibres, aided by optical forces derived from focussed infrared lasers [17, 18]. Surface modification is not required here. However the route is limited by the time taken for tissue development, but this approach is incapable of handling cell migration. Nevertheless this technique does have distinct advantages for studying single cells and cell-to-cell interactions during the development of tissues. Photolithography

---

* **Current address:** Dr. Suwan N. Jayasinghe, Department of Mechanical Engineering, University College London, Torrington Place, London WC1E 7JE, United Kingdom
E-mail: s.jayasinghe@ucl.ac.uk
Fax: +44 207388 0180

Abbreviations: EHDJ, electrohydrodynamic jetting; **AFM,** atomic force microscope

techniques have been used for patterning proteins, and require photosensitive groups on the substrate; patterns are formed by means of selective UV irradiation [19, 20]. This route has been explored for micropatterning cultures and for creating self-assembled monolayers, which create areas of cell adhesion for very high-resolution cell patterns. Atomic force microscope (AFM)-based techniques have also been used for such patterning; dip-pen lithography relies on this technology, successfully creating patterns with features in the range of tens of nanometers [21, 22]. This route is mostly used for creating protein arrays from which cell arrays are fabricated by cells adhering to these proteins. However, all these processing routes are non-jet based techniques, which can restrict their applications.

Ink-jet printing, a jet based processing technology using piezoelectric crystals within a needle, has undergone rapid development in recent years to explore the possibilities of printing cells. The technique when coupled with computational power can direct a print-head to create 2D and 3D cellular architectures, and this technology has made a powerful impact on the field of biomaterials and biotechnology. Hence ink-jets have been used for biosensor development, biochips, DNA synthesis and solid freeform fabrication of scaffolds [23–26]. Although having huge potential, this technology has inherent limitations based on the processing of suspensions containing high volume fractions of cells to fabricate "small" structures with fine features. The limitations stem from the diameter of the needle, which controls droplet size. In practice the deposited droplets give a resolution >100 μm. To try and overcome this, substrate modification has been explored to control the spreading, but this does not help to resolve the problem of processing highly concentrated suspensions.

An emerging technology that is competing successfully with ink-jet printing in the area of jet-based processing sciences, is electric field driven jetting [27–29]. This technique, also known as electrohydrodynamic jetting (EHDJ), is a phenomenon where a multi-phase liquid is passed through a needle at a controlled flow rate; as it passes, it undergoes charging within the needle by being exposed to a high intensity electric field. The field promotes the formation of a jet, which becomes unstable and leads to the formation of droplets. In comparison to ink-jet printing, electrohydrodynamic jetting can process concentrated suspensions having a material loading 20 vol%, from which droplets in the order of a few micrometers can be generated from needles with internal diameters in the range of hundreds of micrometers [30–33]. Furthermore this jetting approach has the capability of forming nanometer sized (<<50 nm) droplets [34].

In this paper we elucidate for the first time the capability of EHDJ to process suspensions containing different cell concentrations under an electric field strength brought about by a potential difference ranging from 10 kV to 30 kV (upper limit of existing equipment). Furthermore we show that such high intensity electric fields have no apparent damaging effects on living cells.

2 Materials and methods

The equipment used for electrohydrodynamic jetting (Figure 1A) consists of a stainless steel needle having an internal diameter of ~500 μm, which is connected to a high precision voltage power supply (FP-30, Glassman Europe Ltd., Tadley, UK). The power supply has the ability to supply a voltage of up to 30 kV. The inlet of this needle was connected via silicone tubing to a syringe (capacity of which could be varied) fitted on a syringe pump (PHD 4400, HARVARD Apparatus Ltd., Edenbridge, UK). The pump has the capability of delivering flow rates in the range 10^{-5} to 10^{-20} m^3/s. A ring-shaped ground electrode made of copper, having an internal and external diameter of 13 and 15 mm respectively, was held approximately 15 mm axisymetrically below the needle. The needle and ground electrode were housed in a sterile tissue culture hood, which was operating at negative pressure. The samples after EHDJ were collected in sterile petri-dishes. EHDJ processing was carried out in an electric field strength ranging from 0.6 to 2 kV/mm for a flow rate regime of 10^{-8} m^3/s.

During the EHDJ of the cellular suspension, an ultra high-speed camera (Phantom V7, Photo-sonics International Ltd, Oxford, UK), in conjunction with a long distance microscope lens (Nikon 50 mm, Oxford Lasers Ltd, Oxford, UK), was triggered simultaneously with a diode laser system (HSI5000, Oxford Lasers Ltd, Oxford, UK), allowing the jetting process to be recorded in real time from needle exit and beyond.

Jurkat cells (ATCC, USA) were grown for 48 hours, in 100 mL of RPMI 1640 growth medium (Invitrogen, UK) with 10% foetal calf serum (Invitrogen, UK), in an incubator (Heraeus BB16, UK) at 37°C and 4% CO_2. Cell viability was assessed by staining with trypan-blue and viable cells were counted using a bright-field-haemocytometer (Sigma), with a phase microscope (Zeiss ID 02, Germany) employing a 10X objective. 2–5 mL of cell suspension containing the high and low concentration of cells were used for each electrospray experiment, respectively. For the controls, similar volumes of the suspension were passed through the needle but without an applied voltage, and collected in petri dishes. The cells were counted immediately after electrospraying and after 24 and 48 hours of incubation. For most of the work cells were used at a concentration of 3×10^5 cells/mL, low concentration, and 2×10^6 cells/mL, high concentration.

The jet processing properties of the cellular suspension were characterized in terms of its electrical conductivity, viscosity, surface tension, relative permittivity and density by using a conductivity meter (HACH SensION™

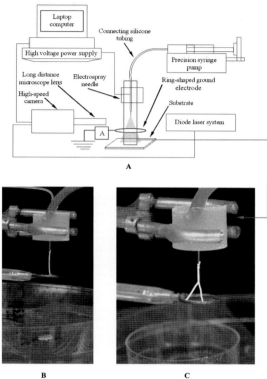

Figure 1. A Schematic representation of the electrohydrodynamic jetting equipment used in this study. **B** A snap shot of the periodic sparking at an applied voltage of 10 kV, and **C** at 30 kV for a corresponding flow rate of 10^{-8} m^3/s.

156 probe), Visco-Easy rotational viscometer, Kruss Tensiometer K9 (Du Novy's ring and plate method), a calibrated cell connected to a high precision multimeter and a standard density bottle, respectively. Electrohydrodynamic jetting of the cells was carried out at applied voltages ranging from 10 kV to 30 kV with a corresponding constant flow rate of 10^{-8} m^3/s.

Droplet size distributions resulting from EHDJ of the cellular suspensions were measured using a Sympatec Helos (helium laser optical spectrometer) Model Vario/KF sizing system (Sympatec Ltd, System-Partikel-Technik, Bury, UK) together with a personal computer, which was used for recording and plotting data. Such measurements made using laser diffraction is based on the observations that droplets passing through a collimated light source scatter light at an angle, which is inversely proportional to their size. The laser system was incorporated in the EHDJ equipment by placing it so that the 2.2 mm diameter laser beam was ~15 mm below the ring. The laser beam was perpendicular to both the needle and ring electrode axis.

In the Sympatec system, the cellular suspension droplets pass through a perpendicular laser beam of wavelength 630 nm. Any scattered light is focused onto a radial array of silicon diode detectors using a 20 mm focal length Fourier transforming lens, which was used to collect the scattering data, allowing the detection of droplets in the size range 10^2 to 10^5 nm. This lens has the property of imaging the scatter from droplets of the same size to the same part of the detector array, regardless of their position within the laser beam and their speed. Subsequently at any given time, light energy distribution across the detector corresponds directly to the size distribution of the droplets, which are present in the laser beam at that moment. The droplet size distribution is estimated by fitting the data obtained to the Fraunhofer scattering model, which is used as it accurately accounts for the scattering and can therefore be used to precisely assess the fine droplet fraction produced. The data acquisition rate was set at 1000 Hz, allowing the dynamics of droplet production to be taken into account. Measurements were synchronized with the appearance of the droplets in the measurement zone by monitoring the decrease in laser light transmission caused by droplet scattering. The average droplet size produced by the EHDJ was obtained from time-resolved data by calculating the volume-weighted average over 10 s. Several separate measurements of the droplet size distribution data were obtained for each applied voltage, using either lens R1, R2 or R3 as required.

3 Results

The cell suspensions containing living human Jurkat cells together with the growth medium were characterized for their electrical conductivity, viscosity, surface tension, density and relative permittivity [35, 36], respectively, and the results are shown in Table 1. These properties were measured as a function of time and found to vary significantly, probably reflecting the complex metabolic interactions occurring between the living cells and medium that would affect these parameters. Hence, once the cell suspensions were prepared and characterized the samples were jetted as soon as possible.

It is clear from Table 1 that the presence of increasing cells decreases the electrical conductivity and increases the viscosity of such bio-suspensions. Media with electrical conductivities and viscosities in the range summarized in Table 1 are rather difficult to stabilize, as the charge within the medium travels rapidly from the core of the suspension to the surface and this would promote instability in the jetting process. Using the EHDJ experimental set-up shown in Figure 1A the samples were jetted and collected into sterile petri dishes. During jetting at 10 kV, 20 kV and 30 kV, sparking was seen between the needle and ring shaped ground electrode. At an applied voltage of 10 kV (Figure 1B) sparking occurred at ~23 sparks per minute and increased to ~57 sparks per minute at 30 kV. At higher voltages, when the field strength reached 2 kV/mm, the spark was seen to fork and exhibit a wish-bone like shape (Figure 1C).

The well established electrohydrodynamic jetting laws [37] state that for EHDJ to take place, t_e, the electrical relaxation time must be much smaller than t_h, the hydrodynamic time,

where $t_e = \dfrac{\beta \varepsilon_0}{K}$ and $t_h = \dfrac{LD^2}{Q}$.

Establishing the inequality: $\dfrac{\beta \varepsilon_0}{K} \ll \dfrac{LD^2}{Q}$

where β is the relative permittivity, ε_0 is the permittivity of free space (8.854 × 10^{-12} F/m), K is the electrical conductivity, L is the axial length between the needle and ground electrode, D the jet diameter, and Q the flow rate. In reality, the jet diameter varies depending on the applied voltage, flow rate and medium properties [38–40]. If we estimate the jet diameter at 30 kV to be ~30µm (Figure 2A–F), then substituting the values from Table 1 into the above inequality, indicates that the process is undergoing EHDJ in the unstable mode.

In EHDJ the stability of the jets is predominantly governed by the applied voltage, flow rate, and medium properties. As far as the properties of the medium are concerned, the electrical conductivity and viscosity are the most important. Because the applied voltage and flow rate were kept constant for a given electric field strength, the major contributor to jet instability in all samples results from the liquid properties, namely electrical conductivity and viscosity. In all samples the conductivity was high and the viscosity was low, characteristics which are known to contribute to jet instability [41].

Laser spectroscopy was used to analyse the droplet sizes and their distributions. The jetted samples at all volt-

Table 1. Characteristics of cell medium and cell suspensions. The table shows the properties of the culture medium and cell suspensions that would affect the formation and stability of cones and jets [14]. The low concentration cell suspension contained 3×10^5 cells/mL, and high concentration cell suspension contained 2×10^6 cells/mL.

Sample	Electrical conductivity S/m	Viscosity mPas	Surface Tension mN/m	Density kg/m^3	Relative permittivity
Medium	~10^{-2}	22	52	900	31
3x 10^5 cells/mL	~10^{-3}	22	52	900	32
2x 10^6 cells /mL	~10^{-3}	23	53	910	32

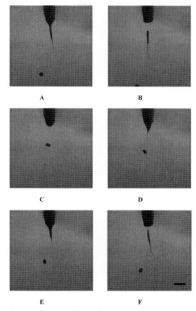

Figure 2. A characteristic high-speed sequence (A–F) depicting the jetting of the Jurkat cell suspension in the unstable jetting mode at 30 kV. The scale bar denotes 810 µm.

Table 2. Statistics of measured and estimated droplet sizes. The table shows the droplet size as measured by laser spectroscopy together with the droplet size as estimated from Refs. 17 and 18. Three applied voltages (10 kV, 20 kV and 30 kV) were used, together with two concentrations of cell suspensions: a low concentration (3×10^5 cells/mL) and a high concentration (2×10^6 cells/mL).

Applied voltage kV	Droplet size range µm a)	Droplet size range µm b)
Low concentration		
10	0.25–48	~2–57
20	0.23–28	~1.8–33
30	0.5–56	~3–64
Applied voltage kV	Droplet size range µm a)	Droplet size range µm b)
High concentration		
10	8–87.5	~10–93
20	0.25–57	~3–61
30	0.25–40	~1–53

a) Measured using laser spectroscopy
b) Estimated as in Refs. 17 and 18

ages exhibited unstable EHDJ giving rise to the polydispersity in the droplet size distributions. Figures 3A–C illustrate the polydispersity in the droplet sizes when the cell medium and suspensions are exposed to an electric field brought about by an applied voltage of 30 kV. The figure also illustrates the profound dependence of droplet size distribution on the presence of cells and actual number of cells present in the medium.

The collected droplet relics at each applied voltage were characterized by measuring their average contact angles and deposit diameters that were used in a volume-equivalence-estimation route for calculating the droplet sizes, as in our previous work [42]. Table 2 summarizes these values.

Ranges of droplet sizes from the droplet distribution plots in Figures 3A–C, obtained through laser spectroscopy, agree with the values using the volume equivalence method from measurements of the collected droplet relics. Comparing in more detail the droplet sizes obtained by these two methods, it is seen that the volume equivalence method gives larger upper and lower limits in all cases, indicating some spreading of the droplets after deposition on the substrate. However in general the values obtained correlate quite well.

Samples were collected after EHDJ for assessing cell survival. Control samples were also collected without the application of an electric field using the same needle.

Jurkat cells were jetted at 10 kV, 20 kV and 30 kV and then incubated for 24 and 48 hours. Cell counts were taken to assess viability and rate of cell division. Controls contained cells that were taken through the same procedure but without the application of an electric field.

Several samples of EHDJ cells were incubated for 24 and 48 hours, and then counted for cell survival (Table 3). The results shown here indicate that this jetting process had no effect on cell mortality and had no adverse affects on the rate of cell division even after jetting at an electric field strength of 2 kV/mm. Optical microscopy of the jetted cells soon after deposition showed that with time the cells underwent normal changes in their morphology, as well as cytokinesis.

Figures 4A–C illustrate low (Figure 4A) and high (Figures 4B–C) magnification optical micrographs of the deposited droplets containing Jurkat cells. Figure 4A shows that jetting can produce lines of droplets and indicates that this technique may have huge potential for forming predetermined architectures with droplets containing cells for patterning two to three dimensional structures.

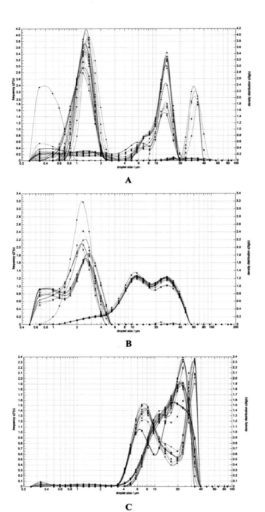

Figure 3. Characteristic droplet size distributions for (A) growth medium, (B) low concentration (3×10^5 cells/mL) and (C) high concentration (2×10^6 cells/mL) cell suspensions that were jetted at an applied voltage of 30 kV and flow rate of 10^{-8} m^3/s.

Table 3. Cell counts for jetting at 10, 20 and 30 kV

Time (h)	Control Jurkats (× 10⁶ cells/mL)	EHDJ at 10 kV Jurkats (× 10⁶ cells/mL)	EHDJ at 20 kV Jurkats (× 10⁶ cells/mL)	EHDJ at 30 kV Jurkats (× 10⁶ cells/mL)	Standard deviation/±
0	2	2.1	1.9	2	2.8×10^4
24	2.7	2.9	3.1	3.1	3.5×10^4
48	3.6	4.3	4.2	4.3	4.9×10^4

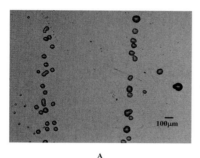

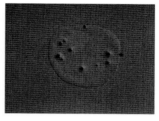

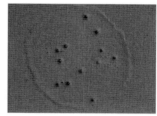

Figure 4. Typical micrographs depicting the collected droplet relics at an applied electric field strength of 2 kV/mm showing unharmed cells (A–C).

4 Discussion

We have uncovered that living Jurkat cells can be jetted at 30 kV, corresponding to an electric field strength of 2 kV/mm, which represented the maximum voltage at which our instrumentation could operate. Even at this extreme, the cells appeared to be undamaged after jetting. Cells jetted under these conditions, when incubated, continued to exhibit normal cellular behaviour, indicating that these conditions of jetting do not appear to impair the cells. This observation considerably extends the range of conditions under which cells can be deposited on to substrates.

EHDJ under applied voltages of 10 kV, 20 kV and 30 kV exhibit jet instability and this is largely due to the properties of the medium, which has a high conductivity because of the ions and molecules needed to maintain the metabolic activities of living cells. The medium also had low viscosity which further contributed to the instability. Clearly the formation of a stable jetting mode is important to achieve if EHDJ is to be developed for processing cells in a controlled manner, and we are pursuing this aspect vigorously.

This investigation demonstrates the EHDJ technique to be a novel, economical and versatile approach for processing living cells. It clearly supersedes its non-jet and jet-based competitors in terms of its ability to process suspensions containing high volume fractions of living cellular materials, therefore offering the possibility of being able to deposit cells within fine droplets (<< 50 μm). Furthermore this bio-fabrication technique is not in any way limited by the concentration of the cells in suspension. Having such a capability, the coupling of this jetting technology with a 2D/3D-patterning device would enable the construction of tissues and other cellular architectures from a very wide range of cell types in suspension.

The realization and potential of this research has consequences in the processing and precise deposition of a range of living cellular materials and biologically related matrices, also for the fabrication of tissues at the micrometer to nanometre level. Thus the electrohydrodynamic jetting technique with its unique potential for handling samples in the form of concentrated biological suspensions with needles of large internal diameter is strongly placed for competing with all other jet-based technologies in the race to develop novel biological tissues.

SNJ gratefully acknowledges funding provided by both The Royal Society (UK) and the Engineering and Physical Sciences Research Council (UK), for research into emerging novel biotechnologies. PAME gratefully acknowledges King's College London for supporting these trial studies. We thank Mr. Marc Simon for taking photographs of the jetting process.

5 References

[1] Lueking, A., Cahill, D.J., Mullner, S., Protein biochips: A new and versatile platform technology for molecular medicine. *Drug Discov. Today.* 2005, *11*, 789–794.

[2] Jain, K.K., Applications of biochips: from diagnostics to personalized medicine. *Curr. Opin. Drug Discov. Devel.* 2004, *3*, 285–289.

[3] Wilson, G.S., Gifford, R., Biosensors for real-time in vivo measurements. *Biosens. Bioelectron.* 2005, *20*, 2388–2403.

[4] Ziegler, K.J., Developing implantable optical biosensors. *Trends Biotechnol.* 2005, *9*, 440–444.

[5] Xu, G., Ye, X., Qin, L., Xu, Y., Li, Y., Li, R., Wang, P., Cell-based biosensors based on light-addressable potentiometric sensors for single cell monitoring. *Biosens. Bioelectron.* 2005, *20*, 1757–1763.

[6] Di Martino, A., Sittinger, M., Risbud, M.V., Chitosan: A versatile biopolymer for orthopaedic tissue-engineering. *Biomaterials* 2005, *26*, 5983–5990.

[7] Hollister, S.J., Porous scaffold design for tissue engineering. *Nat Mater.* 2005, *7*, 518–524.

[8] Sun, W., Starly, B., Nam, J., Darling, A., Bio-CAD modeling and its applications in computer-aided tissue engineering. *Comput.-Aided Des.* 2005, *37*, 1097–1114.

[9] Kim, J., Noskov, V.N., Lu, X., Bergmann, A., Ren, X., Warth, T., Richardson, P., Kouprina, N., Stubbs, L., Discovery of a Novel, Paternally Expressed Ubiquitin-specific Processing Protease Gene through Comparative Analysis of an Imprinted Region of Mouse Chromosome 7 and Human Chromosome 19q13.4. *Genome Res.* 2000, *8*, 1138–1147.

[10] Cooper, A., Bussey, H., Characterization of the yeast KEX1 gene product: a carboxypeptidase involved in processing secreted precursor proteins. *Mol. Cell. Biol.* 1989, *6*, 2706–2714.

[11] Barron, J.A., Krizman, D.B., Ringeisen, B.R., Laser printing of single cells: statistical analysis, cell viability, and stress. *Ann. Biomed. Eng.* 2005, *2*, 121–130.

[12] Barron, J.A., Rosen, R., Meehan, J-J., Spargo, B.J., Belkin, S., Ringeisen, B.R., Biological laser printing of genetically modified Escherichia coli for biosensor applications. *Biosens. Bioelectron.* 2004, *20*, 246–252.

[13] Yeong, W-Y., Chua, C-K., Leong, K-F., Chandrasekaran, M., Rapid prototyping in tissue engineering: challenges and potential. *Trends Biotechnol.* 2004, *22*, 643–652.

[14] Zhang, S.G., Yan, L., Altman, M., Lassle, M., Nugent, H., Frankel, F., Lauffenburger, D.A., Whitesides, G.M., Rich, A., Biological surface engineering: a simple system for cell pattern formation. *Biomaterials* 1999, *13*, 1213–1220.

[15] Kane, R.S., Takayama, S., Ostuni, E., Ingber, D.E., Whitesides, G.M., Patterning proteins and cells using soft lithography. *Biomaterials* 1999, *23–24*, 2363–2376.

[16] Tan, W., Desai, T.A., Microfluidic patterning of cells in extracellular matrix biopolymers: effects of channel size, cell type, and matrix composition on pattern integrity. *Tissue Eng.* 2003, *2*, 255–267.

[17] Odde, D.J., Renn, M.J., Laser-guided direct writing of living cells. *Biotechnol. Bioeng.* 2000, *3*, 312–318.

[18] Bhatia, S.K., Hickman, J.J., Ligler, F.S., New approach to producing patterned biomolecular assemblies. *J. Am. Chem. Soc.* 1992, *11*, 4432–4433.

[19] Liu, V.A., Jastromb, W.E., Bhatia, S.N., Engineering protein and cell adhesivity using PEO-terminated triblock polymers. *J. Biomed. Mater. Res.* 2002, *1*, 126–134.

[20] Piner, R.D., Zhu, J., Xu, F., Hong, S.H., Mirkin, C.A., "Dip-pen" nanolithography. *Science* 1999, *5402*, 661–663.

[21] Lee, K.B., Park, S.J., Mirkin, C.A., Smith, J.C., Mrksich, M., Protein nanoarrays generated by dip-pen nanolithography. *Science* 2002, *5560*, 1702–1705.

[22] Wilson, D.L., Martin, R., Hong, S., Cronin-Golomb, M., Mirkin, C.A., Kaplan, D.L., Surface organization and nanopatterning of collagen by dip-pen nanolithography. *Proc. Natl. Acad. Sci.* 2001, *24*, 13660–13664.

[23] Setti, L., Fraleoni-Morgera, A., Ballarin, B., Filippini, A., Frascaro, D., Piana, C., An amperometric glucose biosensor prototype fabricated by thermal inkjet printing. *Biosens. Bioelectron.* 2005, *20*, 2019–2026.

[24] Bashir, R., BioMEMS: state-of-the-art in detection, opportunities and prospects. *Advanced Drug Delivery Reviews* 2004, *56*, 1565–1586.

[25] O'Donnell-Maloney, M.J., Little, D.P., Microfabrication and array technologies for DNA sequencing and diagnostics. *Genetic Analysis: Biomol. Eng.* 1996, *13*, 151–157.

[26] Tsang, V.L., Bhatia, S.N., Three-dimensional tissue fabrication. *Adv. Drug Delivery Rev.* 2004, *56*, 1635–1647.

[27] Hayati, I., Bailey, A.I., Tadros, Th.F., Mechanism of stable jet formation in electrohydrodynamic atomization. *Nature* 1996, *319*, 41–43.

[28] Rosell-Llompart, J., Fernandez de la Mora, J., Generation of monodisperse droplets 0.3 to 4 µm in diameter from electrified cone-jets of highly conducting and viscous liquids. *J. Aerosol Sci.* 1994, *25*, 1093–1119.

[29] Jaworek, A., Krupa, A., Classification of the modes of EHD spraying. *J. Aerosol Sci.* 1999, *30*, 873–893.

[30] Balachandran, W., Miao, P., Xiao, P., Electrospray of fine droplets of ceramic suspensions for thin-film preparation. *J. Electrost.* 2001, *50*, 249–263.

[31] Jayasinghe, S.N., Edirisinghe, M.J., de Wilde, T., A novel ceramic printing technique based on electrostatic atomization of a suspension. *Mater. Res. Innovations* 2002, *6*, 92–95.

[32] Wang, D.Z., Jayasinghe, S.N., Edirisinghe, M.J., Instrument for electrohydrodynamic print-patterning 3D complex structures. *Rev. Sci. Instrum.*, 2005, *76*, 075105:1-5.

© 2006 Wiley-VCH Verlag GmbH & Co. KGaA, Weinheim
Computer Aided Biomanufacturing, Edited by Roger Narayan and Paul Calvert
© 2011 WILEY-VCH Verlag GmbH & Co. KGaA. Published 2011 by WILEY-VCH Verlag GmbH & Co. KGaA.

[33] Su, B., Choy, K.L., Electrostatic assisted aerosol jet deposition of CdS, CdSe and ZnS thin films. *Thin Solid Films* 2000, *361–362*, 102–106.

[34] Chen, D-R., Pui, D.Y.H., Kaufman, S.L., Electrospraying of conducting liquids for monodisperse aerosol generation in the 4 nm to 1.8 µm diameter range. *J. Aerosol Sci.* 1995, *26*, 963–977.

[35] Hartman, R.P.A., Brunner, D.J., Camelot, D.M.A., Marijnissen, J.C.M., Scarlett, B., Electrohydrodynamic atomization in the cone-jet mode physical modelling of the liquid cone and jet. *J. Aerosol Sci.* 1999, *30*, 823–849.

[36] Hartman, R.P.A., Brunner, D.J., Camelot, D.M.A., Marijnissen, J.C.M., Scarlett, B., Jet break-up in electrohydrodynamic atomization in the cone-jet mode. *J. Aerosol Sci.* 2000, *31*, 65–95.

[37] Ganan-Calvo, A.M., Davila, J., Barrero, A., Current and droplet size in the electrospraying of liquids: scaling laws. *J. Aerosol Sci.* 1997, *28*, 243–275.

[38] Jayasinghe S.N., Edirisinghe, M.J., Electrostatic atomization of a ceramic suspension. *J. Eur. Ceram. Soc.* 2004, *24*, 2203–2213.

[39] Jayasinghe, S.N., Edirisinghe, M.J., Electrostatic atomization of chitosan. *J. Mater. Sci.* 2003, *22*, 1443–1445.

[40] Hartman, R.P.A., Borra, J-P, Brunner, D.J., Marijnissen, J.C.M. and Scarlett, B. The evolution of electrohydrodynamic sprays produced in the cone-jet mode, a physical model. *J. electrost.* 1999, *47*, 143–170.

[41] Jayasinghe, S.N., Edirisinghe, M.J., Effect of viscosity on the size of relics produced by electrostatic atomization. *J. Aerosol Sci.* 2002, *33*, 1379–1388.

[42] Jayasinghe, S.N., Edirisinghe, M.J., Kippax, P.G., Relic and droplet sizes produced by electrostatic atomization of ceramic suspensions. *Appl. Phys. A: Mater. Sci. Process* 2004, *78*, 343–347.

© 2006 Wiley-VCH Verlag GmbH & Co. KGaA, Weinheim
Computer Aided Biomanufacturing, Edited by Roger Narayan and Paul Calvert
© 2011 WILEY-VCH Verlag GmbH & Co. KGaA. Published 2011 by WILEY-VCH Verlag GmbH & Co. KGaA.

5
Inkjet Printing of Bioadhesives

Inkjet Printing of Bioadhesives

Anand Doraiswamy,[1] Timothy M. Dunaway,[2] Jonathan J. Wilker,[2] Roger J. Narayan[1]

[1] Joint Department of Biomedical Engineering, University of North Carolina at Chapel Hill, Chapel Hill, North Carolina 27599-7575

[2] Department of Chemistry, Purdue University, West Lafayette, Indiana 47907-2084

Received 6 February 2008; revised 24 April 2008; accepted 3 June 2008
Published online 19 August 2008 in Wiley InterScience (www.interscience.wiley.com). DOI: 10.1002/jbm.b.31183

> **Abstract:** Over the past century, synthetic adhesives have largely displaced their natural counterparts in medical applications. However, rising concerns over the environmental and toxicological effects of the solvents, monomers, and additives used in synthetic adhesives have recently led the scientific community to seek natural substitutes. Marine mussel adhesive protein is a formaldehyde-free natural adhesive that demonstrates excellent adhesion to several classes of materials, including glasses, metals, metal oxides, and polymers. In this study, we have demonstrated computer aided design (CAD) patterning of various biological adhesives using piezoelectric inkjet technology. A MEMS-based piezoelectric actuator was used to control the flow of the mussel adhesive protein solution through the ink jet nozzles. Fourier transform infrared spectroscopy (FTIR), microscopy, and adhesion studies were performed to examine the chemical, structural, and functional properties of these patterns, respectively. FTIR revealed the piezoelectric inkjet technology technique to be nondestructive. Atomic force microscopy was used to determine the extent of chelation caused by Fe(III). The adhesive strength in these materials was correlated with the extent of chelation by Fe(III). Piezoelectric inkjet printing of naturally-derived biological adhesives may overcome several problems associated with conventional tissue bonding materials. This technique may significantly improve wound repair in next generation eye repair, fracture fixation, wound closure, and drug delivery devices. © 2008 Wiley Periodicals, Inc. J Biomed Mater Res Part B: Appl Biomater 89B: 28–35, 2009
>
> **Keywords:** biomaterials; thin film; bioadhesive; microfabrication

INTRODUCTION

Suturing is the "gold standard" joining technique for many medical procedures. Unfortunately, the use of suture materials requires long operating times as well as significant surgical skill. In addition, use of sutures is associated with several complications, including granulomas, postoperative epithelial ingrowth, postoperative discomfort, infection, and inflammation. Furthermore, sutures may place excess tension on tissues, leading to tissue warping. An alternative joining technique that has gained support over the past few years involves the use of adhesives, which hold tissue together for several weeks while inflammatory and tissue regrowth processes allow the defect to heal. Medical adhesives must perform several functions, which include degrading in order to allow complete healing at the lesion site and providing sufficient tensile strength for the intended application.

Conventional adhesives and techniques suffer from biocompatibility and safety issues. For example, tissue sealants derived from cyanoacrylate esters (Dermabond®, Indermil®, Nexaband®, and Vetbond®) are used in repairing tendon, tooth enamel, cornea, and skin tissues.[1-5] Unfortunately, cyanoacrylate adhesives are nonbiodegradable and permanently remain at the treatment site. As a result, these materials have the potential to induce local inflammation, neovascularization, foreign body reaction, and necrosis.[6-8] In addition, these materials can demonstrate dose-dependent carcinogenic and toxic properties. Fibrin sealants (derived from human blood coagulation factors) have also been considered for use in a variety of surgical and endoscopic applications.[9-11] For example, Beriplast® P is a fibrin sealant that contains Combiset-1 [aprotinin (bovine), factor XIII (human), and fibrinogen (human)] and Combiset-2 (calcium chloride and thrombin (human)); these components are mixed in the operating room. The components obtained from pooled human plasma (fibrinogen, factor XIII, and thrombin) undergo various sterilization, manufac-

Correspondence to: Prof. R. J. Narayan (e-mail: roger_narayan@unc.edu)
Contract grant sponsors: National Science Foundation; National Institutes of Health; Office of Naval Research

© 2008 Wiley Periodicals, Inc.
Computer Aided Biomanufacturing, Edited by Roger Narayan and Paul Calvert
© 2011 WILEY-VCH Verlag GmbH & Co. KGaA. Published 2011 by WILEY-VCH Verlag GmbH & Co. KGaA.

turing, and pasteurization measures. However, there are several safety issues that have limited the use of these materials, including the possibility of disease transmission. For example, the risk of HIV in blood-derived materials screened with the p24 HIV-1 antigen test is currently estimated at 1:700,000.[12] Concerns also exist regarding the transmission of human T-cell lymphotropic virus-1, hepatitis A virus, hepatitis B virus, hepatitis C virus, Parvovirus B19, and spongiform encephalopathy agents from blood-derived materials. Surgeons and their patients require improved tissue joining materials and methods.

Mussel adhesive proteins are natural adhesives secreted by sedentary mollusks (mussels) that inhibit intertidal and subtidal areas. An attachment plaque known as a byssus allows mussels to form strong attachments to underwater surfaces. *Mytilus edulis* (common blue mussel) is one of the most widely studied mussels.[14–23] It produces several unique adhesive proteins, including *Mytilus edulis* foot protein-1 (Mefp-1), *Mytilus edulis* foot protein-2 (Mefp-2), *Mytilus edulis* foot protein-3 (Mefp-3), *Mytilus edulis* foot protein-4 (Mefp-4), and *Mytilus edulis* foot protein-5 (Mefp-5). These proteins contain up to 30 mole percent 3,4-dihydroxyphenyl-L-alanine (DOPA), which is a molecule created by hydroxylation of the aromatic ring in the amino acid tyrosine. It has been suggested that DOPA drives the adhesion of a mussel plaque to an environmental surface by means of hydogen bonding, metal-mediated catechol complexation, and/or weak physical interactions.[14–23]

Rapid prototyping is a technology originally developed approximately thirty years ago for the preparation of machine tool prototypes. One possible application for rapid prototyping technology is microscale processing of biomaterials. Computer aided design (CAD) rapid prototyping techniques such as inkjet printing may allow for high throughput patterning of biological materials for medical applications.[24–26] In piezoelectric inkjet printers, the print head consist of a piezoelectric transducer, nozzle, manifold, pumping chamber, and inlet passage. Piezoelectric printers are categorized based on the deformation mode of the lead zirconate titanate piezoelectric crystal (e.g., squeeze, bend, push or shear). When a voltage is applied to the lead zirconate titanate piezoelectric transducer, the transducer deforms. Mechanical vibrations and acoustic waves are generated. When a given linear velocity is reached by the fluid, it is ejected from the orifice as a droplet. Ink jet printers can dispense fluid droplets with volumes in the picoliter to microliter range. The resolution of patterns fabricated using piezoelectric ink jet printing is determined by several factors, including ink viscosity, ink surface tension, ink droplet size, and printerhead resolution. Unlike thermal inkjet printers, the ink used in piezoelectric inkjet printers does not undergo heating and cooling cycles. We have recently demonstrated that piezoelectric inkjet deposition is a powerful, noncontact, and nondestructive technique for patterning many biological materials, including streptavidin protein, monofunctional acrylate esters, sinapinic acid, deoxyribonucleic acid, and multiwalled carbon nanotube/DNA hybrid materials.[27]

In this study, we have demonstrated CAD patterning of various biological adhesives using piezoelectric inkjet technology. Fourier transform infrared spectroscopy (FTIR), atomic force microscopy, and adhesion studies were performed to examine the chemical, structural, and functional properties of these patterns, respectively. This technique may significantly improve wound repair in next generation eye repair, fracture fixation, wound closure, and drug delivery devices.

MATERIALS AND METHODS

Mussel adhesive proteins (Mefp-1 and Mefp-2) were extracted from marine mussel feet as described in[28] with slight modification. The protein pellets were extracted with water, rather than the reported acetic acid.[28] The extract yields a solution that contains predominantly two proteins, $\sim$80% Mefp-1 and $\sim$20% Mefp-2.[28] The final DOPA concentration in this solution was 0.16 mM, the total protein concentration in this solution was $\sim$2 μM, and the viscosity of this solution was similar to water (density $\sim$1 g/mL). To study iron-induced cross-linking, a FeCl$_3$ solution was prepared in series dilution to obtain ratios of 1:1 Fe:DOPA, 10:1 Fe:DOPA, and 100:1 Fe:DOPA. *N*-Butyl cyanoacrylate (Vetbond®) Tissue Adhesive) was obtained from a commercial source (3M, St. Paul, MN). 2-Octyl cyanoacrylate (Nexaband®) Liquid Topical Tissue Adhesive) was obtained from a commercial source (Abbott Laboratories, North Chicago, IL). Ethyl cyanoacrylate (Loctite®) Quick Set Adhesive) was obtained from a commercial source (Ted Pella, Redding, CA).

The DMP 2800 piezoelectric inkjet printer (FujiFilm Dimatix, Santa Clara, CA) is based on a cartridge printhead system. Fluid was injected into the fluid module. The fluid module was then attached to the jetting module to form a sealed cartridge. The inkjet print head itself consists of a silicon die with sixteen individually addressable jets, which are spaced 254 μm apart. The effective nozzle diameter is 21.5 μm, which provides droplets that are $\sim$10 pL in volume. The waveform pulse shape (amplitude, slew rate, and duration), frequency and voltage were optimized for each adhesive solution independently. The droplet flight (distance traveled) from the nozzle was recorded using an ultra-fast camera. The protein solution was also inkjetted at several voltage values (10, 20, 30, and 40 V) in order to study the effect of voltage on protein structure. The images were recorded at 30 μs intervals at several voltage values.

Approximately 10 μL of the adhesives were inkjetted at a temperature of 25°C and at 40% relative humidity into uniform 1 cm^2 patterns; dispensed volume was determined using the DMP2800 software based on pattern and drop parameters. Adhesives were deposited on Si(111) substrates for optical, AFM, XPS, and contact angle measurements; on full-thickness porcine skin substrates for adhesion test-

Journal of Biomedical Materials Research Part B: Applied Biomaterials

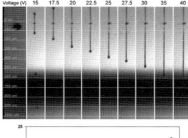

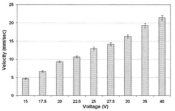

Figure 1. Optical micrograph of mussel adhesive protein solution inkjetted at several voltages (15–40 V) and captured at 30 μs time delay. A corresponding plot of mean velocity of inkjetted solution plotted versus firing voltage is also shown. Bar indicates standard deviation of mean velocity ($p < 0.05$).

ing; and on KCl and AgCl substrates for FTIR measurements. To examine iron-induced cross-linking, mussel adhesive protein solution was inkjetted. A layer of FeCl$_3$ solution (at varying concentrations to reach 1:1, 10:1, 100:1 Fe: DOPA, respectively) was subsequently inkjetted using the identical pattern. Dropcast samples were prepared for the FITR studies.

Fourier transform infrared (FTIR) was performed using a Mattson 5000s spectrometer with 4 cm^{-1} resolution, which was operated in transmission mode. Atomic force microscopy (AFM) was performed using a N-scriptor system (Nanoink, Chicago, IL). Three-dimensional analysis was performed using SPM Nanorule® software (Nanoink, Chicago, IL). X-ray photoelectron spectra was acquired using an LAS-3000 spectrometer (Riber, Rueil-Malmaison, France) with a Mg Kα source ($\lambda = 1254$ eV) and a 1 mm spot size. The take off angle was 75° from the surface, the X-ray incidence angle was 20°, and the X-ray source-analyzer angle was 55°. The base pressure in the analysis chamber was ~10^{-10} Torr. Contact-angle studies were performed using a goniometer consisting of a syringe, an aligned digital zoom camera, and an illumination source. Adhesion studies were performed with butt joints on full-thickness porcine skin substrates using an 8501 uniaxial tensile test system (Instron, Norwood, MA), which has a load range of load range ±10 kN. The adhesion testing was performed on porcine full thickness skin (North Carolina State University College of Veterinary Medicine, Raleigh, NC), which was inkjetted with adhesive over 1 cm^2 area. Loading rates of 0.6 mm/s and sampling rates of 20 s^{-1} were utilized in this study. The tests were carried out six times for each sample, and a statistical analysis was performed using Student's t-test.

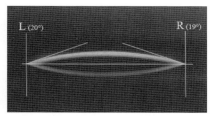

Figure 2. Contact angle image of mussel adhesive protein solution containing 80% Mefp-1 and 20% Mefp-2.

RESULTS AND DISCUSSION

The piezoelectric print head utilizes a voltage waveform input that allows control over volume of solution that is dispensed. The waveform varies as a function of viscosity, surface tension and temperature of the jetted solution. The print head moves the ink solution from the cartridge to the channel. The impedance matching unit allows the solution to move through the descender, where it is ejected through a nozzle. In this study, the mussel adhesive protein solution was processed using piezoelectric inkjetting and dropcasting. Images of the drop dispensed at various voltages (Figure 1) were used to estimate the velocity and volume dispensed. For the mussel adhesive protein solution, an increase in firing voltage resulted in a linear increase in jetting velocity. Contact angle measurements (Figure 2) performed on the mussel adhesive protein solutions that were patterned on Si(111) substrates revealed hydrophilic (contact angle <45°) behavior (Table I). No significant difference in contact angle values ($p < 0.05$) for 1:1 Fe:DOPA, 10:1 Fe:DOPA, and 100:1 Fe:DOPA was observed.

TABLE I. Contact Angle Measurements for Mussel Adhesive Protein Solutions (With Varying Iron Concentration) Examined on Si (111) Substrates

Solution on Si (111) Substrate	Contact Angle[a]
Mefp (0.16 mM DOPA)	20° ± 2.2°
1:1 Fe:DOPA	18.6° ± 2°
10:1 Fe:DOPA	21.3° ± 1.6°
100:1 Fe:DOPA	22.2° ± 1.9°
Deionized water (Control)	13.2° ± 1.6°

[a] Values are expressed as mean ± SD.

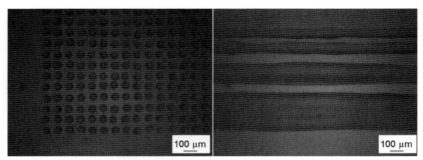

Figure 3. Optical micrographs of mussel adhesive protein solution inkjetted into microarray and line patterns. Scale bar equals 100 μm.

Mussel adhesive protein solutions, $FeCl_3$ solutions, and cyanoacrylate adhesives were successfully deposited in CAD patterns using the piezoelectric inkjet printing system. Inkjetting of mussel adhesive protein solution in microscale patterns with minimum feature size of 50 μm was achieved (Figure 3). Line patterns with widths of ~60, ~90, ~180, and ~300 μm were also fabricated. The typical mammalian cell size is ~10–30 μm. The bonding line-widths of ~60 μm as shown here may be sufficient for microsurgical and other delicate wound closure procedures.

FTIR absorption spectra of inkjetted (at voltages 10, 20, 30, and 40 V) and dropcast mussel adhesive protein materials exhibited similar peak intensity values [Figure 4(A)]. A list of distinct bands for marine mussel adhesive protein materials and their corresponding assignments was previously published by the authors.[17] Amide vibration was observed at ~3250, 1650, 1460, and 1100 cm^{-1} (rocking vibration).[29] C=C stretching was observed at ~1630 cm^{-1} and catechol ring vibration was observed between 1300 and 1100 cm^{-1}.[29] O—H stretching vibration was observed between 3600 and 3300 cm^{-1}. The region from 0 to 1000

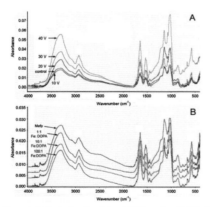

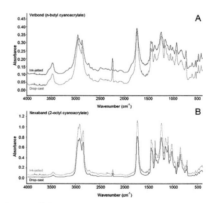

Figure 4. (A) Fourier transform infrared (FTIR) spectra of inkjetted mussel adhesive protein solution (Mefp) as a function of jetting voltage (10–40 V). Control is a dropcast mussel adhesive protein solution. (B) Fourier transform infrared spectra of inkjetted mussel adhesive protein solution (Mefp) as a function of Fe(III) concentration.

Figure 5. (A) Fourier transform infrared (FTIR) spectra of inkjetted and dropcast n-butyl cyanoacrylate (Vetbond®) materials. Relevant structural peaks are labeled. (B) Fourier transform infrared (FTIR) spectra of inkjetted and dropcast 2-octyl cyanoacrylate (Nexaband®) materials. Relevant structural peaks are labeled.

Journal of Biomedical Materials Research Part B: Applied Biomaterials

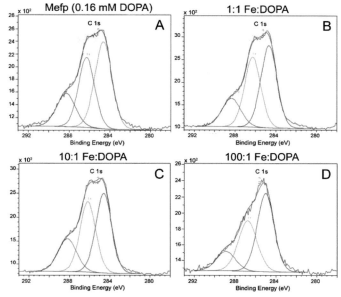

Figure 6. C 1s spectra of inkjetted mussel adhesive protein solutions cured with Fe(III). X-ray photoelectron spectra shown for (A) Mefp (0.16 mM DOPA), (B) 1:1 Fe:DOPA, (C) 10:1 Fe:DOPA, and (D) 100:1 Fe: DOPA. [Color figure can be viewed in the online issue, which is available at www.interscience.wiley.com.]

cm^{-1} contains low-frequency skeletal vibrations, out-of-plane ring deformation, wagging modes of hydrogen atoms, wagging modes of hydroxyl groups on the catechol ring, and wagging modes of carboxylate groups.[29] Significant differences in the absorption peak intensities were observed in materials that were inkjetted at 10, 20, 30, and 40 V. This result may be attributed to the increase in jetting volume that results from an increase in jetting voltage. Similarly, FTIR spectra of inkjetted and dropcast (control) n-butyl cyanoacrylate [Figure 5(A)] and 2-octyl cyanoacrylate [Figure 5(B)] revealed similar peak intensity values. FTIR spectra of inkjetted mussel adhesive protein solutions containing iron (in Fe:DOPA ratios of 1:1, 10:1, and 100:1) and as-prepared mussel adhesive protein solution are shown in Figure 4(B). No significant differences in peak intensity values among these materials were observed. The FTIR spectroscopy data suggest that piezoelectric inkjet printing does not significantly alter the structure of the marine mussel adhesive protein or cyanoacrylate adhesives.

X-ray photoelectron spectra of mussel adhesive protein solutions (Figure 6) revealed C—C bonding (corresponding to 285 eV), C—N bonding (corresponding to 286.1 eV), and N—C=O bonding (corresponding to 288.2 eV). The peaks may be attributed to aliphatic and aromatic carbons in the marine mussel adhesive protein material. Deconvolution of the C 1s peak revealed the concentration of various

TABLE II. C 1s Peak Deconvolution from X-Ray Photoelectron Spectra

Assignment	C—C[a]	C—N[b]	N—C=O[c]
Mefp (0.16 Mm DOPA)	46%	35%	19%
1:1 Fe:DOPA	44	38	18
10:1 Fe:DOPA	42	37	21
100:1 Fe:DOPA	50	36	14

[a] C—C peak corresponds to 285 eV.
[b] C—N peak corresponds to 286.1 eV.
[c] N—C=O peak corresponds to 288.2 eV.

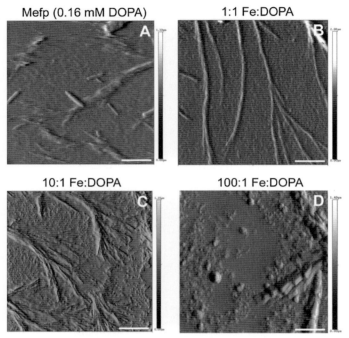

Figure 7. Topography-flattened atomic force micrograph of inkjetted mussel adhesive protein, 1:1 Fe:DOPA, 10:1 Fe:DOPA, and 100:1 Fe:DOPA structures. Scale bar equals 10 μm.

functional groups in inkjetted Fe:DOPA materials (Table II). 1:1 Fe:DOPA and 10:1 Fe:DOPA materials exhibited less C—C bonding than as-prepared Mefp (0.16 mM DOPA) solution. On the other hand, the 100:1 Fe:DOPA material revealed more C—C bonding and less N—C=O bonding than as-prepared Mefp (0.16 mM DOPA) solution. X-ray photoelectron spectra of the inkjetted protein solutions were inconclusive in determining the role of Fe(III) in complex formation. However, the distribution of X-ray photoelectron peaks in the inkjet printed materials was similar to that previously observed in spectra of dropcast mussel adhesive proteins (Mefp) materials.[30]

Atomic force microscopy has previously been used to examine the morphology of DOPA-containing residues.[31] An atomic force microscopy of inkjetted mussel adhesive protein solution (Figure 7) revealed cross-linking upon addition of Fe(III). In the absence of iron, mussel adhesive protein (Mefp) [Figure 7(A)] revealed cross-linking and the presence of some fibrous networks. Precipitation of more complex fiber networks was observed in 1:1 Fe:DOPA and 10:1 Fe:DOPA materials [Figure 7(B,C)]. A higher degree

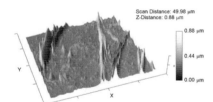

Figure 8. Three-dimensional representation of the surface of mussel adhesive protein solution containing Fe(III) (1:1 Fe:DOPA) obtained using atomic force microscopy. Image was obtained twenty-four hours after curing. [Color figure can be viewed in the online issue, which is available at www.interscience.wiley.com.]

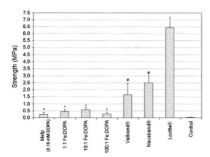

Figure 9. Average strength of bioadhesives inkjetted on full thickness porcine skin. All samples were cured for 24 h. The difference in strength was statistically significant for all except those indicated by "*", "^", and "#" ($p < 0.05$). Bars indicate standard deviation of mean strength.

of cross-linking was observed in the 10:1 Fe:DOPA material than in the 1:1 Fe:DOPA material. Three-dimensional imaging of the surface of the 1:1 Fe:DOPA material revealed high-aspect ratio fibrous network structures (Figure 8). The height of the fibrous networks varied from ~400 to ~800 nm, while the width of fibrous networks varied from ~500 to ~5 μm. The 100:1 Fe:DOPA material revealed islands of cross-linked mussel adhesive protein material (Figure 7D). Small regions of fibrous networks were observed within the inkjetted pattern, which result from nonuniform distribution of mussel adhesive protein in the inkjetted solution. Previous studies have demonstrated iron-induced cross-linking of mussel adhesive proteins using electron paramagnetic, infrared, and ultraviolet-visible absorption spectroscopies.[22,33]

Adhesion characteristics of pure marine mussel extracts have been previously examined under different curing conditions (Figure 9).[34,35] Low humidity and nonoxidative conditions have been shown to be critical in obtaining strong adhesion properties in mussel adhesive proteins. Tensile testing of inkjetted materials on full-thickness porcine skin revealed that mussel adhesive proteins exhibit significantly lower adhesion strength values than cyanoacrylate adhesives (Figure 9). Inkjetted ethyl cyanoacrylate (Quick Set™ Loctite®) showed highest strength among tested adhesives. Inkjetted n-butyl cyanoacrylate (Vetbond®) and 2-octyl cyanoacrylate (Nexaband®) patterns exhibited similar adhesion strength values; however, the toxic effects of these materials are well-documented.[6–8] Addition of Fe(III) to Mefp (0.16 mM DOPA) in 1:1 Fe:DOPA improved adhesion strength. The 10:1 Fe:DOPA and 1:1 Fe:DOPA materials did not exhibit significant differences in adhesion strength. However, the 100:1 Fe:DOPA material exhibited lower adhesion strength values than the 1:1 Fe:DOPA and 10:1 Fe:DOPA materials. This finding suggests that the relatively low adhesion strength of the 100:1 Fe:DOPA material results from a high degree of cross-linking within the mussel adhesive protein material, which limits interaction with the porcine skin substrate. In addition, two different ferric catecholate complexes may be formed at low and high Fe:DOPA ratios.[21] Previous studies have shown that iron (III) can serve as a cross-linking agent for mussel adhesive protein.[36–38] For example, previous electron paramagnetic resonance studies have confirmed iron-induced cross-linking in precursor proteins, which is similar to that observed in intact mussel plaques.[22] The atomic force microscopy images for the 1:1 and 10:1 Fe:DOPA materials contain a relatively high density of fibrous networks. On the other hand, a relatively low density of fibrous networks is observed in the Mefp (0.16 mM DOPA) and 100:1 Fe:DOPA materials. The density of fibrous networks may be correlated with the adhesion strength observed in mussel adhesive protein materials. These results suggest that the extent of cross-linking and precipitation in these inkjetted mussel adhesive protein patterns may be correlated with iron concentration. As discussed earlier, metal-mediated catechol complexation is thought to be responsible for the adhesion properties of mussel adhesive proteins.

CONCLUSIONS

Mussel adhesive proteins could serve as environmentally friendly alternatives to synthetic adhesives in biomedical, electronics, and marine-equipment applications. Fourier transform infrared spectra and X-ray photoelectron spectra have shown that piezoelectric inkjetting is a nondestructive technique that may be successfully used to dispense picoliter amounts of mussel adhesive proteins and other adhesives. Atomic force microscopy and adhesion testing have demonstrated that the adhesive strength in these materials may be correlated with the amount of iron-induced cross-linking. CAD ink-jetting of naturally-derived mussel adhesive proteins such as *Mytilus edulis* foot proteins may overcome several problems associated with conventional medical adhesives. This technology may greatly improve wound repair in next generation eye repair, fracture fixation, wound closure, and drug delivery devices.

REFERENCES

1. Ginsberg SP, Polack FM. Cyanoacrylate tissue adhesive in ocular disease. Ophthalmic Surg 1972;3:126–132.
2. Landegren T, Risling M, Persson JKE. Local tissue reactions after nerve repair with ethyl-cyanoacrylate compared with epineural sutures. Scand J Plast Reconstr 2007;41:217–227.
3. Eskandari MM, Ozturk OG, Eskandari HG, Balli E, Yilmaz C. Cyanoacrylate adhesive provides efficient local drug delivery. Clin Orthop Relat Res 2006;451:242–250.
4. Applebaum JS, Zalut T, Applebaum D. The use of tissue adhesion for traumatic laceration repair in the emergency department. Ann Emerg Med 1993;22:1190–1192.

Journal of Biomedical Materials Research Part B: Applied Biomaterials

5. Vanholder R, Misotten A, Roels H, Matton G. Cyanoacrylate tissue adhesive for closing skin wounds- a double-blind randomized comparison with sutures. Biomaterials 1993;14:737–742.
6. Hauptmann M, Lubin JH, Stewart PA, Hayes RB, Blair A. Mortality from lymphohematopoietic malignancies among workers in formaldehyde industries. J Nat Cancer Inst 2003;95:1615–1623.
7. Pinkerton LE, Hein MJ, Stayner LT. Mortality among a cohort of garment workers exposed to formaldehyde: an update. Occup Environ Med 2004;61:193–200.
8. Leggat PA, Smith DR, Kedjarune U. Surgical applications of cyanoacrylate adhesives: A review of toxicity. Aust NZ J Surg 2007;77:209–213.
9. Dunn CJ, Goa KL. Fibrin sealant—A review of its use in surgery and endoscopy. Drugs 1999;58:863–886.
10. Sierra DH. Fibrin sealant adhesive systems: A review of their chemistry, material properties, and clinical applications. J Biomater Appl 1993;7:309–352.
11. Clark RA. Fibrin glue for wound repair: Facts and fancy. Thromb Haemost 2003;90:1003–1006.
12. Schreiber GB, Busch MP, Kleinman SH, Korelitz JJ. The risk of transfusion-transmitted viral infections. New Engl J Med 1996;334:1685–1690.
13. Lin Q, Gourdon D, Sun C, Holten-Andersen N, Anderson TH, Waite JH, Israelachvili JN. Adhesion mechanisms of the mussel foot proteins mfp-1 and mfp-3. Proc Natl Acad Sci USA 2008;104:3782–3786.
14. Waite JH, Housley TJ, Tanzer ML. Peptide repeats in a mussel glue protein- theme and variattions. Biochemistry 1985;24:5010–5014.
15. Waite JH. Natures underwater adhesive specialist. Int J Adhes Adhes 1987;7:9–14.
16. Olivieri MP, Baier RE, Loomis RE. Surface properties of mussel adhesive protein-component films. Biomaterials 1992;13:1000–1008.
17. Doraiswamy A, Narayan RJ, Cristescu R, Mihailescu IN, Chrisey DB. Laser processing of natural mussel adhesive protein thin films. Mater Sci Eng C. 2007;27:409–413.
18. Waite JH. Adhesion a la Moule. Integr Comp Biol 2002;42:1172–1180.
19. Wiegemann M. Adhesion in blue mussels (Mytilus edulis) and barnacles (genus Balanus): Mechanisms and technical applications. Aquat Sci 2005;67:166–176.
20. Taylor SW, Chase DB, Emptage MH, Nelson MJ, Waite JH. Ferric ion complexes of a DOPA-containing adhesive protein from Mytilus edulis. Inorg Chem 1996;35:7572–7577.
21. Monahan J, Wilker JJ. Specificity of metal ion cross-linking in marine mussel adhesives. Chem Commun 2003;14:1672–1673.
22. Sever MJ, Weisser JT, Monahan J, Srinivasan S, Wilker JJ. Metal-mediated cross-linking in the generation of a marine-mussel adhesive. Angew Chem Int Ed 2004;43:448–450.
23. Waite JH, Andersen NH, Jewhurst S, Sun CJ. Mussel adhesion: Finding the tricks worth mimicking. J Adhes 2005;81:297–314.
24. Lemmo AV, Rose DJ, Tisone TC. Inkjet dispensing technology: applications in drug discovery. Curr Opin Biotechnol 1998;9:615–617.
25. Calvert P. Inkjet printing for materials and devices. Chem Mater 2001;13:3299–3305.
26. Roth EA, Xu T, Das M, Gregory C, Hickman JJ, Boland T. Inkjet printing for high-throughput cell patterning. Biomaterials 2004;25:3707–3715.
27. Sumerel J, Lewis J, Doraiswamy A, Deravi LF, Sewell SL, Gerdon AE, Wright DW, Narayan RJ. Piezoelectric ink jet processing of materials for medical and biological applications. Biotechnol J 2006;1:976–987.
28. Waite JH. Precursors of quinone tanning-dopa-containing proteins. Method Enzymol 1995;258:1–20.
29. Weinhold M, Soubatch S, Temirov R, Rohlfing M, Jastorff B, Tautz FS, Doose C. Structure and bonding of the multifunctional amino acid L-DOPA on Au(110). J Phys Chem B 2006;110:23756–23769.
30. Baty AM, Suci PA, Tyler BJ, Geesey GG. Investigation of mussel adhesive protein adsorption on polystyrene and poly(octadecyl methacrylate) using angle dependent XPS. ATR-FTIR, and AFM. J Colloid Interface Sci 1996;177:307–315.
31. Lee H, Scherer NF, Messersmith PB. Single-molecule mechanics of mussel adhesion. Proc Natl Acad Sci USA 2006;103:12999–13003.
32. Weisser JT, Nilges MJ, Sever MJ, Wilker JJ. EPR investigation and spectral simulations of iron-catecholate complexes and iron-peptide models of marine adhesive cross-links. Inorg Chem 2006;45:7736–7747.
33. Sever MJ, Wilker JJ. Absorption spectroscopy and binding constants for first row transition metal complexes of a DOPA-containing peptide. Dalton Trans 2006;6:813–822.
34. Ninan L, Monahan J, Stroshine RL, Wilker JJ, Shi RY. Adhesive strength of marine mussel extracts on porcine skin. Biomaterials 2003;24:4091–4099.
35. Schnurrer J, Lehr CM. Mucoadhesive properties of the mussel adhesive protein. Int J Pharm 1996;141:251–256.
36. Monahan J, Wilker JJ. Reagents for cross-linking the protein precursor of a marine mussel adhesive. Langmuir 2004;20:3724–3729.
37. Loizou E, Weisser JT, Schmidt G, Wilker JJ. Effects of iron ion cross-linking on biopolymer hydrogels. Macromol Biosci 2006;6:711–718.
38. Hight LM, Wilker JJ. Synergestic effects of metals and oxidation in the curing of marine mussel adhesive. J Mater Sci 2007;42:8934–8942.

6
Laser Microfabrication of Hydroxyapatite-Osteoblast-Like Cell Composites

Laser microfabrication of hydroxyapatite-osteoblast-like cell composites

A. Doraiswamy,[1] R. J. Narayan,[1] M. L. Harris,[2] S. B. Qadri,[2] R. Modi,[2] D. B. Chrisey[2]
[1]Joint Department of Biomedical Engineering, University of North Carolina at Chapel Hill, Chapel Hill, North Carolina
[2]United States Naval Research Laboratory, Washington, District of Columbia

Received 3 November 2005; revised 2 April 2006; accepted 5 June 2006
Published online 18 October 2006 in Wiley InterScience (www.interscience.wiley.com). DOI: 10.1002/jbm.a.30969

Abstract: We have developed a novel approach for layer-by-layer growth of tissue-engineered materials using a direct writing process known as matrix assisted pulsed laser evaporation direct write (MAPLE DW). Unlike conventional cell-seeding methods, this technique provides the possibility for cell-material integration prior to artificial tissue fabrication. This process also provides greater flexibility in selection and processing of scaffold materials. In addition, MAPLE DW offers rapid computer-controlled deposition of mesoscopic voxels at high spatial resolutions. We have examined MAPLE DW processing of zirconia and hydroxyapatite scaffold materials that can provide a medical device with nearly inert and bioactive implant-tissue interfaces, respectively. We have also demonstrated codeposition of hydroxyapatite, MG 63 osteoblast-like cells, and extracellular matrix using MAPLE DW. We have shown that osteoblast-like cells remain viable and retain the capacity for proliferation when codeposited with bioceramic scaffold materials. Our results on MG 63-hydroxyapatite composites can be extended to develop other integrated cell-scaffold structures for medical and dental applications. © 2006 Wiley Periodicals, Inc. J Biomed Mater Res 80A: 635–643, 2007

Key words: laser processing; direct writing; tissue engineering; zirconia; hydroxyapatite

INTRODUCTION

There are many techniques for creating tissue substitutes for use in repairing acute injury, chronic disease, or congenital defects.[1,2] The "gold standard" or best tissue substitute is known as autograft tissue, which is relocated from one site to another within the same person. Use of autograft tissue is associated with many problems. For example, surgery at the donor tissue site can cause infection, inflammation, chronic pain, and the need for additional surgery. In addition, the quantity of material that can be relocated is very limited. Another kind of transplantable tissue is called allograft tissue, which is transferred from one person to another. Twenty-five tissues and organs, including cartilage, cornea, heart, kidney, liver, lung, and pancreas, have been transplanted between different people. Unfortunately, allograft use is also fraught with many problems. The major problem with allograft transplantation is providing a sufficient number of organs for all of the people who need them. There are currently 80,000 people on organ waiting lists in the United States, and over 10,000 people have died over the last 5 years waiting for organs.[3] In addition, the recipient's immune system generates acute vascular rejection and chronic rejection processes that break down transplanted allograft tissue in hours, days, weeks, months, and years after implantation.[4] The immunosuppressive therapy used to counteract the rejection process may itself lead to tumor formation. In addition, there is risk of infection transmission from allograft organ donor to allograft organ recipient. For example, it has been estimated that the possibility of HIV transmission with allograft bone transplant is one case in 1.6 million.[5] One case of hepatitis B transmission and three cases of hepatitis C transmission have been correlated with allograft transplantation.[6]

The continuing limitations of natural graft therapies and the growing demand for tissue substitutes have led to the growth of a field known as tissue engineering. This area was initiated by Robert Langer and Joseph Vacanti at the Massachusetts Institute of

Correspondence to: R. J. Narayan; e-mail: roger_narayan@unc.edu

© 2006 Wiley Periodicals, Inc.
Computer Aided Biomanufacturing, Edited by Roger Narayan and Paul Calvert
© 2011 WILEY-VCH Verlag GmbH & Co. KGaA. Published 2011 by WILEY-VCH Verlag GmbH & Co. KGaA.

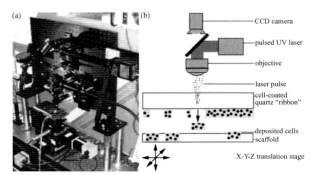

Figure 1. (a) Photograph of experimental apparatus and (b) schematic diagram of the matrix-assisted pulsed laser evaporation-direct write (MAPLE DW) process.

Technology and Harvard University.[7,8] Tissue-engineered materials include living cells, natural materials, and synthetic materials. These structures are fashioned by placing living cells within hydrogel (e.g., poly(vinyl alcohol), resorbable polymer (e.g., poly(lactic acid)), or naturally-derived material (e.g., collagen) scaffolding that guides development. The cell-seeded structures are then placed in bioreactors that provide nutrients and allow cells to multiply within the scaffold, and implanted in the body so that it will resume normal function. Unfortunately, three-dimensional scaffold seeding is very difficult because many cells do not exhibit sufficient multiplication within in vitro bioreactors. Conventional bioreactors simply cannot supply sufficient oxygen and nutrients for cell multiplication. As a result, it is difficult to create structures that possess thicknesses greater than 100 μm (4–7 cell layers).

Solvent-based direct writing techniques for making organic or cellular films (e.g., ink jetting, Langmuir-Blodgett dip coating, and pin arraying) have recently been used to fabricate two-dimensional and three-dimensional cell-seeded scaffolds for use in tissue engineering. However, these solvent-based processes also have several limitations. For example, ink jet processes cannot produce near-monolayer coverage. In addition, film thickness is dependent on dispensed droplet size and surface wetting. Langmuir-Blodgett (L-B) coatings are capable of creating multilayered cell-seeded films; however, increasing L-B film thickness requires repeating the coating procedure for each additional layer. L-B coatings are also limited in the choice of materials used to create these films. Furthermore, the solvent containing the material of interest may dissolve any underlying layers.

These techniques also have limitations in resolution, scale up, speed, and film quality.

A novel process known as matrix-assisted pulsed laser evaporation direct write (MAPLE DW) has been developed for direct writing inorganic material, organic material, and cells.[9] The experimental MAPLE DW setup is shown in Figure 1. The material to be transferred is solvated and evenly coated onto an optically transparent quartz disk, which is referred to as a "ribbon." When low energy laser light is applied to the ribbon, the solute material is driven forward onto a receiving substrate. The resolution of the transferred pattern is controlled by the distance between the ribbon/substrate, the fluence, the spot-size, and the movement of the stage; the current minimum feature size is ~1 μm. Laser-based processing provides several advantages over solvent-based direct writing techniques. These include: (1) enhanced cell–substrate adhesion, (2) deposition can be performed under ambient conditions, (3) deposition of mesoscopic voxels can be performed at rapid deposition rates, and (4) matrix processing allows the amount of transferred material to be quantitatively determined.

We have investigated codeposition of bioceramics, viable mammalian cells, and extracellular matrix (ECM) in mesoscopic patterns using MAPLE DW. We have chosen hydroxyapatite ($Ca_{10}(PO_4)_6(OH)_2$, HA) as a scaffold material. This material is known as a bioactive ceramic, because it is able to form strong chemical bonds with adjacent tissues. Recent studies have shown that osteoblast cells attach, proliferate, and differentiate on hydroxyapatite surfaces.[10,11] These cells secrete osteoid (proteoglycans, glycoproteins, type 1 collagen), enzymes (osteocalcin

Journal of Biomedical Materials Research Part A DOI 10.1002/jbm.a

and alkaline phosphatase), and growth factors (interleukin-1) that mediate *in vivo* bone growth. Hydroxyapatite also exhibits controlled *in vivo* degradation rates, which are dependent on phase, surface area, crystallinity, and ionic substitution.[12,13] In addition, hydroxyapatite acts as a source for calcium, phosphorus, sodium, and magnesium ions necessary for *in vivo* bone growth. We have integrated osteoblasts and hydroxyapatite prior to tissue fabrication to take advantage of its osteoconductive properties. We have also developed scaffolds using zirconia, an inert ceramic that exhibits a stable oxide surface, high hardness, high corrosion resistance, and high wear resistance.[14] Our findings on depositing mesoscopic patterns of cells, ceramics, and ECM composites that possess controlled microstructures will allow the development of novel dental and orthopaedic tissue substitutes.

EXPERIMENTAL PROCEDURE

Matrix assisted pulsed laser evaporation direct write

The MAPLE DW process can be used to transfer materials onto the substrate surface and micromachine channels or other features into the substrate. Figure 1 contains a photograph and a schematic of the MAPLE DW. An ArF pulsed excimer laser ($\lambda = 193$ nm, $f = 10$ Hz, fluence = 0.1–0.3 J/cm^2) was focused onto the ribbon plane using a lens. A biomaterial (hydroxyapatite or zirconia) -coated 1 in. diameter quartz disc is used as a ribbon, which is placed directly above the substrate. The gap between the ribbon and substrate was controlled using a Z-translation stage. Patterns were created using a joystick- or computer program-controlled X–Y translation stage. The diameter of the laser spot on the ribbon was maintained at 70 µm. Laser transfer was observed using an inverted lens camera that was focused on the receiving substrate. These experiments were performed under ambient air and at room temperature (25°C).

MAPLE DW transfer of hydroxyapatite and zirconia

MAPLE DW ribbons of ceramics were created by solvating ceramic powders in glycerol/water matrices, and spin coating these solutions onto quartz ribbons. Hydroxyapatite (average particle size of 500 nm) and zirconia (particle size distribution of 0.33–2.19 µm) powders were ground using a mortar and pestle (Alfa Aesar, Ward Hill, MA). These powders were solvated in 50:50 glycerol:water matrices to create solutions that possessed appropriate viscosities and solubilities for spin coating onto quartz ribbons. Homogeneous ribbons were obtained for hydroxyapatite and zirconia solutions with concentrations of 60 and 70 wt %, respectively. These solutions were spin coated onto 1 in. quartz ribbons at rpm for 10 s. The thickness of the bio-material on the ribbon was ~250 µm. The ribbon was positioned 250 µm above the borosilicate glass substrate. The minimum fluence for ceramic transfer was determined by systematically increasing the laser fluence on the ribbon and observing transfer using the inverted lens camera. The threshold fluences for MAPLE DW transfer of hydroxyapatite and zirconia were observed at 0.22 and 0.18 J/cm^2, respectively. Optical microscopy was used to examine the feature sizes in the mesoscopic patterns. A Hitachi S800 scanning electron microscope (Hitachi High Technologies, Tokyo, Japan) was used to examine the microstructure of the MAPLE DW-transferred ceramic patterns. X-ray diffraction was performed to determine the composition, phase, and crystallinity of the transferred material.

MG 63 osteoblast-like cell culture

The MG 63 human osteosarcoma cell line developed by Billiau et al. is widely used to study the biocompatibility of orthopaedic and dental biomaterials. MG 63 osteoblast-like cells (American Type Culture Collection. Manassas, VA) were subcultured in a Eagle's minimum essential medium (Earle's balanced salt solution) (EMEM (EBSS)) media, which contained 2 mM L-glutamine, 1.5 g/L sodium bicarbonate, 0.1 mM nonessential amino acids, 1.0 mM sodium pyruvate, 10% heat-inactivated fetal bovine serum, and 1% antibiotic syrup. Subconfluent cells were trypsinized and split 1:5 to maintain division of the cell line and avoid differentiation. The cells were stored in a 37°C, 5% CO$_2$ culture incubator.

MAPLE DW transfer of MG 63 osteoblast-like cells

ECM (American Type Culture Collection, Manassas, VA) was used to coat the ribbon and the substrate for the MAPLE DW cell transfer experiments. The properties of ECM are highly conducive to osteoblast growth and proliferation. ECM provides osteoblasts with a hydrophobic surface suitable for cell adhesion.[15] It also contains laminin and type 4 collagen proteins that interact with cellular adhesion receptors and maintain adhesion. In addition, ECM contains growth factor regulators, including heparan sulfate, proteoglycans, TGF-b, EGF, IGF-1, bFGF, and PDGF, that facilitate cell growth at the cell–ECM interface. ECM was slowly warmed from −20°C to 0–4°C to avoid rapid polymerization. ECM (500 µL) was spin coated on sterilized 1 in. quartz ribbons and glass substrates for 10 s at 1000 rpm. The ribbons and substrates were placed in a 37°C, 5% CO$_2$ culture incubator for 30 min to allow complete crosslinking of the ECM.

Sub-confluent MG 63 osteoblast-like cells were removed from a culture flask, trypsinized, and centrifuged for 3 min at 5000 rpm. The resulting concentrated cell pellet was reconstituted with 0.25 mL of EMEM (EBSS) to create a solution that contained ~10^7 cells/mL, which was pipetted onto the ECM-coated ribbon. The cell-seeded ribbon was then placed in the incubator for 10 min to allow cells to attach to ECM prior to transfer. The ribbon was positioned 250 µm above the ECM-coated borosilicate glass substrate. The minimum fluence for osteoblast-like cell transfer was

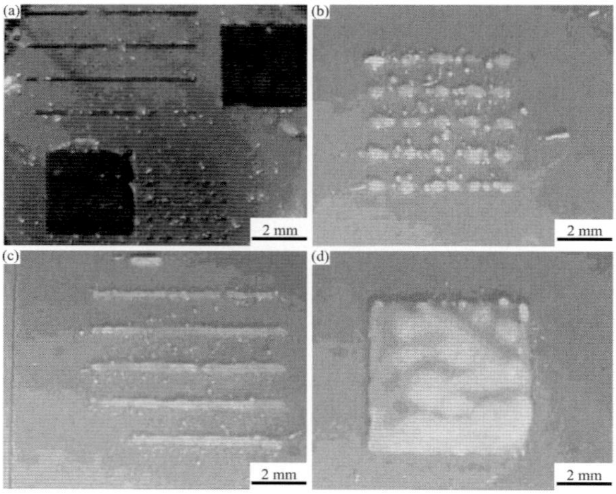

Figure 2. (a) Optical micrograph of MAPLE DW hydroxyapatite ribbon containing regions that have been transferred by the laser. (b)–(d) Optical micrographs of hydroxyapatite patterns on borosilicate glass substrates.

determined by systematically increasing the laser fluence on the ribbon, and observing transfer using the inverted lens camera; the threshold fluence for MAPLE DW transfer of osteoblast-like cells was observed at 0.15 J/cm^2. After MAPLE DW transfer, the ribbon and the substrate were stored in separate Petri dishes containing prewarmed EMEM (EBSS) media. Proliferation of MAPLE DW-transferred cells was examined over several days using optical microscopy. A live/dead stain (Biovision Research Products, Mountain View, CA) was used to examine the MAPLE DW-transferred MG 63 osteoblast-like cells. The staining solution was pipetted over the cells and allowed to incubate for 15 min. The propidium iodide within the staining solution caused nonliving cells to fluoresce a red color, and the Live-dye™ within the staining solution caused living cells to stain a green color. The stained osteoblast-like cells were viewed with an inverted microscope and a digital still camera using an epifluorescence attachment.

MAPLE DW transfer of MG 63-hydroxyapatite composites

The protocols used for MAPLE DW transfer of MG 63-hydroxyapatite composites were similar to those that have been described in earlier sections. Five-hundred microliters of ECM was spin coated onto 1 in. quartz ribbons and borosilicate glass substrates for 10 s at 1000 rpm. Hydroxyapatite powder was ground using a mortar and pestle, and solvated in a 50:50 phosphate buffered saline:ECM solution. This solution was spin coated onto ECM-coated quartz ribbons at 1000 rpm for 10 s. The ribbons and substrates were placed in a 37°C, 5% CO_2 culture incubator for 30 min to allow complete cross-linking of the ECM. Subconfluent MG 63 osteoblast-like cells were trypsinized and centrifuged for 3 min at 5000 rpm. The resulting concentrated cell pellet was reconstituted with 0.25 mL of EMEM (EBSS) to create a solution that contained ~10^7 cells/mL, which was pipetted onto the hydroxyapatite/ECM-coated ribbon. The ribbon was positioned 300 μm above the borosilicate glass substrate. MAPLE DW transfer of MG 63/hydroxyapatite composites was performed using a laser fluence of 0.22 J/cm^2. After MAPLE DW transfer, the ribbon and the substrate were stored in separate Petri dishes containing prewarmed EMEM (EBSS) media. Proliferation of MAPLE DW-transferred cells was examined over several days using optical microscopy and live/dead staining.

RESULTS AND DISCUSSION

MAPLE DW transfer of hydroxyapatite and zirconia

An optical micrograph of the hydroxyapatite ribbon is shown in Figure 2(a). Discrete points, lines,

LASER MICROFABRICATION

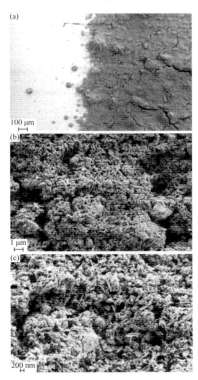

Figure 3. (a–c) Scanning electron micrographs of MAPLE DW-transferred hydroxyapatite at several magnifications.

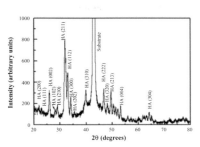

Figure 4. X-ray diffraction of MAPLE DW-transferred hydroxyapatite, which contains peaks that correspond to crystalline hydroxyapatite.

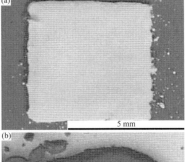

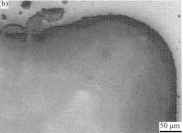

Figure 5. (a–b) Optical micrographs of MAPLE DW-transferred zirconia.

and squares have been transferred by the laser. Figure 2(b–d) contain optical micrographs of hydroxyapatite point, line, and square patterns on a borosilicate glass substrate, respectively. These mesoscopic patterns maintain the dimensions and boundaries seen in the ribbon. Scanning electron micrographs [Figure 3(a–c)] show that MAPLE DW-transferred hydroxyapatite contains a porous mesh-like network. The porosity of MAPLE DW-transferred hydroxyapatite can be tailored to *in vivo* application by controlling the size of the ceramic powder, the amount of solvent used to prepare the ribbon, and the choice of solvent used to prepare the ribbon. The MAPLE DW process also maintained the composition and phase of the target material. Figure 4, an X-ray diffraction

Journal of Biomedical Materials Research Part A DOI 10.1002/jbm.a

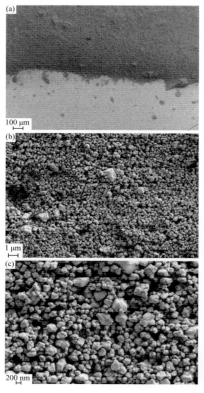

Figure 6. (a–c) Scanning electron micrographs of MAPLE DW-transferred zirconia at several magnifications.

pattern of MAPLE DW-transferred hydroxyapatite reveals the (200), (111), (002), (102), (210), (211), (112), (300), (202), (310), (222), (320), (213), (004), and (304) peaks of crystalline hydroxyapatite.[16] Figure 5(a,b) contain optical micrographs of transferred zirconia square pattern at different magnifications. The splashing near the boundary occurs during the transfer process and can be eliminated using a micromachining technique using the laser system at a higher energy density. Scanning electron micrographs of MAPLE DW-transferred zirconia [Fig. 6(a–c)] reveal the presence of many micrometer-dimen-

sion particles. MAPLE DW is capable of generating materials with a variety of micrometer-dimension surface features as demonstrated in the above patterns.

Reproducible control over surface roughness may provide unique biological functionalities at the tissue/implant interface. For example, osteoblast proliferation, osteoblast differentiation, angiogenesis, and other processes can be modulated by surface roughness.[17] For example, Boyan and coworkers[18] have shown that MG 63 cells respond to increasing surface roughness with increased differentiation and decreased proliferation. Several markers and mediators of cell activity, including alkaline phosphatase, osteocalcin, TGF-β_1, and prostaglandin E_2, are produced in greater amounts on rougher surfaces. In addition, MG 63 cells exhibit enhanced responsiveness to hormones (e.g., 1,25-$(OH)_2D_3$) on rougher surfaces. In addition, Brauker et al. have shown that materials with pores with sizes between 0.8 and

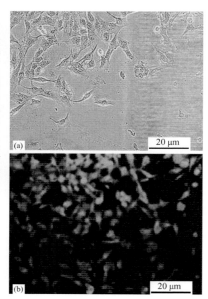

Figure 7. (a) Optical micrograph and (b) fluorescence image of live-dead stained MG 63 osteoblast-like cells 48 h after MAPLE DW transfer. [Color figure can be viewed in the online issue, which is available at www.interscience.wiley.com.]

LASER MICROFABRICATION

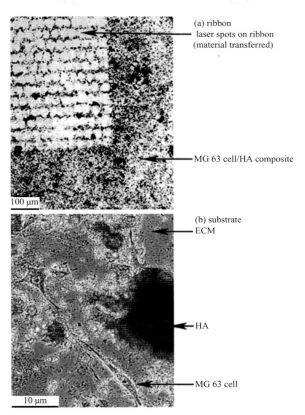

Figure 8. (a) Optical micrograph of MG 63-hydroxyapatite composite MAPLE DW ribbon containing regions that have been transferred by the laser. (b) Optical micrograph of MAPLE DW transferred MG 63-hydroxyapatite composites.

8 μm exhibit increased amounts of cell penetration and neovascularization (blood vessel formation).[19] The interaction among several MAPLE DW deposition parameters, including the laser fluence, laser spot size, ceramic powder size, ribbon-substrate length, amount of solvent used to prepare the ribbon, and choice of solvent used to prepare the ribbon, may provide additional opportunities to create unique surface morphologies and improved tissue/implant interfaces.

MAPLE DW transfer of MG 63 osteoblast-like cells

We have previously demonstrated successful transfers of several cell types, including C2C12 myoblast-like cells and B35 neuroblast-like cells, using MAPLE DW. Transferred cells demonstrate near 100% viability; live/dead, viability, and cytotoxicity assays have shown that cells are not altered by the MAPLE DW process.[20–22] Figure 7(a) contains an

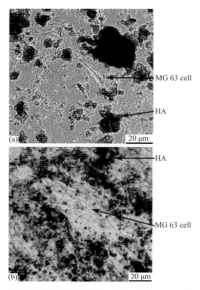

with other cells and the hydroxyapatite matrix. Optical micrographs of MG 63-hydroxyapatite composites at 3 h and 96 h after MAPLE DW transfer are shown in Figure 9(a,b), respectively. The cells continue to proliferate after MAPLE DW transfer, and the numbers of osteoblasts and cytoplasmic extensions appear greater in Figure 9(b) than in Figure 9(a). Live-dead staining of a MG 63-hydroxyapatite composite at 72 h after MAPLE DW transfer [Fig. 10(b)] indicates that the transferred cells remain via-

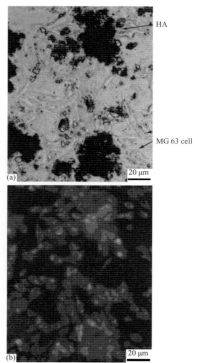

Figure 9. Optical micrographs of MG 63-hydroxyapatite composite taken (a) 3 h and (b) 96 h after MAPLE DW transfer.

optical micrograph of the lower right edge of a square pattern of MAPLE DW transferred MG 63 cells. The osteoblast-like cells exhibited less well defined boundaries than ceramics on borosilicate glass substrates due to cell growth and proliferation after transfer. Figure 7(b) contains live-dead assay results, which revealed that 100% of the osteoblast-like cells remained viable after MAPLE DW transfer. The morphologies of MAPLE DW-transferred cells appear similar to those of cells in the ribbon.

MAPLE DW transfer of MG 63-hydroxyapatite composites

Figure 8(a) is an optical micrograph of MG 63-hydroxyapatite composite ribbon. The square pattern resulted from MAPLE DW transfer of ribbon material. Figure 9(b) contains an optical micrograph of MAPLE DW-transferred osteoblast-like cells and hydroxyapatite particles. MAPLE DW-transferred osteoblast-like cells exhibit cytoplasmic extensions

Figure 10. (a) Optical micrograph and (b) fluorescence image of the live-dead stained MG 63-hydroxyapatite composite 72 h after MAPLE DW transfer. [Color figure can be viewed in the online issue, which is available at www.interscience.wiley.com.]

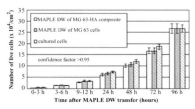

Figure 11. Growth profiles of MG 63 osteoblast-like cells in EMEM (EBSS) media, MAPLE DW transferred MG 63 osteoblast-like cells, and MAPLE DW-transferred MG 63 osteoblast-like cell-hydroxyapatite composites.

ble. Figure 11 contains cell growth curves of MAPLE DW-transferred osteoblast-like cells, MAPLE DW-transferred osteoblast-like cells in MG 63-hydroxyapatite composites, and cultured MG 63 cells over 96 h. The number of live cells per square centimeter and confidence factor is shown at each time interval. The growth rates of MAPLE DW-transferred osteoblast-like cells in MG 63-hydroxyapatite composites, MAPLE DW-transferred osteoblast-like cells, and cultured cells are statistically identical at 0–3, 3–6, 9–12, 24, 48, 72, and 96 h time intervals. No preferential growth of cells was observed.

CONCLUSIONS

MAPLE DW is a versatile technique for creating multilayer, heterogeneous, three dimensional cell-seeded scaffolds for use in tissue engineering. Mesoscopic patterns of inert ceramics, bioactive ceramics, and MG 63 cell-hydroxyapatite composites were created using MAPLE DW. We have shown that osteoblast-like cells remain viable and retain the capacity for proliferation when codeposited with bioceramic scaffold materials. The ability to deposit mesoscopic patterns of cell–ceramic composites offers structural integrity in using two-dimensional layers to build mechanically robust three-dimensional heterogeneous tissue constructs. The versatility of transferring cells along with ceramics to construct CAD/CAM-based patterns makes MAPLE DW unique and very promising for heterogeneous scaffolding. Based on the functionality and structural requirements, this concept can be extended to integrate a variety of cell-lines with most organic/inorganic materials.

References

1. Laurencin CT, Ambrosio AMA, Borden MD, Cooper JA. Tissue engineering: Orthopedic applications. Annu Rev Biomed Eng 1999;1:19–46.
2. Salgado AJ, Coutinho OP, Reis RL. Bone tissue engineering: State of the art and future trends. Macromol Biosci 2004;4: 743–765.
3. Josefson D. AMA considers whether to pay for donation of organs. Br Med J 2002;324:1541.
4. Charlton B, Auchincloss H, Fathman CG. Mechanisms of transplantation tolerance. Annu Rev Immunol 1994;12:707–734.
5. Boyce T, Edwards J, Scarborough N. Allograft bone: The influence of processing on safety and performance. Orthop Clin North Am 1999;30:571–581.
6. Lumelsky A. Transplant tissue: Cryolife human soft tissue implants recalled. J Law Med Ethics 2002;30:474–476.
7. Stock UA, Vacanti JP. Tissue engineering: Current state and prospects. Annu Rev Med 2001;52:443–451.
8. Vacanti CA, Vacanti JP. The science of tissue engineering. Orthop Clin North Am 2000;31:351–356.
9. Barron JA, Ringeisen BR, Kim HS, Spargo BJ, Chrisey DB. Application of laser printing to mammalian cells. Thin Solid Films 2004;453/454:383–387.
10. Okumura M, Ohgushi H, Dohi Y, Katuda T, Tamai S, Koerten HK, Tabata S. Osteoblastic phenotype expression on the surface of hydroxyapatite ceramics. J Biomed Mater Res 1997;37:122–129.
11. Bigi A, Bracci B, Cuisinier F, Elkaim R, Fini M, Mayer I, Mihailescu IN, Socol G, Sturba L, Torricelli P. Human osteoblast response to pulsed laser deposited calcium phosphate coatings. Biomaterials 2005;26:2381–2389.
12. Camire CL, Gbureck U, Hirsiger W, Bohner M. Correlating crystallinity and reactivity in an α-tricalcium phosphate. Biomaterials 2005;26:2787–2794.
13. Suchanek WL, Byrappa K, Shuk P, Riman RE, Janas VF, TenHuisen KS. Preparation of magnesium-substituted hydroxyapatite powders by the mechanochemical-hydrothermal method. Biomaterials 2004;25:4647–4657.
14. Willmann G. Improving bearing surfaces of artificial joints. Adv Eng Mater 2001;3:135–141.
15. Pramatarova L, Pecheva E, Presker R, Pham MT, Maitz MF, Stutzmann M. Hydroxyapatite growth induced by native extracellular matrix deposition on solid surfaces. Eur Cell Mater 2005;9:9–12.
16. Cotell CM, Chrisey DB, Grabowski KS, Sprague JA, Gossett CR. Pulsed laser deposition of hydroxylapatite thin-films on Ti-6Al-4V. J Appl Biomater 1992;3:87–93.
17. Rosa AL, Beloti MM, Van Noort R. Osteoblastic differentiation of cultured rat bone marrow cells on hydroxyapatite with different surface topography. Dent Mater 2003;19:768–772.
18. Schwartz Z, Lohmann CH, Oefinger J, Bonewald LF, Dean DD, Boyan BD. Implant surface characteristics modulate differentiation behavior of cells in the osteoblastic lineage. Adv Dent Res 1999;13:38–48.
19. Brauker JH, Carrbrendel VE, Martinson LA, Crudele J, Johnston WD, Johnson RC. Neovascularization of synthetic membranes directed by membrane. J Biomed Mater Res 1995;29: 1517–1524.
20. Ringeisen BR, Chrisey DB, Pique A, Young HD, Modi R, Bucaro M, Jones-Meehan J, Spargo BJ. Generation of mesoscopic patterns of viable Escherichia coli by ambient laser transfer. Biomaterials 2002;23:161–166.
21. Chrisey DB, Pique A, McGill RA, Horwitz JS, Ringeisen BR, Bubb DM, Wu PK. Laser deposition of polymer and biomaterial films. Chem Rev 2003;103:553–576.
22. Wu PK, Ringeisen BR, Callahan J, Brooks M, Bubb DM, Wu WD, Pique A, Spargo B, McGill RA, Chrisey DB. The deposition, structure, pattern deposition, and activity of biomaterial thin-films by matrix-assisted pulsed-laser evaporation (MAPLE) and MAPLE direct write. Thin Solid Films 2001; 398/399:607–614.

7
Two Photon Polymerization of Polymer–Ceramic Hybrid Materials for Transdermal Drug Delivery

Two Photon Polymerization of Polymer–Ceramic Hybrid Materials for Transdermal Drug Delivery

A. Ovsianikov and B. Chichkov

Laser Zentrum Hannover, Hollerithallee 8, 30419 Hannover, Germany

P. Mente

Joint Department of Biomedical Engineering, North Carolina State University, Raleigh, North Carolina 27695

N. A. Monteiro-Riviere

Center for Chemical Toxicology Research and Pharmacokinetics, and Joint Department of Biomedical Engineering, North Carolina State University, Raleigh, North Carolina 27695

A. Doraiswamy

Joint Department of Biomedical Engineering, University of North Carolina, Chapel Hill, North Carolina 27599

R. J. Narayan*

Department of Materials Science and Engineering, North Carolina State University, Raleigh, North Carolina 27695
Joint Department of Biomedical Engineering, University of North Carolina, Chapel Hill, North Carolina 27599

Three-dimensional microneedle devices were created by femtosecond laser two photon polymerization (2PP) of organically modified ceramic (Ormocer®) hybrid materials. Arrays of in-plane and out-of-plane hollow microneedles (microneedle length = 800 μm, microneedle base diameter = 150–300 μm) with various aspect ratios were fabricated. The fracture and penetration properties of the microneedle arrays were examined using compression load testing. In these studies, the microneedle arrays penetrated cadaveric porcine adipose tissue without fracture. Human epidermal keratinocyte viability on the Ormocer® surfaces polymerized using 2PP was similar to that on control surfaces. These results suggest that 2PP is able to create microneedle structures for transdermal drug delivery with a larger range of geometries than conventional microfabrication techniques.

---

*roger_narayan@unc.edu
© 2007 Blackwell Publishing Ltd.
Computer Aided Biomanufacturing, Edited by Roger Narayan and Paul Calvert
© 2011 WILEY-VCH Verlag GmbH & Co. KGaA. Published 2011 by WILEY-VCH Verlag GmbH & Co. KGaA.

Introduction

Advances in genetic engineering and proteomics have provided protein- and nucleic acid-based treatments for cancer and other chronic diseases.[1,2] Unfortunately, many novel drugs and vaccines cannot be administered in oral or transdermal form, because they may be metabolized by the liver, intestine, kidneys, or lungs before reaching systemic circulation.[3] These agents may be administered intravenously using hypodermic needles; this route provides complete and instantaneous absorption.[4] Hypodermic needles are limited by conventional manufacturing processes to outer diameters of ∼300 μm and wall thicknesses of ∼75 μm. Use of hypodermic needles involves pain to the patient, trauma at the injection site, medical expertise to administer the injection, and difficulty in providing sustained delivery of a pharmacologic agent. In addition, conventional hypodermic needles cannot easily be integrated with portable medical devices.

One emerging option for delivery of pharmacologic agents involves the use of microneedles.[5] These devices, which can take the shape of lancets or miniaturized hypodermic needles, contain at least one dimension that is less than 500 μm in length. By reducing the needle dimensions, pain to the patient and damage at the injection site may be reduced.[6] In addition, administration of pharmacologic agents via microneedles requires no specialized medical training. Hollow microneedles may allow diffusion- or pressure-driven transport of pharmacologic agents through the needle bore to be adjusted over an extended period of time.

There are several requirements for the development of effective microneedles. Microneedles for drug delivery must penetrate the outermost 15 μm of epidermis (stratum corneum layer), which contains keratinized dead cells and serves as a barrier against drug transport through the skin.[7] The pharmacologic agents may diffuse from the inner epidermal layers into the dermis blood vessels. Microneedle shafts for drug delivery are greater than 100 μm in length and are generally 300–400 μm in length, as the stratum corneum exhibits thickness values that vary with age, location, and skin condition. Microneedles for withdrawal of blood must exceed lengths of 700–900 μm in order to penetrate the dermis, which contains blood vessels, Meissner's corpuscles, Pacinian corpuscles, and nerve endings. Most importantly, microneedles must not fracture during skin penetration. The ratio between microneedle fracture and skin insertion force is highest for needles exhibiting large wall angles, large wall thicknesses, and small tip radii. Finally, arrays of microneedles provide injection or extraction over a wider area and at higher rates than solitary needles. Having several needles provides redundancy in case individual needles are obstructed or fractured during insertion.[8] In addition, arrays of needles possess a greater possibility of directly reaching dermal blood vessels for extraction. Microneedle arrays are also less prone to fracture if exposed to shear force, because the shear force is distributed over a wider area.[9]

Several investigators have demonstrated individual microneedles and microneedle arrays using conventional microelectronics fabrication technologies, including chemical isotropic etching, injection molding, reactive ion etching, surface micromachining, bulk micromachining, polysilicon micromolding, and lithography-electroforming-replication.[10–14] Wise et al. created in-plane microneedles by combining anisotropic wet etching of a silicon substrate with use of deep-diffused boron etch stops. In these devices, the density of needles that could be obtained was limited, and only one row of needles was fabricated per chip; however, many blood analysis techniques require high needle densities in order to achieve sufficient liquid flow. McAllister et al. and Kobayashi and Suzuki. have demonstrated electroplated shell structures, which exhibited thin microneedle walls and large radii of curvature.[15,16] These devices did not exhibit sufficient skin penetration or fracture properties for widespread clinical use. Chun et al. have demonstrated fabrication of microcapillaries using deep reactive ion etching, which exhibit relatively small radii of curvature.[17] However, the needle length is limited by the aspect ratio of a single deep reactive ion etching step. In addition, the number of needles per unit area is limited by the isotropy of the etch step and the mask structure. Griss et al. and Gardeniers et al. have demonstrated single-crystal silicon microneedle arrays; however, the openings in these needles were positioned far away from the tip.[8,9] As a result, the needles must be inserted deeper within the skin. Microneedles prepared using conventional silicon, steel, or titanium microfabrication processes have not been employed in widespread clinical use.

We have used two photon polymerization (2PP) to create microneedle arrays for transdermal drug delivery. The 2PP process involves both temporal and spatial overlap of photons to induce chemical reactions leading to photopolymerization and material hardening within well-defined highly localized volumes.[18–26] Near simultaneous absorption of two photons creates a so-called virtual state for several femtoseconds. This electronic excitation is analogous to electronic excitation by a single photon with a much higher energy. Absorption of laser pulses breaks chemical bonds on starter photoinitiator molecules within a small focal volume. The radicalized starter molecules react with monomers and create radicalized polymolecules. The desired three-dimensional structure is produced by polymerizing the material along the laser trace, which is moved in three dimensions using a galvano-scanner and a micropositioning system. On the other hand, the material outside the desired region does not participate in the reaction and can be washed away with an appropriate alcohol solution.

The two photon absorption process exhibits a quadratic dependence on the incident intensity. The minimum resolution is defined by the smallest polymerized volume. This value is determined by the exposure dose, which is in turn determined by the pulse energy and scanning speed. The highest lateral resolution achieved in previous studies using this technique is 100 nm.

2PP provides several advantages over conventional processing for scalable mass production of microneedles. A large variety of inexpensive ceramics, polymers, and other photosensitive materials may be used for 2PP. In addition, 2PP can be set up in a conventional "dirty" manufacturing environment that does not contain cleanroom facilities. Furthermore, the 2PP process may be readily scaled up for industrial use. Finally, 2PP of microneedles is an extremely rapid, straightforward, single-step process, as opposed to conventional multiple step fabrication techniques.

2PP may be used to create three-dimensional devices from Ormocer® (organically modified ceramic; Fraunhofer-Gesellschaft, Munich, Germany) materials. These amorphous organic–inorganic hybrid materials were originally developed by the Fraunhofer-Institut für Silicatforschung, and are prepared by sol–gel processes from liquid precursors. These materials include urethane- and thioether (meth)-acrylate alkoxysilanes, and contain strong covalent bonds between the ceramic and polymer components.[27] The cross-linking of both organic and inorganic components creates a three dimensional network, which prevents separation of the material into separate phases and provides Ormocer® material with exceptional chemical and thermal stability. In previous studies, we have demonstrated using X-ray diffraction that Ormocer® surfaces created using 2PP exhibit an amorphous structure, and that there is no separation between the inorganic and organic phases in the polymerized Ormocer® material.[28,29] The Young's modulus values for Ormocer® materials (11–17,000 MPa) may be varied between those of ceramics and those of polymers by modifying the concentration of organic and inorganic network modifying elements, the lengths of the groups that attach the organic and the inorganic crosslinking sites, and the concentration of filler materials.[30] Ormocer® materials have recently received increased interest from the medical device community. Biological assays, including the ISO 10933-5 cytotoxicity assay, have shown that Ormocer® materials are nontoxic and biologically inert.[31] Ormocer®-based matrix components (Definite™, Degussa, Hanau, Germany) and Ormocer®-based light-curable dental composites (Admira™ Degussa, Hanau, Germany) have been used in restorative dentistry since 1988.

In this study, we have fabricated in-plane hollow microneedles, which contain flow channels that are positioned on-center with respect to the needle tip, and out-of-plane hollow microneedles, which contain flow channels that are positioned off-center with respect to the needle tip. Griss et al. have shown that out-of-plane microneedles created using a multistep reactive ion etching/passivation process do not suffer from obstructions caused by loose skin, which is generated during the microneedle insertion process.[9] Compression load testing was performed in order to examine the effect of the needle geometry on application-specific mechanical properties. The 3-(4,5-dimethylthiazol-2-yl)2,5-diphenyl tetrazolium bromide (MTT) assay was performed in order to compare cell growth on polymerized Ormocer® surfaces with that on control surfaces. Our results suggest that 2PP is able to create hollow Ormocer® microneedles with a larger range of sizes and shapes than conventional microfabrication techniques.

Materials and Methods

Three-dimensional microneedle arrays were produced by 2PP of Ormocer® US-S4. Ormocer® US-S4 is a UV sensitive hybrid material that exhibits a refractive index at 589 nm of 1.520. The Irgacure® 369 initiator (Ciba Specialty Chemicals, Basel, Switzerland) has an absorption peak at around 320 nm. Femtosecond laser pulses (60 fs, 94 MHz, <450 mW, 780 nm) from

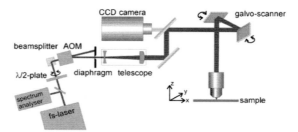

Fig. 1. A schematic of the two photon polymerization system used for fabrication of microneedle arrays.

a titanium: sapphire laser (Kapteyn-Murnane, Boulder, CO) were focused using a 10 × conventional plan achromat microscope objective into a small focal volume within the photosensitive resin (Fig. 1).[31,32] The laser pulses passed through the out-of-focus region and did not interact with the material. On the other hand, nonlinear absorption of laser pulses broke chemical bonds on starter photoinitiator molecules within a small focal volume. The radicalized starter molecules reacted with monomers and created radicalized polymolecules. The reactions were terminated when two radicalized polymolecules reacted with one other.

The desired structures were fabricated by moving the laser focus in three dimensions. Polymerization of the device occurred along the trace of the laser focus. A combination of three C-843 linear translational stages (Physik Instrumente, Karlsruhe, Germany) was used in order to change the position of the laser focus in three dimensions. In addition, a HurrySCAN galvo-scanner (Scanlab AG, Puchheim, Germany) was used to change the position of the laser focus in the XY plane.

Square arrays of 25 identical microneedles (needle-needle distance = 500 μm) were fabricated on glass coverslip substrates. A computer-aided design program was used to prepare in-plane and out-of-plane microneedles with various geometries. The fabrication time for a single microneedle was approximately 2 min. In this study, no special efforts were made to reduce the fabrication time. It is anticipated that the fabrication time may be significantly reduced in future studies. The microneedles exhibited length values of 800 μm, and base diameter values of 150–300 μm.

After the processing, the samples were immersed into a 50:50 blend of 4-methyl-2-penthanone and 2-propanol for a few minutes in order to remove non-irradiated resin. Finally, the samples were rinsed with 2-propanol and cured using ultraviolet light. In an earlier nanoindentation study, the nanohardness and Young's modulus values for an Ormocer® surface processed using 2PP were found to be 0.185 ± 0.031 and 7.011 ± 0.873 GPa, respectively.[28,29]

Microneedles undergo several forces during insertion into the skin, including compressive forces, bending forces, shear forces, buckling forces, and skin resistance.[33] Fracture testing and penetration testing of microneedle arrays was determined using an ELF 3200 compression load testing (Bose EnduraTEC Systems Group, Minnetonka, MN). In these studies, 50 and 500 g load cells were driven at 0.008 mm/s displacement rate against polytetrafluoroethylene (duPont, Wilmington, DE) and cadaveric porcine adipose tissue. Cadaveric porcine material was chosen for this study because porcine epidermal and dermal layers closely resemble their human counterparts. A live video capture device was used to monitor the microneedle penetration behavior and determine the mode of failure.

Cell proliferation on Ormocer® surfaces processed using 2PP was examined using human epidermal keratinocytes. The 3-(4,5-dimethylthiazol-2-yl)MTT test was performed using a modification of the method described by Mossman.[34] This assay is based on reduction of a yellow tetrazolium salt (MTT) to a purple formazan dye by mitochondrial succinnic dehydrogenase. The Ormocer® was placed between two 18 mm × 18 mm coverslips. This construct was carefully wedged apart with a razor blade, and the polymer adhered to one of the coverslips. The remaining coverslips were used as control surfaces. Three wells in the plate contained control coverslips, and three wells in the plate contained the polymer. The Ormocer® materials and the control materials were placed in plastic Petri dishes and exposed to ultraviolet-B light on both sides in order to sterilize the surfaces. They were briefly rinsed in keratinocyte growth medium-2 (KGM-2) and placed in 6-well plates. Two microlitres of KGM-2 cell culture medium was placed in each well. Human epidermal keratinocytes (100,000) were seeded in each medium-containing well. The medium was changed after 24 h. The cells were then grown for an additional 48 h. The controls and the polymers were transferred to new 6-well plates. The MTT medium (2 mL; 0.5 mg/mL KGM-2 cell culture medium) was placed on the human epidermal keratinocytes for 3 h. The tetrazolium metabolized within the mitochondria of viable cells was extracted with isopropanol. The extracted solution in each well pipetted into a new 96-well plate (in duplicate), and absorbance was determined spectrophotometrically at 550 nm using a Multiskan RC microplate reader (Labsystems, Helsinki, Finland).

Results and Discussions

The flexibility of the 2PP process allows rapid fabrication of microneedles with different designs. In-plane hollow microneedle arrays and out-of-plane hollow microneedle arrays in various geometries were fabricated using 2PP. Figures 2a–2c contain computer aided design images used for fabrication of in-plane and out-of-plane microneedles with different aspect ratios. Figures 2d–2f contain scanning electron micrographs of Ormocer® microneedles that exhibit the geometries shown in Figs. 2a–2c, respectively. The microneedles taper linearly from the base to the tip. In addition, ripple-like features were observed on the walls of the needles. These ripple-like features were attributed to the layer-by-layer fabrication approach, and can be eliminated by increasing the number of the layers in these structures and reducing the distance between the layers in these structures. The length of the microneedles (800 μm) would enable use for both delivery of pharmacologic agents and drawing of blood and/or interstitial fluids. Off-center microneedles were fabricated by adjusting the position of the channel relative to the central symmetry axis. The aspect ratio of the microneedle was modified by altering the diameter of the microneedle base. The diameter of the channel was

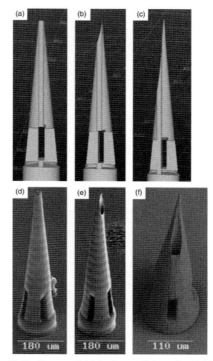

Fig. 2. Computer-aided design diagrams of microneedles with (a) 0 μm, (b) 1.4 μm, and (c) 20.4 μm pore–needle center displacement values. Scanning electron micrographs of Ormocer® microneedles with (d) 0 μm, (e) 1.4 μm, and (f) 20.4 μm pore–needle center displacement values.

maintained at a constant value for all of the microneedles. The four openings visible at the base of the needle were connected to the channel. These openings were included in the microneedle design in order to promote the rapid removal of the non-cross-linked material from the channel during the fabrication step, as one end of the needle was blocked by the glass coverslip.

The microneedle arrays were tested against cadaveric porcine adipose tissue in order to examine

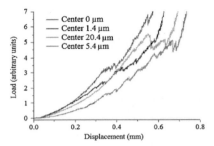

Fig. 3. Load versus displacement data for microneedle arrays with several pore–needle center displacement values.

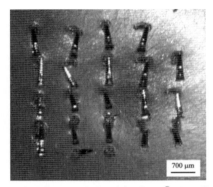

Fig. 4. Light micrograph of out-of-plane Ormocer® microneedle array (5.4 μm pore–needle center displacement) after mechanical testing against flat polytetrafluoroethylene surface.

penetration and fracture properties. Although cadaveric porcine adipose tissue is softer than whole porcine skin, cadaveric porcine adipose tissue exhibits a homogeneous, uniform surface that is appropriate for mechanical testing. Microneedle–cadaveric porcine adipose tissue interaction was examined using a 50 g load cell. Figure 3 contains load-displacement curves for in-plane and out-of-plane hollow microneedle arrays with several flow channel–microneedle tip displacement values. Similar load versus displacement curves were observed for needles with different base diameters. These results indicate minimal dependence between geometry and skin penetration properties for Ormocer® microneedles processed using 2PP. The tips of the microneedles exhibited bending during the compression loading studies; this elastic behavior was attributed to the presence of methacrylate groups in the organically modified ceramic material. The increase in the resistance to penetration during compression testing was attributed to this bending process.

The slopes on the curves can be divided into three regimes. Initially, the needles came into contact with the porcine adipose tissue material but did not puncture the surface. The local maximum values indicate the points at which the load threshold was reached. At these values, the porcine adipose tissue was punctured by one or microneedles in the microneedle array. Local minimum values were observed immediately adjacent to these local maximum values. Henry et al.[35] demonstrated that the pressure required before skin puncture exceeds the pressure required after skin puncture, and attributed this finding to physical and/or chemical forces between the penetrating microneedle and the surrounding tissue. The final displacement value was attributed to contact between the cadaveric porcine adipose tissue and the coverslip substrates. At this value, microneedles were entirely immersed in the cadaveric porcine adipose tissue. The 20.4 μm off-center microneedles exhibited the sharpest needle tips and the lowest penetration threshold values among the out-of-plane microneedles. It has been suggested that microneedles with high aspect ratios and small radii of curvature require lower forces for skin penetration.[33]

The in-plane and out-of-plane microneedles were also examined using polytetrafluoroethylene surfaces (Fig. 4). In these studies, the microneedles with smaller base diameters exhibited failure as a result of bending and fracture from the glass substrate during mechanical testing. On the other hand, microneedles with larger base diameter values primarily demonstrated fracture during mechanical testing. In addition, higher load values were required to fracture microneedles with larger base diameter values. Henry et al.[35] demonstrated that microneedles are highly susceptible to bending and shear forces. For example, bending of the needle shaft caused a maximum stress concentration at the needle base. In addition, shear forces may result from perpendicular movement of the microneedle. These results suggest that microneedles

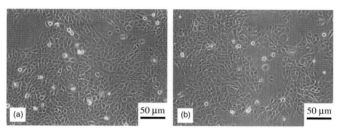

Fig. 5. Light micrograph of human epidermal keratinocytes on (a) control surface and (b) Ormocer® surface.

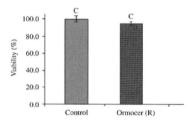

Fig. 6. MTT viability of human epithelial keratinocytes on Ormocer® and control substrates.

with larger base diameters possess greater mechanical stability than microneedles with smaller base diameters. The mechanical properties of microneedles processed using 2PP may be improved by subjecting the devices to a post-bake processing step, which may increase cross-linking between the polymer groups in the inorganic-organic hybrid material.

Cell growth on control surfaces and the Ormocer® polymer surfaces was examined using an inverted microscope, and was shown to be 65%–80% confluency. Both the control surface (Fig. 5a) and Ormocer® surface (Fig. 5b) were shown to support human epidermal keratinocyte growth. The MTT human epidermal keratinocyte viability results for control surfaces and Ormocer® surfaces are shown in Fig. 6. These results indicate that human epidermal keratinocyte growth on the Ormocer® surfaces was similar to that on control surfaces (>95%). In addition, these growth values were not significantly different ($P<0.05$). These results suggest that Ormocer® materials processed using 2PP do not impair cell viability or cell growth.

Conclusions

2PP is a novel technique for processing hybrid organic–inorganic materials. Our results suggest that 2PP is able to create in-plane and out-of-plane hollow Ormocer® microneedles with a larger range of geometries than conventional microfabrication techniques. Human epidermal keratinocyte growth on the Ormocer® surfaces polymerized using 2PP was similar to that on control surfaces. In addition, Ormocer® microneedle arrays penetrated porcine tissue surfaces without fracture. We envision future work that will involve integration of control systems with pumping systems in order to provide patient or healthcare provider with improved management over blood extraction, drug delivery, and other device functions. For example, microneedles may be integrated with micropumps and biosensors to provide autonomous sampling of blood, analysis, and drug delivery capabilities for treatment of chronic disease. For example, integrated microneedle devices may provide continuous blood glucose monitoring and insulin delivery for treatment of diabetes mellitus, a metabolic disease that results from defects in insulin action or secretion. In this integrated device, one needle/pump/sensor unit would assay the glucose level in interstitial fluid and another needle/pump/drug delivery unit would deliver insulin in a continuous or programmed manner. Maintenance of blood glucose levels within the euglycemic physiologic range using an integrated blood glucose testing and insulin treatment device would result in fewer ophthalmic, cardiovascular, nephrologic, and neurologic complications.

Acknowledgment

The authors acknowledge A. O. Inman, Center for Chemical Toxicology Research and Pharmacokinetics, North Carolina State University, for his assistance with cell growth studies.

References

1. G. J. Opiteck and J. E. Scheffler, "Target Class Strategies in Mass Spectrometry-Based Proteomics," *Expert Rev. Proteom.*, 1 [1] 57–66 (2004).
2. V. G. Zarnitsyn, M. R. Prausnitz, and Y. A. Chizmadzhev, "Physical Methods of Nucleic Acid Delivery into Cells and Tissues," *Biologicheskie Membrany*, 21 [5] 355–373 (2004).
3. R. O. P. Potts and R. A. Lobo, "Transdermal Drug Delivery: Clinical Considerations for the Obstetrician-Gynecologist," *Obs. Gynecol.*, 105 [5] 953–961 (2005).
4. M. R. Prausnitz, "Microneedles for Transdermal Drug," *Adv. Drug Delivery Rev.*, 56 [5] 581–587 (2004).
5. M. R. Prausnitz, S. Mitragotri, and R. Langer, "Current Status and Future Potential of Transdermal Drug Delivery," *Nat. Rev. Drug Discovery*, 3 [2] 115–124 (2004).
6. S. Kaushik, A. H. Hord, D. D. Denson, D. V. McAllister, S. Smitra, M. G. Allen, and M. R. Prausnitz, "Lack of Pain Associated with Microfabricated Microneedles," *Anesth. Analg.*, 92 502–504 (2001).
7. R. K. Sivamani, B. Stoeber, G. C. Wu, H. B. Zhai, D. Liepmann, and H. Maibach, "Clinical Microneedle Injection of Methyl Nicotinate: Stratum Corneum," *Skin Res. Technol.*, 11 [2] 152–156 (2005).
8. H. J. G. E. Gardeniers, R. Luttge, E. J. W. Berenschot, M. J. de Boer, S. Y. Yeshurun, M. Hefetz, R. van't Oever, and A. van den Berg, "Silicon Micromachined Hollow Microneedles for Transdermal Liquid," *J. Microelectromech. Syst.*, 12 [6] 855–862 (2003).
9. P. Griss and G. Stemme, "Side-Opened Out-of-Plane Microneedles for Microfluidic Transdermal Liquid Transfer," *J. Microelectromech. Syst.*, 12 [3] 296–301 (2003).
10. J. H. Park, M. G. Allen, and M. R. Prausnitz, "Biodegradable Polymer Microneedles: Fabrication, Mechanics and Transdermal Drug Delivery," *J. Control. Rel.*, 104 [1] 51–66 (2005).
11. B. Stoeber and D. Liepmann, "Arrays of Hollow Out-of-Plane Microneedles for Drug Delivery," *J. Microelectromech. Syst.*, 14 [3] 472–479 (2005).
12. S. P. Davis, W. Martanto, M. G. Allen, and M. R. Prausnitz, "Hollow Metal Microneedles for Insulin Delivery to Diabetic Rats," *IEEE Trans. Biomed. Eng.*, 52 [5] 909–915 (2005).
13. M. Yang and J. D. Zahn, "Microneedle Insertion Force Reduction Using Vibratory Actuation," *Biomed. Microdevices*, 6 [3] 177–182 (2004).
14. S. J. Moon, S. S. Lee, H. S. Lee, and T. H. Kwon, "Fabrication of Microneedle Array Using LIGA and Hot Embossing Process," *Microsyst. Technol.-Micro Nanosyst.-Informat. Storage Proc. Syst.*, 11 [4–5] 311–318 (2005).
15. D. V. McAllister, P. M. Wang, S. P. Davis, J. H. Park, P. J. Canatella, M. G. Allen, and M. R. Prausnitz, "Microfabricated Needles for Transdermal Delivery of Macromolecules and Nanoparticles: Fabrication Methods and Transport Studies," *Proc. Natl. Acad. Sci. USA*, 100 [24] 13755–13760 (2003).
16. K. Kobayashi and H. Suzuki, "A Sampling Mechanism Employing the Phase Transition of a Gel and its Application to a Micro Analysis System Imitating a Mosquito," *Sensor Actuator B-Chem.*, 80 [1] 1–8 (2001).
17. K. Chun, Q. Hashiguchi, H. Toshiyoshi, and H. Fujita, "Fabrication of Array of Hollow Microcapillaries Used for Injection of Genetic Materials into Animal/Plant Cells," *Jpn. J. Appl. Phys.*, 38 [3A] 279–281 (1999).
18. R. Houbertz, "Laser Interaction in Sol-Gel Based Materials- 3-D Lithography for Photonic Applications," *Appl. Surf. Sci.*, 247 [1–4] 504–512 (2005).
19. F. K. Te, E. Koch, J. Serbin, A. Ovsianikov, and B. N. Chichkov, "Three-Dimensional Nanostructuring with Femtosecond Laser Pulses," *IEEE Trans. Nanotechnol.*, 3 [4] 468–472 (2004).
20. J. Serbin, A. Ovsianikov, and B. Chichkov, "Fabrication of Woodpile Structures by Two-Photon Polymerization and Investigation of their Optical Properties," *Optics Express*, 12 [21] 5221–5228 (2004).
21. J. Serbin, A. Egbert, A. Ostendorf, B. N. Chichkov, R. Houbertz, G. Domann, J. Schulz, C. Cronauer, L. Frohlich, and M. Popall, "Femtosecond Laser-Induced two-Photon Polymerization of Inorganic-Organic Hybrid Materials for Applications in Photonics," *Optics Lett.*, 28 [5] 301–303 (2003).
22. K. D. Belfield, K. J. Schafer, Y. U. Liu, J. Liu, X. B. Ren, and E. W. Van Stryland, "Multiphoton-Absorbing Organic Materials for Microfabrication, Emerging Optical Applications and Non-Destructive Three-Dimensional Imaging," *J. Phys. Org. Chem.*, 13 [12] 837–849 (2000).
23. M. T. Gale, C. Gimkiewicz, S. Obi, M. Schnieper, J. Sochtig, H. Thiele, and S. Westenhofer, "Replication Technology for Optical Microsystems," *Optics Lasers Eng.*, 43 [3–5] 373–386 (2005).
24. S. Obi, M. T. Gale, C. Gimkiewicz, and S. Westenhofer, "Replicated Optical MEMS in Sol-Gel Materials," *IEEE J. Selected Topics Quant. Electron.*, 10 [3] 440–444 (2004).
25. R. Houbertz, G. Domann, J. Schulz, B. Olsowski, L. Frohlich, and W. S. Kim, "Impact of Photoinitiators on the Photopolymerization and the Optical Properties of Inorganic-Organic Hybrid Polymers," *Appl. Phys. Lett.*, 84 [7] 1105–1107 (2004).
26. S. H. Park, I. Krejci, and F. Lutz, "Consistency in the Amount of Linear Polymerization Shrinkage in Syringe-Type Composites," *Dental Mater.*, 15 [6] 442–446 (1999).
27. M. Rosin, A. D. Urban, C. Gartner, O. Bernhardt, C. Splieth, and G. Meyer, "Polymerization Shrinkage-Strain and Microleakage in Dentin-Bordered Cavities of Chemically and Light-Cured Restorative Materials," *Dental Mater.*, 18 [7] 521–528 (2002).
28. A. Doraiswamy, C. Jin, R. J. Narayan, P. Mageswaran, P. Mente, R. Modi, R. Auyeung, D. B. Chrisey, A. Ovsianikov, and B. Chichkov, "Two Photon Polymerization of Microneedles for Drug Delivery," *Acta Biomateri.*, 2 [3] 267–275 (2006).
29. R. J. Narayan, C. Jin, A. Doraiswamy, I. N. Mihailescu, M. Jelinek, A. Ovsianikov, B. N. Chichkov, and D. B. Chrisey, "Laser Processing of Advanced Bioceramics," *Adv. Eng. Mater.*, 7 [12] 1083–1098 (2005).
30. K. H. Haas and H. Wolter, "Synthesis, Properties and Applications of Inorganic–Organic Copolymers," *Curr. Opinion Solid State Mater Sci.*, 4 [6] 571–580 (1999).
31. A. S. Al-Hiyasat, H. Darmani, and M. M. Milhem, "Cytotoxicity Evaluation of Dental Resin Composites and their Flowable Derivatives," *Clin. Oral Invest.*, 9 [1] 21–25 (2005).
32. R. Janda, J. F. Roulet, M. Kaminsky, G. Steffin, and M. Latta, "Color Stability of Resin Matrix Restorative Materials as a Function of the Method of Light Activation," *Eur. J. Oral Sci.*, 112 [3] 280–285 (2004).
33. S. P. Davis, B. J. Landis, Z. H. Adams, M. G. Allen, and M. R. Prausnitz, "Insertion of Microneedles into Skin: Measurement and Prediction of Insertion Force and Needle Fracture Force," *J. Biomech.*, 37 [8] 1155–1163 (2004).
34. T. Mossman, "Rapid Colorimetric Assay for Cellular Growth and Survival: Application to Proliferation and Cytotoxicity Assays," *J. Immunol. Methods*, 65 [1–2] 55–63 (1983).
35. S. Henry, D. V. McAllister, M. G. Allen, and M. R. Prausnitz, "Microfabricated Microneedles: A Novel Approach to Transdermal Drug," *J. Pharm. Sci.*, 87 [8] 922–925 (1998).

8
Simultaneous Immobilisation of Bioactives During 3D Powder Printing of Bioceramic Drug-Release Matrices

www.MaterialsViews.com

www.afm-journal.de

Simultaneous Immobilization of Bioactives During 3D Powder Printing of Bioceramic Drug-Release Matrices

By Elke Vorndran, Uwe Klammert, Andrea Ewald, Jake E. Barralet, and Uwe Gbureck*

The combination of a degradable bioceramic scaffold and a drug-delivery system in a single low temperature fabrication step is attractive for the reconstruction of bone defects. The production of calcium phosphate scaffolds by a multijet 3D printing system enables localized deposition of biologically active drugs and proteins with a spatial resolution of approximately 300 μm. In addition, homogeneous or localized polymer incorporation during printing with HPMC or chitosan hydrochloride allows the drug release kinetics to be retarded from first to zero order over a period of 3–4 days with release rates in the range 0.68%–0.96% h^{-1}. The reduction in biological activity of vancomycin, heparin, and rhBMP-2 following spraying through the ink jet nozzles is between 1% and 18%. For vancomycin, a further loss of biological activity following incorporation into a cement and subsequent in vitro release is 11%. While previously acknowledged as theoretically feasible, is its shown for the first time that bone grafts with simultaneous geometry, localized organic bioactive loading, and localized diffusion control are a physical reality. This breakthrough offers a new future for patients by providing the required material function to match patient bone health status, site of repair, and age.

1. Introduction

Rapid prototyping enables the layer-by-layer creation of near net shape 3D objects in a variety of materials. The general underlying principle is spatial control of powder bonding by methods such as localized laser sintering and liquid solvent or binder application to form a "green body" prior to sintering. Recently, custom made scaffolds for bone repair and tissue engineering have been created

[*] Dr. U. Gbureck, E. Vorndran, Dr. A. Ewald
Department for Functional Materials in Medicine and Dentistry
University of Würzburg. 97070 Würzburg (Germany)
E-mail: uwe.gbureck@fmz.uni-wuerzburg.de
Dr. U. Klammert
Department of Cranio-Maxillo-Facial Surgery
University of Würzburg (Germany)
Dr. J. E. Barralet
Faculty of Dentistry, McGill University
Strathcona Anatomy & Dentistry Building
Montreal, Quebec H3A 2B2 (Canada)

DOI: 10.1002/adfm.200901759

by selective laser sintering[1] or slip casting,[2] and in the production of porous polyethylene implants for craniofacial recontouring.[3] The performance of porous scaffolds made by these approaches has recently been reviewed.[4] Many of these procedures involve a heat treatment step such that the incorporation of organic, biologically active, or hydrated molecules within the bulk of the implant is impossible. Recently, we reported the development of a rapid 3D printing technique that utilized a calcium phosphate cement setting reaction to create bioceramic implants at ambient temperature.[5–7] This one nozzle system could precisely control liquid deposition such that hitherto impossible geometries could be fabricated with the formation of precisely defined channels for controlled tissue growth.[8]

Biomaterials with precise composition and bioactive concentration gradients can help exploit cell chemotaxis and haptotaxis, attachment, and differentiation to optimize healing.[9–13] Localized delivery of therapeutic substances can reduce the dose required to achieve a biological response compared with systemic delivery. In this way, both the risk of side effects[14] and cost of treatment can be significantly reduced. By using a multijet 3D rapid prototyping machine we report the first low temperature synthesis of bioceramic implants while simultaneously depositing bioactive compounds with high spatial accuracy for localized delivery. Three-dimensional macroporous architectures and discrete drug modification of the implants was achieved following the strategy summarized in Figure 1.

Initially we sought to determine the compatibility and accuracy of the multijet printing system with bioactives; recombinant bone morphogenic protein 2 (rhBMP-2), heparin (a model polysaccharide), and vancomycin (an antibiotic glycopeptide) were evaluated. Secondly, the activity of the bioactives was determined following immobilization onto the calcium phosphate implant during the setting reaction. In addition, the effect of bioactive localization within the implant structure and polymer modification on the ceramic on bioactive release kinetics was investigated. Biocompatible polymers were incorporated by either using a blend of hydroxypropylmethylcellulose (HPMC) and tricalcium phosphate (TCP) powders to result in a homogeneous polymer

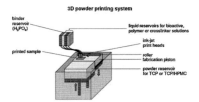

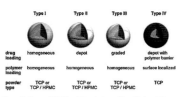

Figure 1. The multijet 3D printing strategy of brushite-based bioceramic implants with controlled bioactive loading. Bioactives were either dispersed homogeneously through the ceramic (Type I), concentrated in the center (Type II and IV) or dispersed along a concentration gradient from a high concentration in the center to low at the exterior (Type III). Polymer modification was achieved either by mixing tricalcium phosphate (TCP) powder with hydroxypropylmethylcellulose (HPMC) or by printing chitosan polymer solutions directly onto TCP powder, either homogeneously or localized to the surface to create a polymer barrier (Type IV). Colors represent: orange-yellow: bioactive (color intensity indicates drug concentration), blue: polymer barrier.

distribution (types I–III), or by simultaneously printing chitosan and crosslinker solutions during implant fabrication and drug deposition for a surface localized polymer modification (types IV).

2. Results

The fabrication of brushite samples by 3D powder printing is based on the hydraulic setting reaction of TCP powder and a phosphoric acid binder solution according to Equation (1):

$$Ca_3(PO_4)_2 + H_3PO_4 + 6H_2O \rightarrow 3CaHPO_4 \cdot 2H_2O \quad (1)$$

Printed samples consisted predominately of the crystalline phase brushite (CaHPO$_4 \cdot$ 2H$_2$O, 51%) and contained a smaller proportion of monetite (CaHPO$_4$, 12%) and unreacted α/β-

TCP (Ca$_3$(PO$_4$)$_2$, 37%) with a total porosity of 45.5% and a median pore size of 27 μm as previously established.[5,8] The deviation of the printed structure dimension was less than ± 5% and we observed that this resulted from the liquid binder bleeding through the porous calcium phosphate (CaP) matrix slightly. This bleeding presented a problem for the defined deposition of bioactives. The printable accuracy of liquid additives was compared by printing a parallel series of fine lines (200–1000 μm) with colored solutions on polymer-modified and unmodified samples. Polymer modification was either performed homogeneously by mixing TCP and HPMC powders, or locally by printing chitosan simultaneously with the colored lines on both TCP and TCP that contained HPMC (Fig. 2). Pure brushite samples showed the highest dimensional deviation (Fig. 2a) with a line width of 1523 ± 130 μm compared with the intended 200 μm (Fig. 2b-I), followed by chitosan-modified brushite (Fig. 2b-II) with a line width of 1238 ± 133 μm, and HPMC/brushite with a line width of 440 ± 46 μm (Fig. 2b-III), and the best results were achieved with HPMC and chitosan-modified brushite that showed a line width of 272 ± 19 μm (Fig. 2b-IV). Lines of 350 μm thickness or more were faithfully reproduced for the latter material combination.

The in vitro release kinetics of spherical (11 mm diameter) polymer-modified and pure brushite samples loaded with vancomycin according to loading strategies Type I–IV was determined for up to 100 h (Fig. 3). Table 1 shows the fitting parameters of the experimental data with the Korsemeyer–Peppas Equation (2):[15]

$$M_t/M_\infty = k \cdot t^n \quad (2)$$

where M_t/M_∞ is the cumulative amount of released drug [%], k [% s^{-1}] is the release constant, and n is the release exponent that indicates the release process. In the case of spherical samples, $n \leq 0.43$ indicates Fickian diffusion processes, while $0.43 < n < 0.85$ characterizes a combination of diffusion and swelling controlled (anomalous) transport.[16] Drug release of Type I homogeneously loaded samples (Fig. 3a,d,f) agreed well with the Korsemeyer–Peppas model, which indicates a diffusion controlled process ($n = 0.31$–0.45) with an initial burst and a total release within 7 days for pure brushite samples ($n = 0.33$; Fig. 3d) and 9 days for chitosan-modified brushite samples ($n = 0.31$; Fig. 3f). The release from HPMC-modified brushite samples

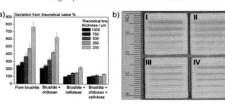

Figure 2. a) Degree of bleeding of colored lines of different thicknesses for polymer-modified and pure brushite cuboids ($n = 6$). b) Printed samples with colored lines: I: pure brushite, II: brushite with co-printed chitosan, III: brushite with homogeneously distributed HPMC, and IV: brushite with both chitosan and HPMC modifications.

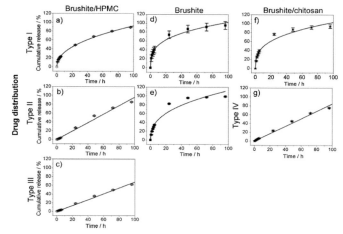

Figure 3. Cumulative release of vancomycin from polymer-modified and brushite spherical samples depending on polymer modification and drug loading. Type I homogeneously loaded samples (a: brushite/HPMC, d: pure brushite, f: brushite/chitosan) and Type II depot loaded brushite structures (e) followed the Korsemeyer–Peppas equation, while Type II depot loaded brushite/HPMC (b), Type VI depot-chitosan barrier (g), and Type III graded brushite/HPMC structures (c) showed a linear release.

(Fig. 3a) showed anomalous transport ($n = 0.45$) and was completed within 7 days. Pure brushite samples with Type II depot loading (Fig. 3e) also followed the Korsemeyer–Peppas equation ($n = 0.38$), however, polymer-modified structures showed a zero-order release with a constant release rate (a) of 0.96% h^{-1} (Fig. 3b) for up to 3–4 days. Inclusion of a polymer barrier (Type IV loading) decreased the release rate to 0.84% h^{-1} (Fig. 3g); zero-order release over a period of 4 days was also be achieved by Type III graduated loading of HPMC/brushite samples with a constant release rate of 0.68% h^{-1} (Fig. 3c). By graduating the deposition of vancomycin in brushite/HPMC, the total release time was extended from 7 to 11 days (Fig. 3a and c). The deviation between experimental data and fitting curves resulted from the limited area of validity (60% cumulative release) of the Korsemeyer–Peppas model.

Physical and chemical stresses imposed on bioactives during printing include high shear, the potential for partial thermal evaporation during purging through the print-head, as well as contact with the phosphoric acid binder during hardening of the structures (Fig. 4a). However, bulk drug activity was found to be retained after the purging of liquids through the print head, which demonstrated good resilience to this process (Fig. 4b). In comparison to the control solutions, the biological activity of the purged solutions were reduced to 82% ± 1% for heparin, 91% ± 18% for rhBMP-2, and 99% ± 7% for vancomycin. Furthermore, the vancomycin activity after printing and in vitro

Table 1. Fitting parameters of the experimental data of Figure 3 with the Korsemeyer–Peppas model $M_t/M_\infty = k \cdot t^n$ or linear fit $M_t/M_\infty = a \cdot t$.

Model	Brushite/polymer	Vancomycin distribution type	n	a
Korsemeyer–Peppas (first-order release)	Brushite	Homogeneous I	0.33 ± 0.03	
	Brushite	Depot II	0.38 ± 0.05	
	Brushite/cellulose	Homogeneous I	0.45 ± 0.01	
	Brushite/chitosan	Homogeneous I	0.31 ± 0.02	
Linear fit (zero-order release)	Brushite/cellulose	Depot II		0.96 ± 0.04
	Brushite/cellulose	Graded III		0.68 ± 0.02
	Brushite/chitosan barrier	Depot IV		0.84 ± 0.02

www.afm-journal.de

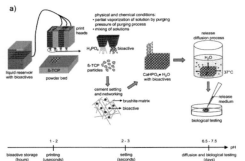

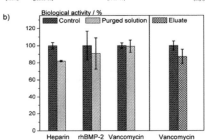

Figure 4. a) Physical and chemical stresses that have the potential to deteriorate the biological activity of additives from the fabrication process of brushite samples to biological testing. b) Biological activities of heparin, rhBMP-2, and vancomycin after the printing process and after release of brushite sample for vancomycin. The biological activity of heparin was defined by activated partial thromboplastin times (aPTT) [s]: standard human plasma: 37.67 ± 1.45, control: 70.27 ± 2.61, and printed solution: 57.57 ± 0.47. The biological activity of rhBMP-2 was defined by ALP activity expressed as $\times 10^{-6}$ M of p-nitrophenol produced per minute per well: control: 15.53 ± 2.60 and printed solution: 14.11 ± 2.56. The biological activity of vancomycin was defined by the diameter of the bacterial inhibition zone [mm]: control solution: 26.20 ± 0.84, printed solution: 26.00 ± 1.87, and eluate: 21.33 ± 2.08.

release from homogeneous-loaded scaffolds was quantified. The eluate of vancomycin obtained after performing the whole printing process followed by in vitro release showed an activity of 87% ± 9% (Fig. 4b).

3. Discussion

The ever growing and inextricable link between medicine and modern technology has had far reaching consequences for biomaterials science, which traditionally revolved around a microstructure–property–cost balance and now is increasingly directed by advances in the knowledge of cell–protein–material surface interactions. Regenerative products based on tissue induction prompted by protein release from polymeric matrices are now a reality in the field of bone and periodontal surgery.[16–18] Three-dimensional printing combined with calcium phosphate cement chemistry enables the preparation of low temperature, microporous calcium phosphate bioceramics, which can be adapted to irregular bone defects using computed tomography (CT) scan data from a patient[19] and can now also release biologically active substances in a controlled manner.

3.1. Polymer Modification

The theoretically achievable resolution of the printer used 600 × 540 dpi (spot sizes: 42.33 μm × 47.04 μm), however, this degree of resolution was not attained when printing liquid bioactives on pure brushite samples because the bioactive solution diffused within the TCP powder. By mixing TCP powder with HPMC or printing chitosan hydrochloride, bioactive diffusion through the cement powder was greatly reduced as a result of polymer swelling, and drug localization was retained. Powders used for 3D printing must fulfill two crucial criteria, firstly they must allow the formation of thin powder layers 100–200 μm in thickness with a smooth surface (to obtain high printing quality) and secondly they must harden with the binder solution or not interfere with the setting reaction of TCP with acid during printing. The first criterion is associated with the particle size distribution of the powder, it has been demonstrated by our group that ideal particle sizes are in the range of 20–50 μm with the absence of small particle fractions <5 μm.[5] The limiting factors for applicable polymeric printing solutions are the compatibility of the solution to the print-head and purging process as well as a fast gelling reaction. In order to purge a solution through thin channels (∼20 μm) of the print heads, a low viscosity (< 5 mPa s, approx. 1 wt% chitosan hydrochloride) is crucial. To act as an efficient diffusion inhibitor the gelling reaction has to take place within seconds to avoid diffusion of bioactive substances in the structures as well as to develop a water-soluble gel. Low viscosity chitosan hydrochloride solutions fulfill this role since they undergo a fast gelling reaction by the reaction of negatively charged polymers and polyanions in contact with an aqueous environment (Fig. 5).[20–22]

By modifying printed brushite samples with HPMC and/or chitosan hydrochloride, the liquid printing resolution was

© 2010 WILEY-VCH Verlag GmbH & Co. KGaA, Weinheim
Computer Aided Biomanufacturing, Edited by Roger Narayan and Paul Calvert
© 2011 WILEY-VCH Verlag GmbH & Co. KGaA. Published 2011 by WILEY-VCH Verlag GmbH & Co. KGaA.

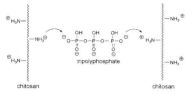

Figure 5. Scheme of ionotropic crosslinking between chitosan and tripolyphosphate.

improved as demonstrated by the deposition of toluidine blue solution in defined line thicknesses (Fig. 2a and b) such that lines of 350 μm thickness or more were faithfully reproduced. The highest resolution was obtained with a HPMC-modified TCP powder in addition to chitosan hydrochloride printing. Only a marginally lower resolution was obtained by HPMC modification alone, which indicated that the resolution was mainly improved by the high water uptake of the HPMC powder. Modification of brushite samples with chitosan hydrochloride alone resulted in only a marginally higher resolution than pure brushite because of the limited water uptake ability of the locally applied gel.

3.2. Dependency of Release Profile and Drug/Polymer Modification

By discrete bioactive localization and printing of graded drug distributions in the structures it was possible to control the release kinetics. Investigations of the release kinetics included pure and polymer-modified brushite spheres with a Type I homogeneous, Type II and IV depot, or Type III graded vancomycin distribution (Fig. 1). Unmodified brushite samples with different bioactive loading strategies showed no considerable differences in release kinetics (Fig. 3d and e) because of unhindered drug diffusion within the structures during the printing process. Modification of brushite with HPMC led to a delayed drug release, whereas the release kinetics were strongly dependant on the drug localization (Fig. 3a–c). Release from Type I-loaded brushite/HPMC (Fig. 3a) or brushite/chitosan (Fig. 3f) structures showed first-order kinetics. In comparison to Type I-loaded pure brushite the release is retarded as a result of polymer swelling that forms a diffusion barrier. This is also indicated by the release exponent n, which characterizes the release as a diffusion and swelling controlled process (Table 1). Zero-order release was achieved from Type II and III loaded HPMC/brushite structures (Fig. 3b and c). According to Ficks first law, drug diffusion depends on both the concentration gradient and matrix properties. In the case of Type II loading (Fig. 3b), diffusion is limited by polymer swelling, and since drug diffusion through a drug free polymer barrier occurs before release, the drug concentration gradient is decreased in comparison to Type I-loaded scaffolds. In contrast, graded drug release depends predominantly on the creation of a drug concentration distribution tapered towards the periphery (Type III),

which reduces the concentration gradient and hence the release rate. A zero-order release was also obtained by creating a diffusion barrier with chitosan in depot-loaded brushite structures (Type IV, Fig. 3g). The variation of drug amount and local drug concentration in homogeneously polymer-modified structures by graded or depot drug modification or a local polymer modification by printing polymer solution was beneficial to adjust the release rate as well as the total release time. Furthermore, simultaneous modification of bioceramic scaffolds with different drugs that induce, for example, specific biological reactions in different regions of the implant would be possible. Stimulation of osteointegration would be feasible by modifying the implant surface with osteoinductive additives such as bone morphogenic protein (BMP)[23–25] and promoting vascularization in scaffolds by loading with angiogenic factors such as vascular endothelial growth factor (VEGF)[26] or copper ions.[27,28]

3.3. Biological Activity of Printed Drugs

To remain biologically active, printed drugs must be resilient to the printing process (Fig. 4a). The slight loss of biological activity observed in printed bioactives is likely a result of the heat developed during (thermal) purging through the narrow print heads, whereby a small fraction of the printing liquid is evaporated. Encouragingly, the bulk activity (>82%) of drug solutions was retained during the printing process even for heat-sensitive proteins like rhBMP-2 (Fig. 4b). Of course, the printing process also includes further steps such as acid treatment for the setting reaction, which may also lower the biological activity of rhBMP-2 or heparin and have to be tested in further studies. The activity of vancomycin was only reduced by a further ∼12% following the complete printing process, which indicates this effect may only be minor.

4. Conclusions

Polymer modification of brushite samples reduced the diffusion of drug solutions within the structures during the printing process and enabled faithful reproduction of micrometer-scale features. Consequently release kinetics can be controlled by locally modifying drug loading within the structures by 3D printing, which results in a zero-order release with release rates in the range of 0.68%–0.96% h^{-1}. Bioceramic scaffolds produced by multijet 3D printing now allow the discrete deposition of pharmaceutical agents. Using these strategies it should now be possible to induce localized biological reactions to enhance healing since there was only a marginal loss in biological activity of the bioactive additive following printing.

5. Experimental

Tricalcium phosphate (TCP) was synthesized by heating a 2:1 molar mixture of anhydrous dicalcium phosphate (DCPA, CaHPO$_4$, monetite) and calcium carbonate (both Merck, Darmstadt, Germany) followed by quenching to room temperature. The sintered cake was crushed with a pestle and mortar, passed through a 160 μm sieve and ground for 10 min in a ball mill.

Printing of cement samples was performed with a multicolor 3D-powder printing system (spectrum Z510, Z-Corporation, Burlington, USA) using TCP powder (polymer-modified or unmodified) and a binder solution of 20% phosphoric acid (Merck, Darmstadt, Germany). For the printing parameters, a thickness of 125 μm per layer was chosen and a binder/volume ratio of 0.371. Polymer modification of printed samples was performed either by blending TCP powder with a) 5 wt% of HPMC (Fluka, Buchs, Switzerland) or b) by printing with pure TCP powder and applying a polymer solution of 1 wt% chitosan hydrochloride (Kraeber GmbH & Co, Ellerbek, Germany) in water that was crosslinked with 0.5 wt% trisodiumpolyphosphate (TPP, Sigma–Aldrich, Steinheim, Germany) through two different print heads.

The binder solution was stored in the first liquid reservoir that is linked to the inkjet print head 0 (white) and was always involved to the printing process at a certain percentage rate. For the additives three color reservoirs (yellow, magenta, cyan) are available. The drug solutions (5% vancomycin hydrochloride in distilled water (Abbott, Wiesbaden, Germany), 0.1% toluidine blue in water, 5×10^{-6} M rhBMP-2 (Department of Physiological Chemistry II, Biocenter, University of Wuerzburg, Germany) [29] or 10 IU mL^{-1} of heparin (Meduna GmbH, Isernhagen, Germany)) were applied through print head 1 (yellow), while chitosan hydrochloride solution was printed with print head 3 (cyan) and TPP was printed with print head 2 (magenta). Structure geometries were designed using Think3design (thinkiD Design Xpressions for Windows 2000/XP/Vista Version 2007.1.106.49 SP2, think3 Inc., USA) software. To demonstrate the achievable resolution a cuboid ($h = 2$ mm, $l = 20$ mm) with 5 colored lines of different width (1000, 750, 500, 350, and 200 μm) were printed with HPMC-modified and pure TCP powder.

The release kinetics of vancomycin were studied on polymer-modified or pure brushite spherical samples ($r = 5.56$ mm), whereas the structures were modified with vancomycin according to Figure 1: homogeneous, depot, or graded. For graded modification, the amount of printed drug solution was tapered towards the periphery. The amount of drug in the printed samples was determined by dissolving the loaded samples in 2.4 M HCl following absorbance measurements against standard solutions at 237 nm using an UV/vis spectrometer (Cary 13, Varian, Australia). The drug desorption kinetics were measured after immersion of the loaded samples ($n = 3$) in double distilled H$_2$O (10 mL) at 37 °C for up to 18 days and changing the immersion liquid after 1 h, the first 5 h, and after 1, 2, 3, and 4 days, and then every third day up to 18 days. The possible influence of interfering polymer compounds was accounted for by using unloaded polymer-modified samples as reference. Adsorption and desorption profiles were modelled using the Korsmeyer–Peppas equation or by linear fitting as pharmaceutical release models.

The biological activity after the thermal purging process through the print-head was analyzed for vancomycin, heparin, and rhBMP-2. Furthermore, the biological activity of vancomycin after the whole printing process and in vitro release was analyzed. Therefore, vancomycin-loaded cylindrical ($h = 5$ mm, $r = 4$ mm) scaffolds (2.5 mg sample^{-1}) were submerged and eluted in static conditions for 2 h in H$_2$O (1 mL) in a 15 mL centrifuge tube. The eluate was exposed to gram positive *Staphylococcus epidermidis* (strain RP62A) in an agar diffusion assay. Agar (1%) was suspended in LB medium (1% w/v tryptone, 0.5% w/v yeast extract, 0.5% w/v NaCl) and autoclaved (120 °C, 20 min). The hot agar solution was poured into sterile Petri dishes. *S. epidermidis* from an over night culture (100 μL) was plated onto the solidified agar by the use of sterile glass spheres. A freshly prepared 5% (4 μL) and a 0.1% (50 μL) vancomycin solution as well as a 5% (4 μL) vancomycin solution purged through the print head and the eluate (50 μL) were placed onto a filter piece (1 cm in diameter). This was placed on top of solidified agar on which *S. epidermidis* had been plated. Each test sample was prepared five-fold. The Petri dishes were incubated at 37 °C for 48 h. After this time the diameter of the zone of inhibition was determined by using a sliding rule. The average and standard deviations were calculated. Statistical analysis was performed by using the Anova *t*-test.

The anti-coagulation activity of heparin was analyzed after printing a 10 IU mL^{-1} heparin solution and purging through a print head. The original 10 IU mL^{-1} heparin solution (5 μL) as well as the purged heparin solution (5 μL) were mixed with standard human plasma (250 μL; Siemens, Marburg, Germany) and the activated partial thromboplastin time (aPTT) was measured with a coagulation analyzer (Sysmex CA-540, Siemens, Marburg, Germany), $n = 3$.

The biological activity of the purged 5×10^{-6} M rhBMP-2 solution was determined by alkaline phosphatase (ALP) activity. Therefore, cells of the mouse myoblast cell line C2C12 [30] were maintained in growth medium consisting of Dulbecco's modified eagle medium (DMEM) supplemented with 10% fetal calf serum (FCS) at 37 °C in a humidified atmosphere of 5% CO$_2$. Cells were seeded into 96-well microtiter plates at a concentration of 5×10^4 cells per well (to survey the rhBMP-2 solutions) and cultured with growth medium (200 μL). After 48 h, the growth medium was removed and replaced with equivalent low nitogen medium (DMEM supplemented with 5% FCS). Simultaneously 10% of a rhBMP-2 solution (5×10^{-6} M, non-treated and treated by purging through the print head) was added. After incubation for a further 72 h the ALP activity was measured. Therefore, the cell layers were washed with PBS. Next the lysis buffer 1 (0.1 M glycine (Carl Roth, Karlsruhe, Germany), 1×10^{-3} M MgCl$_2$ (Merck, Darmstadt, Germany), 1×10^{-3} M ZnCl$_2$ (Sigma–Aldrich, Taufkirchen, Germany), 1% Nonidet P40 Substitute (Sigma–Aldrich, Taufkirchen, Germany)) was added (96-well plates: 100 μL per well) and incubated at room temperature for one hour in a shaker. Afterwards an equivalent quantity of lysis buffer 2 (0.1 M glycine (Carl Roth, Karlsruhe, Germany), 1×10^{-3} M MgCl$_2$ (Merck, Darmstadt, Germany), 1×10^{-3} M ZnCl$_2$ (Sigma–Aldrich, Taufkirchen, Germany), *p*-nitrophenyl phosphate (pNPP) 20 mg per mL of H$_2$O (Sigma–Aldrich, Taufkirchen, Germany)) was added in the ratio of 1:10 immediately prior to use. The enzymatic conversion of pNPP to *p*-nitrophenol was measured photometrically at 405 nm after 5 min. Data were normalized by a standard curve using various concentrations of *p*-nitrophenol. The protein content of the cell cultures was determined using the DC Protein Assay (Biorad, Munich, Germany) following the producer's manual and using various concentrations of BSA (bovine serum albumin) as the standard. The ALP activity was expressed as $\times 10^{-6}$ M of *p*-nitrophenol produced per minute per well. The biological activity of the printed solution was compared with the activity of the control solution.

Acknowledgements

The authors sincerely thank the Deutsche Forschungsgemeinschaft (DFG GB1/7-1), the Quebec-Bavarian support grant from the Ministère Dévelopement économique, innovation et Exportation of Quebec, Canada and the Canadian research chair (JB) for their financial support. The company Kraeber GmbH is acknowledged for providing the chitosan material and the Department of Physiological Chemistry II, Biocenter, University of Wuerzburg, for providing the rhBMP-2.

Received: September 17, 2009
Revised: January 23, 2010
Published online: April 6, 2010

[1] Z. Sadeghian, J. G. Heinrich, F. Moztaradeh, *CFI, Ceram. Forum Int.* **2004**, *81*, E39.
[2] C. E. Wilson, J. D. de Bruijn, C. A. van Blitterswijk, A. J. Verbout, W. J. A. Dhert, *J. Biomed. Mater. Res.* **2004**, *68A*, 123.
[3] J. K. Liu, O. N. Gottfried, C. D. Cole, W. R. Dougherty, W. T. Couldwell, *Neurosurg. Focus* **2004**, *16*, 1.
[4] S. J. Hollister, *Nat. Mater.* **2005**, *4*, 518.
[5] U. Gbureck, T. Hölzel, U. Klammert, K. Würzeler, F. A. Müller, J. E. Barralet, *Adv. Funct. Mater.* **2007**, *17*, 3940.
[6] E. Vorndran, M. Klarner, U. Klammert, L. M. Grover, S. Patel, J. E. Barralet, U. Gbureck, *Adv. Eng. Mater.* **2008**, *10*, B67.
[7] U. Gbureck, E. Vorndran, F. A. Müller, J. E. Barralet, *J. Controlled Release* **2007**, *122*, 173.
[8] U. Gbureck, T. Hölzel, C. J. Doillon, *Adv. Mater.* **2007**, *19*, 795.

[9] W. J. Rosoff, R. McAllister, M. A. Esrick, G. J. Goodhill, J. S. Urbach, *Biotechnol. Bioeng.* **2005**, *91*, 754.
[10] L. Formigli, G. Fiorelli, S. Benvenuti, A. Tani, G. E. Orlandini, M. L. Brandi, S. ZecchiOrlandini, *Cell. Tissue Res.* **1997**, *288*, 101.
[11] M. D. McKee, A. Nanci, *Microsc. Res. Tech.* **1996**, *33*, 141.
[12] J. E. Barralet, S. Aldred, A. J. Wright, A. G. A. Coombes, *J. Biomed. Mater. Res.* **2002**, *60*, 360.
[13] B. G. Chung, L. A. Flanagan, S. W. Rhee, P. H. Schwartz, A. P. Lee, E. S. Monuki, N. L. Jeon, *Lab Chip* **2005**, *5*, 401.
[14] P. Wu, D. W. Grainger, *Biomaterials* **2006**, *27*, 2450.
[15] J. Siepmann, N. A. Peppas, *Adv. Drug Delivery Rev.* **2001**, *48*, 139.
[16] M. Boakye, P. V. Mummaneni, M. Garrett, G. Rodts, R. Haid, *J. Neurosurg. Spine* **2005**, *2*, 521.
[17] A. R. Vaccaro, T. Patel, J. Fischgrund, D. G. Anderson, E. Truumees, H. N. Herkowitz, F. Phillips, A. Hilibrand, T. J. Albert, T. Wetzel, J. A. McCulloch, *Spine* **2004**, *29*, 1885.
[18] L. Heijl, G. Heden, G. Svardstrom, A. Ostgren, *J. Clin. Periodontol.* **1997**, *24*, 705.
[19] U. Gbureck, T. Hölzel, R. Thull, F. A. Müller, J. E. Barralet, *Cytotherapy* **2006**, *8*, 14.
[20] S. Chen, M. Liu, S. Jin, B. Wang, *Int. J. Pharm.* **2008**, *349*, 180.
[21] X. Z. Shu, K. J. Zhu, *Int. J. Pharm.* **2002**, *233*, 217.
[22] F. L. Mi, H. W. Sung, S. S. Shyu, C. C. Su, C. K. Peng, *Polymer* **2003**, *44*, 6521.
[23] K. K. Huang, C. Shen, C. Y. Chiang, Y. D. Hsieh, E. Fu, *J. Periodont. Res.* **2005**, *40*, 1.
[24] R. S. Thies, M. Bauduy, B. A. Ashton, L. Kurtzberg, J. M. Wozney, V. Rosen, *Endocrinology* **1992**, *130*, 1318.
[25] T. Katagiri, A. Yamaguchi, T. Ikeda, S. Yoshiki, J. M. Wozney, V. Rosen, E. A. Wang, H. Tanaka, S. Omura, T. Suda, *Biochem. Biophys. Res. Commun.* **1990**, *172*, 295.
[26] T. J. Poole, E. B. Finkelstein, C. M. Cox, *Dev. Dyn.* **2001**, *220*, 1.
[27] C. K. Sen, S. Khanna, M. Venojarvi, P. Trikha, E. C. Ellison, T. K. Hunt, S. Roy, *Am. J. Physiol. Heart Circ. Physiol.* **2002**, *282*, H1821.
[28] D. Rajalingam, T. K. Kumar, C. Yu, *Biochemistry* **2005**, *44*, 14431.
[29] N. R. Kuebler, J. F. Reuther, G. Faller, *Int. J. Oral Maxillofac. Surg.* **1998**, *27*, 307.
[30] H. M. Blau, C. P. Chiu, C. Webster, *Cell* **1983**, *32*, 1171.

9
Structural and Mechanical Evaluations of a Topology Optimized Titanium Interbody Fusion Cage Fabricated by Selective Laser Melting Process

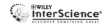

Structural and mechanical evaluations of a topology optimized titanium interbody fusion cage fabricated by selective laser melting process

Chia-Ying Lin,[1,2,3] Tobias Wirtz,[4] Frank LaMarca,[1] Scott J. Hollister[2,3,5,6]

[1]Spine Research Laboratory, Department of Neurosurgery, The University of Michigan, Ann Arbor, Michigan
[2]Scaffold Tissue Engineering Group, The University of Michigan, Ann Arbor, Michigan
[3]Department of Biomedical Engineering, University of Michigan, Ann Arbor, Michigan
[4]Fraunhofer Institute of Laser Technology, Aachen, Germany
[5]Department of Mechanical Engineering, University of Michigan, Ann Arbor, Michigan
[6]Department of Surgery, University of Michigan, Ann Arbor, Michigan

Received 31 January 2006; revised 25 August 2006; accepted 9 December 2006
Published online 5 April 2007 in Wiley InterScience (www.interscience.wiley.com). DOI: 10.1002/jbm.a.31231

Abstract: A topology optimized lumbar interbody fusion cage was made of Ti-Al6-V4 alloy by the rapid prototyping process of selective laser melting (SLM) to reproduce designed microstructure features. Radiographic characterizations and the mechanical properties were investigated to determine how the structural characteristics of the fabricated cage were reproduced from design characteristics using micro-computed tomography scanning. The mechanical modulus of the designed cage was also measured to compare with tantalum, a widely used porous metal. The designed microstructures can be clearly seen in the micrographs of the micro-CT and scanning electron microscopy examinations, showing the SLM process can reproduce intricate microscopic features from the original designs. No imaging artifacts from micro-CT were found. The average compressive modulus of the tested caged was 2.97 ± 0.90 GPa, which is comparable with the reported porous tantalum modulus of 3 GPa and falls between that of cortical bone (15 GPa) and trabecular bone (0.1–0.5 GPa). The new porous Ti-6Al-4V optimal-structure cage fabricated by SLM process gave consistent mechanical properties without artifactual distortion in the imaging modalities and thus it can be a promising alternative as a porous implant for spine fusion. © 2007 Wiley Periodicals, Inc.
J Biomed Mater Res 83A: 272–279, 2007

Key words: interbody fusion cage; topology optimization; titanium alloy; selective laser melting; porous tantalum

INTRODUCTION

The use of interbody fusion cages as an adjunct to spinal arthrodesis has become prevalent for a variety of pathological spine disorders in the last decade. Clinical outcome has been successful after short-term follow-up evaluation. However, many still agree that the long-term effects of cage devices on the motion segment still remain unclear despite these initial good results.[1–7] The role of conventional interbody fusion cages has been mainly focused on providing immediate strength to maintain disc height and shielding bone grafts from large mechanical forces within the cage to allow for bony healing. Therefore, conventional designs for cage devices are either cylindrical or wedge shaped with thick shells as outer walls and a hollow interior space that contains grafting materials.[8] However, excessive cage rigidity may be associated with increased incidence of postoperative complications such as stress-shielding, the migration or dislodgement of the cage, pseudoarthrodesis, or combined adverse symptoms.[5] The stress-shielded environment due to excessive stiffness of metallic cage devices compared to the motion segments and vertebral bodies allow lower intracage pressure propagation,[9] which leads to subsequent decreased mineralization, bone resorption, and significant bone mineral density decrease in long term.[10]

Enormous progress has been made in the development of biodegradable osteosyntheses to offer

Correspondence to: C.-Y. Lin; e-mail: lincy@umich.edu
Contract grant sponsor: NIH; contract grant numbers: DE13608 (Bioengineering Research Partnership), DE13416

© 2007 Wiley Periodicals, Inc.
Computer Aided Biomanufacturing, Edited by Roger Narayan and Paul Calvert
© 2011 WILEY-VCH Verlag GmbH & Co. KGaA. Published 2011 by WILEY-VCH Verlag GmbH & Co. KGaA.

numerous major advantages over traditional metallic implants, one of which is the reduction of stress-shielding because of material compliance so that functional forces can be transferred to regenerate bone tissue to achieve a better healing.[11,12] However, many still believe that metallic biomaterials can withstand physiological loads in both short and long term and thus they are more suitable for the development of implants for load bearing applications such as spine arthrodesis. To better match bone stiffness for avoidance of stress shielding, and to deliver osteobiological materials, high porosity is required in processing metallic biomaterials. One example of a material designed to meet this need is porous tantalum. Porous tantalum is fabricated via a chemical vapor infiltration (CVI) process that forms a reticulated vitreous carbon (RVC) skeleton, which is then encased by the precipitation of tantalum metal.[13,14] The material is comprised of 75–85% void space and is characterized by interconnected unit cells that possess dodecahedron geometry. Despite this breakthrough, for processing a metallic biomaterial, significant batch-by-batch variation of mechanical properties of porous tantalum were recently found from the mechanical testing because of differences in morphology and processing.[14] This inconsistency can be attributed to the less precise control on microstructural features such as thickness and structural arrangement. Porous Nitinol has also aroused recent interest for medical device applications, but more research may be required to better understand its nature for physical performance.[15]

We reported previously our development for a new design approach for lumbar spine interbody fusion cages by using topology optimization algorithms to define the structural layout and inner microstructures.[16] A suitable design for spinal fusion cages needs to address three major criteria: (1) limited displacements for stability, (2) sufficient strain energy density transfer to ingrown bone to reduce stress shielding, and (3) desired porosity for tissue ingrowth and biofactor delivery. Conventional designs[1,2,9] may not be able to meet the multiple design requirements necessary to achieve sufficient rigidity, reduced stress shielding, and large porosity for biofactor delivery. Topology optimization[17,18] is a design technique that provides optimal distribution of material under applied force to satisfy the objective of maximal stiffness with desired porosity, under constraints of the three design criteria. This approach addresses the conflicting design issues of having sufficient stability while at the same time having enough porosity to deliver biofactors like cells, genes, and proteins and impart sufficient mechanical strain to maintain developing tissue. The interior architecture consists of microstructures with reserved channel spaces for potential cell-based therapies and drug delivery. The interconnected microstructural struts form a network of load transmission so that the strain energy is absorbed by appositional bone at the cage/body interface as well as by regenerate tissue inside the cage. Thus, the three major design criteria considered were providing initial stability, reducing long-term stress shielding, and providing porosity for biofactor delivery.

In the present study, we demonstrate the capability to carry out the topology optimized design for lumbar interbody fusion cages made of Ti-6Al-4V alloy by utilizing a rapid prototyping process, selective laser melting (SLM), to achieve the designed spatial arrangement of material and reproduction of designed features of microstructures. In addition, radiographic and imaging characterizations as well as the mechanical properties from both compression test and finite element analysis (FEA) are conducted and the data are compared with those from previous clinical investigations using porous tantalum implants for spine interbody fusion.

MATERIALS AND METHODS

Overview of integrated topology optimization design

Topology optimization algorithms[17,19,20] generate an optimized material distribution for a set of loads and constraints within a given design space, defined by solid finite elements. The topology optimization algorithm determines the material layout that gives the stiffest structure possible under both volume fraction and displacement constraints. Two rectangular block design spaces were used to represent the location of the implanted cages between vertebrae. Multi-directional physiological loads including compression, lateral bending, torsion, and flexion-extension were applied to the entire vertebral model as mentioned previously.[16] This hierarchical macroscopic or first scale topology optimization solution that provides the general density and location of material within the design domain is then discretized into finite elements, and each element will contain a predicted material density between 0 and 1. A material density value of 0 indicates void space while a value of 1 indicates complete material; values in between indicate partial material with the corresponding volume fraction. The resolution of the global topology design is too coarse, however, to give the specific microstructure that will be located within that point of the scaffold. Furthermore, since we would like the microstructure to have specific elastic properties at a fixed porosity, homogenization based topology optimization is used to design the microstructure.[21,22] The microscopic or second scale topology optimization approach gives the specific microstructure design that achieves a desired compliance while matching the predicted volume fraction of the macroscopic or 1st level topology optimization.

Journal of Biomedical Materials Research Part A DOI 10.1002/jbm.a

Selective laser melting process for cage fabrication

The selective laser melting (SLM) process (Fraunhofer ILT, Aachen, Germany) has been developed in recent years to overcome the limitation of the powder bed based generative manufacturing processes (so called rapid prototyping) that use a specific material or material composition resulting in insufficient mechanical properties. The material used in SLM is a single component metal powder like stainless steel X2CrNiMo17-13-2, tool steel X38CrMoV5-1, Titanium GdII or Titanium Ti-6Al-4V. In addition, the physical process is complete melting of a powder layer with metallurgical bonding between layers, which yields densities close to 100% in one step. These characteristics enlarge the field of applications for this technology from Rapid Prototyping to the Rapid Manufacturing of functional parts such as the intricate spinal cage presented from the design of integrated topology optimization.[23]

In the current investigation, Ti-6Al-4V powder was selected with a particle size of 25–45 μm as basic material to conduct the designed spine cage fabrication. The image data of the designed cage were converted to a surface representation in stereolithography format (.STL). Like all other generative manufacturing processes, the 3-D computer aided design (CAD) model was then sliced into layers with defined thickness. In this case, the dimension of our designed cage is 24.5 mm (L) by 14 mm (W) by 14 mm (H), which is composed of 3.2 mm by 3.2 mm by 3.2 mm microstructures with the minimal feature size of 500 μm. Using the commercial software (VisCam SLM v1.97, Paderborn, Germany), the CAD model of the cage was raised up 2 mm high and then was supported by thin wall structures to enable the cage to be released from the substrate after its build-up. It was then sliced into 534 layers. The layer thickness used for the fabrication of the spinal cage was 30 μm that provides a reasonable balance between geometric accuracy, surface quality, and fabrication time. The actual parts were generated on a modified F&S (Fockele & Schwarze) fabrication system by repeating the process of applying new material layers and subsequently scanning the area and the contour with the laser beam from Nd:YAG-solid state laser system offering 130 W optical power onto overlapping tracks (Fig. 1).

Radiographic and imaging characterizations

Five samples with volume fracations of 52% were fabricated, scanned, and characterized by a MS-130 high resolution Micro-CT Scanner (GE Medical Systems, Toronto, Canada) at 27.2 μm resolution using 2 × 2 binning (120 kVp, 100 mA). Volumes of each fabricated cage were measured using MicroView v 1.1.1 (GE Medical Systems, London, Ontario) and the scanned features were also compared with the original design by registering corresponding 3-D reconstructed images from standard micro-CT DICOM slides in a commercialized image process software, Analyze 5.0 (Biomedical Imaging Resource, Mayo Foundation, Rochester, MN). Macrostructural topology, microstructural

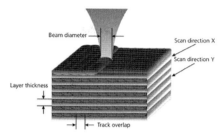

Figure 1. Schematic process of selective laser melting (SLM) fabrication technique.

features, and morphology of Titanium Alloy Ti-6Al-4V were also investigated by scanning electron microscopy (SEM).

Mechanical testing

Axial compression tests were performed to measure construct stiffness. A 4.45 N preload was applied followed by a compressive test to failure at a crosshead speed of 1 mm/min [American Society for Testing and Materials (ASTM) D695-02a] using a MTS Alliance RT30 Electromechanical Test Frame (MTS Systems, MN). The compression test was continued, until the set break point of 20,462 N was met in the real-time compressive load-displacement curve, since the failure load of tested samples made of Ti-6Al-4V alloy was estimated beyond the maximum load of 22,261 N of the default load cell of the testing system that is mainly designated for the biological tissue testing. Load versus deflection was continuously monitored and recorded, and stress-strain curve was generated based on geometrical parameters of samples. Effective compressive moduli defined as the slope of the linear region at the stress-strain curve were then calculated by the system.

To further characterize the ultimate compressive strength of the designed cage, two cages were subjected to more destructive loads at a rate of 0.25 mm/min until they reached catastrophic failure using an Instron Floor Model Testing System (Instron, MA) with 150 kN loading capacity.

Microhardness test was also conducted on a sandblasted cross section of the fabricated cages with a static indentation made with the load of 9.81 N. The Vickers diamond pyramid indenter and precision microscopes (magnifications 10× and 40×) in a microhardness tester (Buehler, Lake Bluff, IL) were used to measure the indentations for the calculation of the hardness.

Image-based finite element analysis

An image-based approach was used to deal with the enormously large-scale problem generated by complex 3-D geometries of the designed cages for the FEA simulating

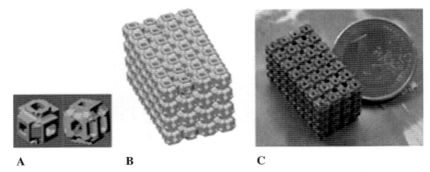

Figure 2. A: Designed microstructures by the topology optimization with volume fractions of 35% (left) and 55% (right). B: The three-dimensional volumetric image represented in .STL format of Optimal-Structure (OS) cage with total volume fractions of 52% and the dimension of 14 mm by 14 mm by 24.5 mm. C: The fabricated titanium alloy cage.

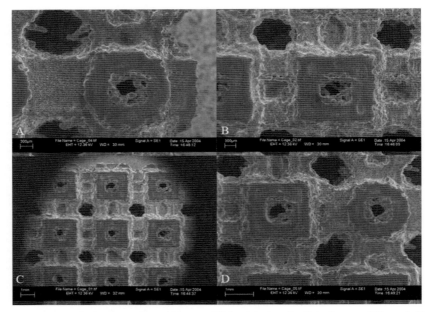

Figure 3. Micrographs showing microstructural features of fabricated titanium alloy Optimal-structure (OS) cage. A: The microstructure of a single unit cell with a volume fraction of 35%. B: The microstructure of a single unit cell with a volume fraction of 55%. C: The periodic interconnected microstructures of the design for 55% volume fraction. D: The connected microstructures with different designs.

Journal of Biomedical Materials Research Part A DOI 10.1002/jbm.a

the compression test in the present study. Image-based approaches allow very accurate replication of the design details, a characteristic not possible with the coarser traditional meshes. The concept of image-based FEA is simply to first convert the designed cage model in .STL format into a three-dimensional voxel dataset and then convert the voxels to finite elements. After the assignment of the material properties according to the grayscale levels to respective components and definition of the boundary conditions for cases of interest, the resulting model is solved using large-scale iterative algorithms. In this case, a Young's modulus of 118 GPa for post-SLM annealed Ti-6Al-4V based on a previous report [24] was assigned in the model and the fixed end was applied to the inferior surface of the cage, while a 1-mm displacement was applied on the superior surface. All aspects of the voxel finite element modeling process, including pre/post processing and analysis were performed using the commercial voxel finite element package Voxelcon (Quint, Tokyo, Japan).

RESULTS

The corresponding microstructures for volume fractions of 35 and 55% [Fig. 2(A)] as reported previously [16] were assigned to the global density layouts to complete the final design. The three-dimensional volumetric .STL image of the topology optimized design denoted as the optimal-structure (OS) cage with total volume fractions of 52% is shown in Figure 2(B). The fabricated cage shown in Figure 2(C) demonstrates the final product from the original design with dimensions of 14 mm by 14 mm by 24.5 mm. The designed microstructures can be clearly seen in representative micrographs of the SEM examination of fabricated cages shown in Figure 3. Figure 3(A,B) show the microstructures of a single unit cell with volume fractions of 35 and 55, respectively. Figure 3(C) shows the periodic interconnected microstructures of the design for 55% volume fraction. Note that features of the microstructures are preserved from the design, giving an interconnected porosity resulting from integration of the designed local microstructure with the macroscopic density layout. Even between different designed microstructures, a bonded connection is seen, eliminating concern of weak interfaces commonly existing in materials with multi-phasic properties [Fig. 3(D)]. The reticulated micro-architecture of the tantalum implant on the other hand presented a well interconnection among each cell that constituted the porous structure within the global domain [Fig. 4(A)]. However, the pore size, volume fraction, and geometry varied due to the CVI process [Fig. 4(B)].

When registered with the original design, the micro-CT scanned images from fabricated cages showed that the designed features were able to be reproduced by the SLM process, but the variation

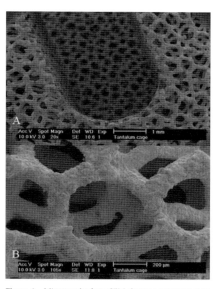

Figure 4. Micrographs from SEM showing microstructure of a tantalum cervical implant. A: Reticulated micro-architecture constituted with unit cells processed by chemical vapor infiltration. B: Microstructures with varied pore size, volume fraction, and geometry.

compared to the original design was also obvious (Fig. 5). The minimal feature size of the cage is 500 μm at the finest struts of the designed microstructure, and these struts were reproduced successfully. However, the pore size of the designed channels within both microstructures is around 1000 μm, but the actual sizes of these pores from the fabricated cages were reduced to ~700 μm. The rims of the pores were thickened in the range of 150 μm, which was caused by excessive sintering of Ti-6Al-4V powder during SLM process. The pores remained continuous, but the inner surface of the pores appeared irregular with some structural protrusion into the pore lumens, as shown consistently in a previous study.[24] The result was also reflected on the volume in which the average volume of the fabricated cages was 2840.68 ± 100.78 mm^3 taking (59.16 ± 0.02)% volume fraction, which was higher than the design volume of 2497.04 mm^3 taking 52% volume fraction. In all, the image characterization indicates that the fabrication of OS cage by SLM process was considered successful and the process can reproduce intricate microscopic features from the original designs,

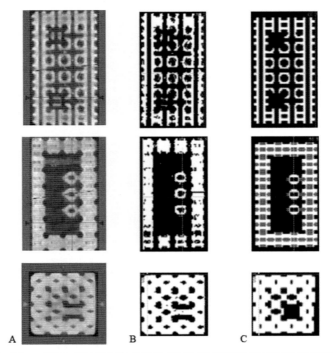

Figure 5. Comparisons of image slices from the designed cage (A) the micro-CT scan and (B) the registered scanned images with (C) the original design (top to bottom: X-, Y-, and Z-axis).

even with complex architecture such as optimized topology.

The modulus for compression testing of fabricated cages was given by the slope of the stress-strain curve on the testing samples (Fig. 6). The stress-strain curve showed that the compressive moduli of the tested cages were consistent, indicating the fabrication process could achieve constant reproduction of the designed features and retain the consistency of mechanical performance of the designed implants. The average compressive modulus of the tested OS cage was 2.97 ± 0.90 GPa, and the ultimate compressive load that caused the destructive failure of cages was 88.94 ± 1.28 kN and the ultimate compressive strength of tested cages 794.07 ± 11.42 MPa. However, the computed effective compressive modulus from the FEA of the compression simulation is 5.5 GPa, which is almost as twice that calculated from the actual compression test.

The average Vickers hardness obtained from microhardness tests on the blasted surface of the fabricated cage is 303.461 ± 16.019 Hv, which is ~87% of the range (349 Hv) of the medical grade, annealed Ti-6Al-4V alloy according to ASTM standards.[25]

DISCUSSION

Metallic implants have been frequently used in the spine to enhance segmental stability, correct deformity, and deliver graft materials. Postoperatively, high-quality image examinations are required to investigate the effectiveness of the implantation such as the position of the implants and evaluate the developing status of surrounding anatomic structures. To this point, it is necessary to notice whether the materials used will interfere with the visualiza-

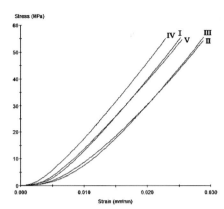

Figure 6. The stress-strain curves correspond to the testing samples (I to V) of fabricated titanium alloy Optimal-Structure (OS) cages ($n = 5$).

tion and assessment of the degree of arthrodesis and the integrity of the spinal canal and neural foramina because of the artifact generated on MR imaging and CT scanning.

Tantalum, a rare heavy metal with an atomic number of 73 and an atomic weight of 180.95, has been used for a variety of medical applications for over 50 years for high biocompatibility, high mechanical performance, resistance to corrosion, and biological inertness.[26–28] Porous tantalum composed of 98% tantalum and 2% vitreous carbon has been recently introduced in orthopaedic applications and direct osseous apposition with the metal are observed, resulting in a strong bone-metal interface.[29] However, it was also noticed that tantalum spinal implants can produce a large amount of streaking, starburst-type metal artifact on the CT imaging under standard clinical settings.[30,31] The image distortion, therefore, intervenes in the radiographic assessment of bony ingrowth and surrounding segmental structures. No substantial artifacts were observed in MR imaging.

Titanium alloy consisting of titanium, aluminum, and vanadium (Ti-6Al-4V) shows a comparable amount of artifact on magnetic resonance imaging, but provides much clearer images in computed tomographic scans.[30,31] In the current study, we were able to fabricate porous Ti-6Al-4V OS cages with designed topology optimized features by the SLM process. The internal architecture can be clearly viewed from the micro-CT imaging without artifactual distortion, suggesting that the segmental integrity and the bony ingrowth of the construct can be assessed after surgery. With these advantages to acquire high-quality examination of imaging modalities, the porous Ti-6Al-4V OS cage demonstrates a better option as a porous metallic implant for spine fusion, compared to porous tantalum cages with the aspect for patients' follow-ups.

The porous titanium alloy Ti-6Al-4V OS cages fabricated by SLM process also gave consistent mechanical properties. The average elastic compressive modulus is 2.97 ± 0.09 GPa, which is comparable with the reported porous tantalum modulus of 3 GPa and falls between that of cortical bone (15 GPa) and trabecular bone (0.1 GPa).[32] The actual compressive modulus of the fabricated cage was lower than the computationally predicted modulus. This may be attributed to the slight disparity of the reproduced microstructures from the design. Even though most of the design features remained intact after the fabrication, the topological distribution of material was not perfectly identical with the original design. We know that the bulk properties of the design are the overall expression of individual microstructures. Therefore, the global properties are sensitive to the proximity of the manufactured microstrucutures to the designed ones, as well as to the reciprocal micro-to-micro and micro-to-macro structural interactions. Nonetheless, the design still gives a consistent layout for material deposited by SLM. Even though there was difference of material properties for the fabricated cages from the design, the properties of individuals remained very similar.

Porous tantalum, however, even though it has **good mechanical properties, experiences significant** deviations in the properties because of the variability of the foam structure and carbon strut dimensions coupled with variability in the layers structure and thickness due to the random pore distribution and interconnectivity generated by CVI process.

In general, metallic biocompatible materials are still a preferable in high load bearing sites like fusion cages in spine arthrodesis and acetabular cups in hip arthroplasty. However, the high stiffness of these materials compared to surrounding tissues will induce unfavorable complications related to the stress-shielding. Porous metal, such as porous tantalum, decreases the strength and stiffness dramatically by creating highly porous structures. The new techniques of integrated topology optimization design approach and SLM process are introduced in the present study as an option to create porous metallic implants with more precise control over mechanical properties that meet the requirements from various applications, for example, the aforementioned titanium alloy OS cage for interbody fusion. The design **domain can be defined with arbitrary shapes** according to the implant size, anatomic geometry, and/or disease/injury requirement.

In all, the titanium alloy OS cage presents comparable stiffness to porous tantalum, providing sufficient compressive strength without excessive stiffness for maintaining spine segmental integrity. It is also better for CT imaging providing fewer artifacts than porous tantalum. Future work of biomechanical testing on spine segments and preclinical *in vivo* studies are warranted to investigate the efficacy of the proposed titanium-based spinal fusion device.

The authors thank Mr. Ali Kasemkhani and Ms. Colleen Flanagan for help in mechanical testing, and Ms. Erin Wilke and Ms. Leena Jongpaiboonkit for micro-computed tomographic (micro-CT) scan and scanning electron microscopy (SEM).

References

1. Brantigan JW, Steffee AD. A carbon fiber implant to aid interbody lumbar fusion. Two-year clinical results in the first 26 patients. Spine 1993;18:2106–2107.
2. Kuslich SD, Ulstrom CL, Griffith SL, Ahern JW, Dowdle JD. The Bagby and Kuslich method of lumbar interbody fusion. History, techniques, and 2-year follow-up results of a United States prospective, multicenter trial. Spine 1998;23:1267–1278. Discussion 1279.
3. McAfee PC, Regan JJ, Geis WP, Fedder IL. Minimally invasive anterior retroperitoneal approach to the lumbar spine. Emphasis on the lateral BAK. Spine 1998;23:1476–1484.
4. Ray CD. Threaded titanium cages for lumbar interbody fusions. Spine 1997;22:667–679. Discussion 679–680.
5. van Dijk M, Smit TH, Burger EH, Wuisman PI. Bioabsorbable poly-L-lactic acid cages for lumbar interbody fusion: Three-year follow-up radiographic, histologic, and histomorphometric analysis in goats. Spine 2002;27:2706–2714.
6. van Dijk M, Smit TH, Sugihara S, Burger EH, Wuisman PI. The effect of cage stiffness on the rate of lumbar interbody fusion: An in vivo model using poly(L-lactic Acid) and titanium cages. Spine 2002;27:682–688.
7. van Dijk M, Tunc DC, Smit TH, Higham P, Burger EH, Wuisman PI. In vitro and in vivo degradation of bioabsorbable PLLA spinal fusion cages. J Biomed Mater Res 2002;63:752–759.
8. Weiner BK, Fraser RD. Spine update lumbar interbody cages. Spine 1998;23:634–640.
9. Kanayama M, Cunningham BW, Haggerty CJ, Abumi K, Kaneda K, McAfee PC. In vitro biomechanical investigation of the stability and stress-shielding effect of lumbar interbody fusion devices. J Neurosurg 2000;93:259–265.
10. Cunningham BW, Ng JT, Haggerty CJ. A quantitative densitometric study investigating the stress-shiedling effects of interbody spinal fusion devices: Emphasis on long-term fusions in thoroughbred racehorses. Trans Orthop Res Soc 1998;23:250.
11. Laftman P, Nilsson OS, Brosjo O, Stromberg L. Stress shielding by rigid fixation studied in osteotomized rabbit tibiae. Acta Paediatrica Scand Suppl 1989;60:718–722.
12. Tonino AJ, Davidson CL, Klopper PJ, Linclau LA. Protection from stress in bone and its effects. Experiments with stainless steel and plastic plates in dogs. J Bone Joint Surg Br 1976;58: 107–113.
13. Bobyn JD, Stackpool GJ, Hacking SA, Tanzer M, Krygier JJ. Characteristics of bone ingrowth and interface mechanics of a new porous tantalum biomaterial. J Bone Joint Surg Br 1999;81:907–914.
14. Zardiackas LD, Parsell DE, Dillon LD, Mitchell DW, Nunnery LA, Poggie R. Structure, metallurgy, and mechanical properties of a porous tantalum foam. J Biomed Mater Res 2001;58:180–187.
15. Shabalovskaya SA. Surface, corrosion and biocompatibility aspects of Nitinol as an implant material. Biomed Mater Eng 2002;12:69–109.
16. Lin CY, Hsiao CC, Chen PQ, Hollister SJ. Interbody fusion cage design using integrated global layout and local microstructure topology optimization. Spine 2004;26:1747–1754.
17. Bendsoe MP, Kikuchi N. Generating optimal topologies in structural design using a homogenization method. Comput Methods Appl Mech Eng 1988;71:197–224.
18. Kikuchi N. Design optimization method for compliant mechanisms and material microstructure. Comput Math Appl Mech Eng 1998;151:401.
19. Arora JS, Haug EJ. Methods of design sensitivity analysis in structural optimization. AIAA J 1979;17:970–974.
20. Suzuki K, Kikuchi N. A homogenization method for shape and topology optimization. Comput Methods Appl Mech Eng 1991;93:291–318.
21. Hollister SJ, Maddox RD, Taboas JM. Optimal design and fabrication of scaffolds to mimic tissue properties and satisfy biological constraints. Biomaterials 2002;23:4095–4103.
22. Lin C, Kikuchi N, Hollister SJ. A novel method for internal architecture design to match bone elastic properties with desired porosity. J Biomech 2004;37:623–636.
23. Lin CY, Hsiao CC, Chen PQ, Hollister SJ. Interbody fusion cage design using integrated global layout and local microstructure topology optimization. Spine 2004;29:1747–1754.
24. Hollander DA, von Walter M, Wirtz T, Sellei R, Schmidt-Rohlfing B, Paar O, Erli HJ. Structural, mechanical and in vitro characterization of individually structured Ti-6Al-4V produced by direct laser forming. Biomaterials 2006;27:955–963.
25. Annual Book of ASTM Standards. Medical devices and services, Section 13, Vol. 13.01, 2004.
26. Black J. Biological performance of tantalum. Clin Mater 1994;16:167–173.
27. Lewis RJS. Hawley's Condensed Chemical Dictionary, 12th ed. Ban New York:Nostrand Reinhold; 1993.
28. Lide DR. CRC Handbook of Chemistry and Physics, 76th ed. Boca Raton, FL:CRC Press; 1995.
29. Pfluger G, Plenk H, Bohler N, Grandschober F, Schider S. Experimental studies on total knee and hip joint endoprosthesis made of tantalum. In: Winder GD, Gibbons DF, Plenk HJ, editors. Biomaterials. Chichester: Wiley; 1980. p 161–167.
30. Levi AD, Choi WG, Keller PJ, Heiserman JE, Sonntag VK, Dickman CA. The radiographic and imaging characteristics of porous tantalum implants within the human cervical spine. Spine 1998;23:1245–1250. Discussion 1251.
31. Wang JC, Yu WD, Sandhu HS, Tam V, Delamarter RB. A comparison of magnetic resonance and computed tomographic image quality after the implantation of tantalum and titanium spinal instrumentation. Spine 1998;23:1684–1688.
32. Wigfield CC, Robie BH. Porous tantalum for spinal interbody fusion. In: Lewandrowski KU, Wise DL, Trantolo DJ, Yaszemski MJ, White AA, editors. Advances in Spinal Fusion. Basel, NY: Marcel Dekker; 2004. p 775–781.

10
Monitoring Muscle Growth and Tissue Changes Induced by Electrical Stimulation of Denervated Degenerated Muscles with CT and Stereolithographic 3D Modeling

Monitoring Muscle Growth and Tissue Changes Induced by Electrical Stimulation of Denervated Degenerated Muscles With CT and Stereolithographic 3D Modeling

*Thórdur Helgason, *Paolo Gargiulo, *Fjóla Jóhannesdóttir, †Páll Ingvarsson,
†Sigrún Knútsdóttir, †Vilborg Gudmundsdóttir, and †Stefán Yngvason

*Department of Research and Development, HTS, Landspitali-University Hospital; and †Department of Rehabilitation Medicine, Landspitali-University Hospital, Reykjavik, Iceland

Abstract: In the frame of the EU-funded RISE project, patients with lower motor neuron lesion and denervated and degenerated muscles are treated with electrical stimulation, with the aim of restoring muscle mass and force. Spiral computer tomography from the hip joint down to the knee joint is used to gather three-dimensional data on the upper leg tissue. These data are analyzed in order to monitor tissue changes induced by the electrical stimulation treatment. Especially the data representing muscle tissue and bone tissue were isolated for measurement purposes. Computer models and models made with rapid prototyping methods were used to display and demonstrate changes in muscle shape and size, as well as position relative to bone. Results showed that time and spatial dependencies of muscle growth can be monitored and studied quantitatively and qualitatively with the aid of a three-dimensional data set displayed on the computer screen or in the form of plastic models. These first results indicate muscle growth and an increase in bone density.
Key Words: Modeling—Electrical stimulation—Denervated degenerated muscle—Lower motor neuron lesion—Rehabilitation.

As part of the RISE project three paraplegic patients with fully denervated and to a great extent degenerated muscles in the lower extremities were treated with electrical stimulation (1,2). These patients with long-term flaccid paraplegia have no hope of regaining their muscle function with traditional treatment. Moreover, in comparison with patients with a spastic paraplegia, they often suffer more from several disturbing complications, e.g., decubitus ulcers, reduced bone density with a high risk of fractures, severe muscle atrophy with decreased circulation, lower metabolism, etc. The goal of the electrical stimulation is to restore muscle fibers, mass, and function in order to make the patients able to stand up and maintain a standing posture, e.g., in bars, with the aid of electrical stimulation. The muscle force should enable the legs to bear the patients weight. Building up mass, force, and function of denervated and degenerated muscles has been shown to be possible with long-term electrical stimulation treatment (1,3). The muscles are stimulated for up to two hours per day, six days a week, for two years. During that time the muscle is expected to gain considerably in mass and size and thus its ability to perform work. The treatment effects on the patients are monitored, e.g., by morphological and histochemical analysis of muscle biopsies as well as by clinical neurological, neurophysiological mechanical, and radiological methods (2,3). To follow changes in size and shape of the quadriceps muscle, computer tomography (CT) scans are taken at 10 cm intervals from the trochanter major to the knee (1). A comparison of two scans taken at two different times at the same level shows the muscle growth in that specific place during the time period between the two scans. Comparing five scans, taken at 10 cm intervals, yields an estimate of the total muscle growth and changes in fat and bone tissue. However, it does not show the growth of the whole muscle—data from only 10 scans is not

Received February 2005.
Address correspondence and reprint requests to Dr. Thórdur Helgason, Department for Research and Development, HTS, Landspitali-University Hospital, 101 Reykjavik, Iceland. E-mail: thordur@landspitali.is

enough to make a three-dimensional model of the muscle, bone, or other tissue.

In this article we describe a different approach, where stereolithographic 3D modeling is applied on data from repeated serial CT scans of three RISE study participants, in an attempt to monitor changes in the shape of muscle or bone, as well as to make geometrical measurements and 3D calculations of current distribution in the leg.

MATERIALS AND METHODS

Spiral CT

A spiral CT is taken every four months on the Icelandic subgroup of three patients with a complete spinal cord injury of flaccid type that were included in the RISE study. Within the two-year treatment period of the on-going RISE project, seven examinations in total are planned, three of which are done. The serial CT scan starts above the head of the femur and continues down to the knee joint, with both legs covered by one scan. The scans are taken with a pitch of 0.8 mm, which results in a total of about 750 CT slices, depending on the patient's size. Each slice has 512×512 pixels, and each pixel has a gray value in the Hounsfield scale of 4096 gray scale values, meaning that it is represented with a 12-bit value. A total data set from a single scan is therefore $512 \times 512 \times 750 \times 12 = 2.36$ GBit or around 300 MB. This data set gives a complete three-dimensional description of the tissue, including the muscles and bones in both upper legs. See the example of muscle and bone tissue from the upper right of one patient on three examinations in Fig. 1.

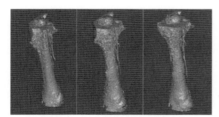

FIG. 1. Three-dimensional models of right upper leg muscles and femur. The leftmost image is from dataset 1 and shows the leg just before the stimulation treatment was stopped. The image in the middle is from dataset 2 and shows the leg immediately after treatment had begun again, and the image on the right, from dataset 3, shows the leg after an additional 4 months of electrical stimulation treatment.

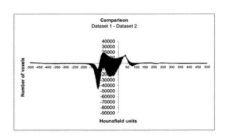

FIG. 2. The results of subtracting the histogram values of dataset 2 from the histogram values from dataset 1. The horizontal axis is the Hounsfield unit scale, representing different tissue types. The vertical axis shows the difference in number of voxels of each data set. Solid areas are where adjacent HU values are associated with very different voxel numbers. Since dataset 2 is taken at a later point of time values above the Hounsfield unit axis represent a decrease of corresponding tissue type and values below the Hounsfield unit axis represent an increase of corresponding tissue type in the time period between dataset 1 and 2. During this time no therapy was given and it is obvious that there has been a decrease in muscle tissue (peak at 40 HU), an increase in fat tissue (negative peak at −120 HU) but no changes can be seen in bone tissue.

Data analysis

Each spiral CT scan gives one data set. A histogram was made for each leg showing the number of voxels (volume elements) belonging to each Hounsfield unit value and hence the tissue type distribution at the time of the scan. The Hounsfield unit (HU) scale is calibrated on water (= 0 HU) and air (= 1000 HU). This gives a reading for fat in the range of −300 to −100 HU, for muscle in the 10–70 HU range, while bone has a density of >100 HU. By subtracting the values of the histogram at one point of time from the values of a histogram made from a data set taken at a later point of time, changes in tissue type distribution can be shown. An example of this is shown in Figs. 2 and 3, which is the same example as is shown in Fig. 1. A male subject (54 years old), seven years post injury had been treated with electrical stimulation for four months when treatment had to be stopped due to plastic surgery operations on old pressure sores. The data set 1 (see Fig. 2) was taken before and data set 2 (see Figs. 2 and 3) after this three-month period. After another four months of electrical stimulation treatment, data set 3 (see Fig. 3) was taken. Thus, Fig. 2 shows the change in tissue type distribution during a nontreatment period while Fig. 3 shows the change induced by treatment with electrical stimulation (3). See the figure legends.

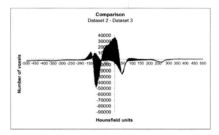

FIG. 3. During the period between dataset 2 and 3, electrical stimulation therapy was given. The comparison of the datasets shows an increase in muscle tissue (negative peak at 42 HU), an increase in bone tissue (negative peak at 263 HU), an increase in fat tissue (negative peak at 108 HU), and a decrease in fat and muscle tissue containing water (positive values between –75 to 25 HU).

Tissue differentiation, display, and measurements

The data sets were loaded into a computer program used to extract the tissue of interest. By defining the HU of interest, the area of interest, and some other properties which the object to be displayed has to fulfill, bone can easily be separated from muscle and muscle from fat. However, as all muscles have the same HU values the location of the boundaries between the muscles or muscle parts are not easily detectable, and it has not been possible to separate the different muscles or different muscle parts from each other.

Once the tissue of interest has been extracted, it can be displayed as a 3D object on a computer screen. The 3D models of both bone and muscles in Fig. 1 illustrate how different tissue types can be put together in the same image.

In order to monitor treatment effects, clinical evaluation of the muscle and other tissue can be made with the 3D models and with measurements. Measurements are made with the help of the data representing the isolated muscle tissue and its portion of total tissue in a single slice. Slice area, muscle volume, muscle mass, and density are examples of parameters that can be measured or estimated. This will be done in due time to assess muscle growth and other tissue changes.

Stereolithography models

Solid models of various materials have been made for the muscles of the upper leg and the associated femur bone, for clinical assessment of the muscles and for demonstration purposes. These models are made in different colors so that bone tissue is clearly distinguished from muscle tissue. Such models will be made for every measurement instance, resulting in a row of models from the three patients showing each patient's progress throughout the treatment.

RESULTS

The first results achieved with stereolithography using data from the first three spiral CTs of the right leg of one of the three patients in the ongoing RISE study, are shown (see Figs. 1–3, and the Methods section above). Even at this early stage of analysis, interesting changes in tissue type and distribution were seen, as demonstrated in Figs. 2 and 3. The method is tissue specific, so that increases or decreases in muscle, bone, fat, or other tissue types can be evaluated independently. The sensitivity of the method is limited by the spatial resolution of the X-ray CT scan and by the HU scale used.

DISCUSSION

Three-dimensional computer models of denervated degenerated upper leg muscles of paraplegic patients have been made. These models are the first in a series to monitor the outcome of the RISE electrical stimulation treatment regime. In due time they will show muscle growth throughout the whole treatment period. Since the models of this ongoing project were—and will be—made with data taken periodically every four months, they will show the muscle growth rate as a function of time. They also show the spatial distribution of the muscle growth, which can be unequal along the length of a muscle that is treated with electrical stimulation.

Comparison of the data and results from a more detailed analysis in this subgroup of three patients with data from the large RISE group of about 24 patients will hopefully be an aid to understanding and evaluating treatment effects of the group, as these patients are representative for different patient subgroups with short (10 month), moderate (5 year) and long (7.5 year) duration since their injury.

In further work, other data sampling modalities than CT—e.g., MRI and ultrasound—will be investigated. This gives hope of solving the problem of isolating separate muscles from one another or separating muscle parts.

In conclusion, a method to monitor changes in tissue type distribution, especially muscle growth and bone density, has been demonstrated. It is fast and uncomplicated and delivers tissue-specific and exact results. This method can be used to monitor electrical stimulation treatment of denervated and degenerated muscles.

Acknowledgments: This work has been supported by Health Technology Venue (HTV, http://www.htv.is) and The Icelandic Student Innovation Fund.

REFERENCES

1. Kern H, Hofer C, Mödlin M, Forstner C, Mayr W, Richter W. Functional electrical stimulation (FES) of long-term denervated muscles in humans: clinical observations and laboratory findings. *Basic Appl Myol* 2002;12:291–9.
2. Mayr W, Hofer C, Bijak M, et al. Functional electrical stimulation (FES) of denervated muscles: existing and prospective technological solutions. *Basic Appl Myol* 2002;12:287–90.
3. Kern H, Boncompagni S, Rossini K, et al. Long-term denervation in humans causes degeneration of both contractile and excitation-contraction coupling apparatus, which is reversible by functional electrical stimulation (FES): a role for myofiber regeneration? *J Neuropath Exp Neurol* 2004;63:919–31.

Update

Monitoring Muscle Growth and Tissue Changes Induced by Electrical Stimulation of Denervated Degenerated Muscles with CT and Stereolithographic 3D Modeling

Thordur Helgason, Paolo Gargiulo, Sigrun Knutsdottir, Vilborg Gudmundsdottir, Helmut Kern, Ugo Carraro, Stefan Yngvason, and Pall Ingvarsson

1
Introduction

Monitoring human tissue *in vivo* is done in many ways. The method of choice strongly depends on the tissue type, its position in the body, and the aspect of interest. In this work, we use spiral computer tomograpy (CT) scans or images as data acquisition method to gather 3D data of the thigh, especially its muscles and bones [1]. The information gathered is the X-ray attenuation property of the tissue as the ray passes through. This property is expressed in Hondsfield values (Hu) where higher values mean higher attenuation, more of the X-ray energy is stuck in the tissue and less passes through. These data are then processed to isolate or segment the tissue of interest such as single muscle bellies or bones. Once segmented, analysis of volume and density can be made.

In the frame of the research project RISE (QLG5-CT-2001-02191), the patients were monitored with additional methods such as histological examination of muscle tissue [2], including electron microscopy [3], neurological and muscle functional examinations [4], bone density measurements, blood examination, and measurement of mechanical properties of the knee joint and patella tendon stiffness. These additional monitorings give data that can be correlated with the CT scans and muscle biopsy morphometry.

Patients with conus cauda lesion, which is a spinal column injury below and to the distal end of the spinal cord, suffer from the consequences of lower motor neuron (LMN) lesion. The absence of a functioning LMN means that the muscle is never getting a nerve action potential, that is, a signal from the spinal cord, and is therefore almost always inactive, meaning never contracting. This leads to a long-term muscle degeneration process with a severe loss of contractile proteins in the muscle fibers and to thinner muscles. In about a decade, this process can go as far

Computer Aided Biomanufacturing, Edited by Roger Narayan and Paul Calvert
© 2011 WILEY-VCH Verlag GmbH & Co. KGaA. Published 2011 by WILEY-VCH Verlag GmbH & Co. KGaA.

as leaving no contractile elements in the muscle fibers. In the complex process of degeneration, the muscle takes on different consistency. Degenerating muscle fibers and the muscle tissue is infiltrated by fat, which has lower Hu value than the healthy muscle tissue, that is, it is less dense. Therefore, it lowers the overall density of the muscle, even though it takes up volume. This fat migration is seen as both the lower density of the muscle tissue in a CT scan and fat clusters throughout the muscle volume. As the degeneration proceeds, the boundaries of the muscle bellies shrink losing their content and lowering the volume of the muscle. The shape can be altered. The rectus femoris we have investigated in this work is normally in a straight line from its fixation on the hip bone down to the patella. Since the denervated rectus femoris muscle is longer than a normal innervated muscle, in our subjects it therefore makes an arc toward the inner thigh. Bone mineral density (BMD) measured in mg/cm^3 decreases in subjects with denervated muscles [3]. This raises the risk of bone fracture. Both the cortical and the trabecular bone are affected. The decrease of density can be down to below 40% of the original bone density [5].

Electrical stimulation of the muscle fibers can stop or even reverse the degeneration process of a denervated muscle [3]. It is the only therapy that addresses the muscle regeneration and hence all the positive effects on other tissue types associated with that.

2
Material and Methods

2.1
Subjects

Three subjects participated in our part of the RISE project. They are all males and victims of accidents. They all suffer from a spinal cord injury at the lower thoracic or lumbar level. Table 1 gives an overview of the patients. They are of different age and the time elapsed from injury to the beginning of therapy, called degeneration time, was very different. They all have similar therapy time as they started the therapy almost at the same time.

Table 1 Percentage of muscle volume.

	Muscle tissue normal density	Muscle tissue low density	Connective tissue	Fat
Healthy control person	64	17	14	5
P2, 4-year denervation, no stimulation	45	24	23	8
P2, 8-year denervation, 4-year stimulation	60	20	16	5
P3, 7-year denervation, no stimulation	41	31	20	8

2.2
Electrotherapy

The home-based functional electrotherapy (h-bFES) aims at the recovery of the quadriceps muscle of the thigh. Two big electrodes (12 cm × 15 cm) were put on the surface of the skin of each thigh. Each electrode pair forms one stimulating channel. Electrical pulses are conducted through the electrodes to the underlying muscles for the depolarization of the muscle fibers that in turn contract. The recruitment of the muscles is such that first the muscles or muscle fibers nearest to the electrodes and the gap between the electrodes contract. As the intensity of the stimulating pulse is increased, the deeper muscles and those farther away from the electrodes are stimulated.

The therapy protocol starts relatively mildly. The patients are supposed to stimulate with a warm-up mode (single twitch) for 3 min. After the warm-up period, the main stimulation period is of about 4–5 min with pulse burst of 2 s and a pause of 2 s in between. Training is done with 20 Hz, followed by single twitch stimulation of approximately 2 Hz for 15 min. Total stimulation time for each muscle group was about 35 min daily. This is done 6 days a week and needs to be done as long as the muscles are to be kept in form. The progressive stimulation protocols of h-bFES are detailed in Refs [6, 7].

From the three subjects, one (P1) was not therapy compliant. As can be seen from Table 1, he started relatively soon after injury, only 10 months. Monitoring of his muscles, therefore, shows a history of muscle degeneration. The second subject (P2) started therapy more than 4 years after the injury. He has been rather therapy compliant with the result that the volume of his rectus femoris muscle has increased about 80%. The third subject (P3) and the oldest one of the three started therapy very late – almost 8 years after the injury – that reduces his chances of muscle rehabilitation. Besides these constraining factors, he also had some complications reducing his possibilities of therapy. Monitoring of his muscles shows an increase of muscle mass in some periods but a reduction of the same in the next period.

2.3
Data Acquisition

The data acquisition with a spiral computer tomography was described in our former article [1]. Here the calibration will be outlined. For the analysis of tissue density with CT scans made at different points of time, calibration of the Hounsfield (Hu) values becomes inevitable. The data were acquired over a period of more than 6 years, using the same CT scanner all the time. However, the X-ray tube, the sensors, the compositions of the patients, and some other factors have changed. In order to keep the Hu values comparable, every scan was made with three rods within the images. Two of them are solid plastic but of different diameter. The third one is a plastic pipe filled with water. These rods could easily be put alongside the thigh each time they were scanned. The Hu values of the rods were scanned and compared with two calibration phantoms. One of the phantoms is specially made for calibration of measurement of bone mineral density. It is made of three square bars of reference material, that is, three types of material with different concentration of calcium hydroxyapatite [5]. The second phantom was a normal image quality assessment phantom for CT scanner. It has several materials with known Hu values to mimic different types of tissues such as muscle, fat, and bone. With this comparison, drift and noise in the CT images could be evaluated and density values from different times compared.

2.4
Segmentation

Extracting the tissue of interest from a CT scan data set, that is, segmenting muscle, bone, or other tissue from the spiral CT scan is done with special software called Mimics. As bone, muscles, and fat have very different Hu values, they can normally be separated from each other easily. Difficulties arise when adjacent muscles or single muscle bellies have to be segmented from each other. They have the same density, that is, same Hu values and the resolution of the CT is not enough to show the boundaries between the different bellies. In denervated and degenerated muscle, this becomes all the more difficult as the normal anatomy of the muscle is not there anymore. In addition, fat migrates into the muscle lowering its density far below the normal muscle values. In this study, we have focused on the rectus femoris muscle. This muscle was more distinguished from other thigh muscles and could be segmented with a special method developed in this study [8]. First, the muscle tissue of the whole thigh is segmented choosing Hu values from -37 to 129 Hu [9]. Then, a CT slice is chosen where the boundaries of the rectus femoris muscle are clear. The part of the slice belonging to the muscle is marked with a different color and put into a special storage or masks and given a name. Next, this muscle slice is projected on to the adjacent slice of the muscle. If it fits the adjacent slice, it gets the same color and is a part of the mask. If it does not fit, corrections are done manually and the new slice gets the color and is put into the mask. This process is repeated for every slice until the whole muscle is covered. At this point, the mask is a three-dimensional object describing the muscle and defining what voxels belong to the muscle. Now it can be used further for analysis of changes in the muscle structure such as volume and density. As the boundaries for the denervated degenerated rectus femoris muscle are more or less clear, this method enables its segmentation but it does not work for the other thigh muscles as they are not distinguishable from each other.

2.5
Muscle Volume Measurement

Once the muscle has been segmented, the voxels (volume element) representing him are also defined. Each voxel has a defined position in space and one density value measured in Hu. They can be thought of as small rectangular cubes having defined length, width, and height and so a defined volume. Therefore, the volume measure-

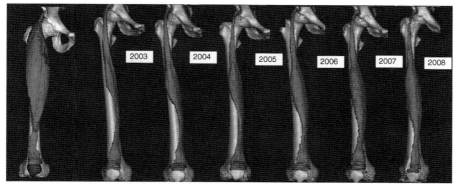

Normal   Denervated in electrical stimulation treatment

Figure 1 The figure shows a model of the left leg of a healthy control subject to the left and a time series of left leg of P2 (six models). The rectus femoris muscle, the femur bone, the patella, and a part of the hip bone are modeled. The rest of the soft tissue has been removed. The row shows the development of the rectus femoris muscle from the beginning of electrical stimulation therapy in the year 2003 until 2008 (10,6; 13,7; 10,4; 16,2; 16,1; 17,0 cm^3, respectively). It can clearly be seen how the muscle gains volume in the middle and straightens up. But in comparison to the control subject, the denervated muscle is far from its form.

ment becomes a task of counting the voxels inside the muscle mask. Errors arise at the boundary between the muscle and other tissues. Here the question arises whether a voxel should be counted as a part of the muscle or as a part of the surrounding tissue since in reality it is only partially inside the muscle. This phenomenon is known as partial volume effect. It is counted being inside the muscle if its density value is in the interval defined for that particular mask. Otherwise, it is outside. The software we use has two algorithms to compensate for the partial volume effect. One is called "contour interpolation" and the other "gray value interpolation." The former takes into account the geometry of the surrounding voxels belonging to the muscle, while the latter takes into account the gray values of the surrounding elements.

The volume of the rectus femoris muscle in all the subjects was measured regularly, from the beginning of the treatment in 2003 until 2008. An example of the results is shown in Figure 1.

2.6
Muscle Density Analysis

Density of the muscles was analyzed principally in two ways, in a geometrical density distribution and in a statistical way.

The mean density of each CT slice of the muscle was plotted as a function of the length [10]. In this way, the density distribution along the length of the muscle is visualized and it can be seen where and where not the muscle is gaining in density.

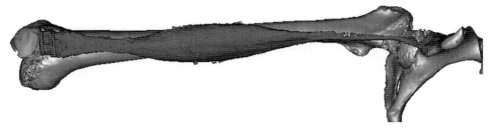

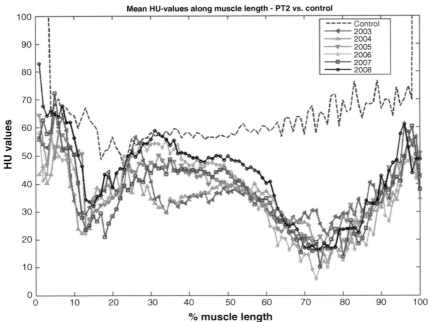

Figure 2 The upper part is a model of the left thigh of P2 in 2008, the same as the rightmost model in Figure 1 The diagram below shows the tissue density in the rectus femoris muscle as a function of the normalized length of the muscle, one curve for each year from the beginning of the therapy in 2003 until 2008. As can be seen, the density of the muscle tissue is highest in the middle of the muscle, where the stimulating electrodes meet, and hence most frequent stimulation can be expected. Toward the upper end, the muscle is not stimulated and the lower end is mostly tendon tissue. It can also be seen that in the middle of the muscle, the tissue density rises during the therapy period from its lowest value in 2003 to its highest value in 2008.

The plot is shown in Figure 2 along with the muscle, patella, and the femur bone. The length is plotted as percentage of the total length.

The voxels in the rectus femoris were classified according to the density value in four groups and color coded [11]. The range of density values of fat is -200 to -6 Hu, connective tissue -5 to 20 Hu, atrophic muscle 21–40 Hu, and normal muscle 41–135 Hu. (Some work was done with the following density values: fat -200 to -30 Hu, loose connective tissue -23 to -10 Hu, atrophic muscle 11–30 Hu, normal muscle 31–80 Hu, connective tissue 81–139 Hu.) Each of these tissue types is imaged in front of the femur bone showing its distribution. Comparing images made this way show the changes in tissue composition of the muscle throughout the therapy period in one case but the degeneration of another that was not therapy compliant.

Statistical analysis of the whole thigh tissue was described in Ref. [1]. Statistical analysis of the rectus femoris muscle was done in a way that the volume of each density was plotted against the density [12]. This was done for one data set a year showing one curve for each treatment year. In a therapy compliant subject, the volume increases and the density of the muscle is shifted to higher values, meaning denser tissue, more muscle, and less fat.

2.7
Muscle Shape

The mask from a segmented muscle was used to monitor the shape of the muscle. Figure 1 shows the development of the muscle throughout the therapy time. There are two obvious changes. First, the muscle is clearly growing in the middle. This is where the two stimulating electrodes meet on the skin above the muscle. Second, the denervated rectus femoris develops an arc toward the inner thigh. This arc was analyzed quantitatively in Refs [8, 13] by measuring the curvature of the central line of the muscle.

2.8
Bone Density Analysis

Bone density loss can be seen on X-ray equipment several months after the injury. But calcium and other chemicals released during bone breakdown can be measured in blood soon after the injury [14]. The density of the two bones, the femur bone and the patella, were analyzed [5, 8, 15]. Bone mineral density distribution was analyzed and the surface density was mapped as a color code on a 3D model of the femur. Then, for a region of interest, the central part of the femur, the density was divided into several intervals and the volume of bone in each interval was measured. The third analysis was done on the patella bone [8, 16]. The patella is connected to all four parts of the quadriceps muscle. As the muscle pulls the load, it is transferred to the patella. This is the only load on the patella in a SCI patient with peripheral lesion. Also, the influence of electrical current is excluded as the patella lies outside the current path of the stimulating current.

3
Results

Results from the volume measurement show a considerable increase in the volume of the rectus femoris muscle of the therapy compliant subject (from $88.000 \, mm^3$ in

2003 to 160.000 mm^3 in 2008). This is an increase of about 80%. The other two were not therapy compliant or had complications that prevented stimulation. It is worth stressing that the development of the volume correlates with the changes in density. This can be seen in Figure 2 for the most compliant subject P2. Above the graph, the rectus femoris muscle is shown in front of the femur bone. It is connected to the patella (left end) and to the hip bone (right end). The graph shows the mean density of the muscle in the corresponding slice measured in Hu. The dotted line shows the density of a healthy control person. The other lines show the density of the muscle from different years. It is clear that the density of the muscle has been rising but only in a part of the muscle. It is the same part where the volume has been increasing. Above this part, the muscle volume and the density have been slightly decreasing. This may be explained by recognizing that the muscle has a pennatus (feather-like) structure. The muscle fibers pass from the middle to the outskirts and not from one end to the other. This means that electrodes placed on top of the skin above the muscle is bound to stimulate more often the muscle fibers in the middle than those at the end because they are where the stimulating electrical current has the highest intensity. At the end of the muscle, the electrodes will not cover the muscle and they probably do not get any stimulation and in fact they are still degenerating. If this is the case, it means that the same muscle can be growing and increasing in its volume and density as well as degenerating, that is, losing volume and density at the same time.

The tissue composition analysis of the muscle also shows a correlation with the volume changes. Table 1 shows four measurements [11]. The first one is made on a healthy control person as reference. The second row shows P2 4 years after the injury and at that time without electrical stimulation treatment. The third row again shows P2 8 years after the injury and 4 years of stimulation treatment. The last row shows P3 7 years after the injury and without stimulation treatment.

Table 1 shows that P2 gains almost the same tissue distribution as the control person after 4 years of electrical stimulation treatment. P2 had almost the same tissue distribution after 4 years of muscle degeneration as P3 after 7 years of muscle degeneration. This suggests that degeneration is faster in the beginning but slows down later. The recovery that these numbers represent shows that the degenerated muscle can regain its tissue composition and volume as discussed above.

The shape of the muscle shown in Figure 1 in 2003 is a curvature toward the inner thigh. This means that the muscle is longer than it would have been if it was in a straight line from its fixation on the hip bone down to the patella. As it is treated, the curvature decreases but it does not disappear in 5 years of treatment. This is evident when compared with the muscle of the control person (leftmost image in Figure 1). An explanation for the curvature could be that since the muscle is not contracting but is stretched when the knee is bent, it stays in a prolonged position. As it is treated, the stimulated parts get straight but the other parts, above and below, do not. This still keeps the curvature.

Bone density analysis showed an increase and a decrease in the surface layer of the femur bone in the same period of time [5]. When the volume was divided into intervals, the decrease in the second most dense interval of the bone was equal to the increase in the most dense interval of the bone. This suggests that the loading of the bone through electrical stimulation of the muscles was increasing the density of the trabecular femur bone. The analysis of the patella showed a slowing down of the mineral loss in a subject treated with electrical stimulation compared to a subject with no treatment [8].

4
Discussion

Our data show that h-bFES can be an effective home therapy to counteract muscle atrophy/degeneration after complete LMN denervation due to conus cauda lesions. The h-bFES device stimulates muscle fibers in the absence of nerve endings and after prolonged denervation, enabling (i) recovery of muscle mass and fiber size, (ii) recovery of tetanic contractility, and (3) restoration of muscle fiber ultrastructure [6, 7, 17, 18].

Up to now, the muscles of affected extremities in these paraplegic patients are commonly not treated with FES because it is widely accepted that long-term and completely denervated muscles cannot be effectively stimulated. On the other hand, studies in animal models and humans indicate that (i) severe atrophy does not occur in rats for at least 3–4 months; (ii) in rabbit, the degeneration of muscle tissue does not appear during the first year of denervation; and (iii) in humans, muscle tissue degeneration starts from the third year onward. Our recent findings that the long-term denervated rat muscle maintains L-type Ca_2^+ current and gene expression of the related proteins longer than the functional contractile machineries provide the molecular, structural, and functional rationale of a rehabilitation training for human permanently denervated muscles that was developed as a result of empirical clinical observations [19].

This leaves a window of opportunity to initiate muscle stimulation and avoid muscle degeneration and infiltration. For people with permanent lower motor neuron lesion, there is no other therapy that will keep their muscle volume and ability to develop force than home-based functional electrical stimulation. Other therapy modalities do not address muscle atrophy, although they seem to influence occurrence of side effects such as decubitus ulcers and infections. In the project described here, it has been demonstrated that the muscle not only gains volume but also approaches its normal tissue composition. Detailed light and electron microscopy analyses of muscle biopsy from a larger study group (the European RISE study) support this conclusion [6, 7, 20].

Furthermore, a new ultrasound approach for the analyses of structure, function, and perfusion characteristics of the permanently denervated muscles submitted to h-bFES allows the follow-up and optimization of the stimulation protocols [17, 21, 22].

On the other hand, the therapy has to be refined so that all denervated muscles in the lower limb and all muscle fibers in each muscle can be stimulated. As there are no nerve fibers that spread the electric-induced action potential to all muscle fibers (thus enabling them to contract in synchrony), the stimulating electrical current has to be brought in an adequate intensity to each muscle fiber. This is a difficult goal still to be fully addressed. The modeling of tissue, its geometrical form, and its electrical, mechanical, and other properties play a central role in enhancing our understanding of the muscle and bone tissue and their responses to electrical (and also to mechanical and other) stimulation. Monitoring a therapy and documenting with real-world models give additional information and insight into the therapy process.

In this work, however, the muscle growth can be seen as a function of time by comparing the models (Figure 1).

In order to design and test neural prosthesis for applying on denervated muscles, both mathematical models and models made of materials are used. The mathematical models allow the relatively cost-effective computer simulations of different properties, whereas the real models allow the testing of a prototype in the real world. For this, testing models of different materials with different electrical and mechanical properties are used.

In conclusion, our findings strongly support the RISE rehabilitation protocol as a method to improve the mass and contractility of LMN denervated muscles. These benefits could be extended to patients with similar lesions especially to determine whether h-bFES can reduce secondary complications related to disuse and impaired blood perfusion (reduction in bone density, risk of bone fracture, decubitus ulcers, and pulmonary thromboembolism).

References

1 Helgason, T., Gargiulo, P., Jóhannesdóttir, F., Ingvarsson, P., Knútsdóttir, S., Guðmundsdóttir, V., and Yngvason, S. (2005) Monitoring muscle growth and tissue changes induced by electrical stimulation of denervated degenerated muscles with CT and stereolithographic 3D modelling. *Artif. Organs,* **29** (6), 440–443.

2 Carraro, U., Rossini, K., Mayr, W., and Kern, H. (2005) Muscle fiber regeneration in human permanent lower motoneuron denervation: relevance to safety and effectiveness of FES-training, which induces muscle recovery in SCI subjects. *Artif. Organs,* **29**, 187–191.

3 Kern, H., Rossini, K., Boncompagni, S., Mayr, W., Fanó, G., Zanin, M.E., Pokhorska-Okolow, M., Protasi, F., and Carraro, U. (2004) Long-term denervation in humans causes degeneration of both contractile and excitation–contraction coupling apparatus, which is reversible by functional electrical stimulation (FES): a role for myofiber regeneration? *J. Neuropathol. Exp. Neurol.,* **63**, 919–931.

4 Kern, H., Mödlin, M., and Forstner, C. (2004) The rise patient study: FES in the treatment of flaccid paraplegia. Proceedings of the 8th Vienna International Workshop on Functional Electrical Stimulation, September 10–13, Vienna, Austria.

5 Johannesdottir, F. (2006) Bone: use it or lose it. MS thesis. University of Iceland.

6 Kern, H., Carraro, U., Adami, N., Biral, D., Hofer, C., Forstner, C., Mödlin, M., Vogelauer, M., Boncompagni, S., Paolini, C., Mayr, W., Protasi, F., and Zampieri, S. (2010) Home-based functional electrical stimulation (h-bFES) recovers permanently denervated muscles in paraplegic patients with complete lower motor neuron lesion. *Neurorehabil. Neural Repair,* **24** (8), 709–721.

7 Kern, H., Carraro, U., Adami, N., Biral, D., Hofer, C., Loefler, S.,

Vogelauer, M., Mayr, W., Rupp, R., and Zampieri, S. (2010) One year of home-based functional electrical stimulation (FES) in complete lower motor neuron paraplegia: recovery of tetanic contractility drives the structural improvements of denervated muscle. *Neurol. Res.*, **32**, 5–12.

8 Gargiulo, P. (2008) 3D modelling and monitoring of denervated muscle under functional electrical stimulation treatment and associated bone structural changes. PhD thesis. The Technical University of Vienna.

9 Gargiulo, P., Helgason, T., Ingvarsson, P., Knútsdóttir, S., Guðmundsdóttir, V., and Yngvason, S. (2007) Morphological changes in rectus femoris muscle: advanced image processing technique and 3-dimensional visualization to monitor denervated and degenerated muscles treated with functional electrical stimulation. *Basic Appl. Myol.*, **17** (3–4), 133–136.

10 Helgason, T., Gargiulo, P., Vatnsdal, B., Yngvason, S., Gudmundsdottir, V., Knútsdóttir, S., and Ingvarsson, P. (2009) Density distribution of denervated degenerated rectus femoris muscle in electrical stimulation treatment. *IFMBE Proc.*, **25** (IX), 370–373.

11 Gargiulo F P., Kern, H., Carraro, U., Ingvarsson, P., Knutsdottir, S., Gudmundsdottir, V., Yngvason, S., Vatnsdal, B., and Helgason, T. (2010) Quantitative colour three-dimensional computer tomography imaging of human long-term denervated muscle. *Neurol. Res.*, **32** (1), 13–19.

12 Helgason, T., Gargiulo, P., Halldorsdottir, G., Vatnsdal Palsson, B., Ingvarsson, P., Knutsdottir, S., Gudmundsdottir, V., and Yngvason, S. (2008) Comparing muscle and bone density changes in denervated and degenerated muscle treated with electrical stimulation. *Biomed. Tech.*, **53** (Suppl. 1), 259–261.

13 Gargiulo, P., Vatnsdal, B., Ingvarsson, P., Yngvason, S., Gudmundsdottir, V., Knutsdottir, S., and Helgason, T. (2008) Denervated and degenerated muscle stimulation: advanced image processing techniques and 3-dimensional rendering to monitor muscles restoration. *Biomed. Tech.*, **53** (Suppl. 1), 408–410.

14 Reiter, AL., Volk, A., Vollmar, J. et al. (2007) Changes of basic bone turnover parameters in short-term patients with spinal cord injury. *Eur. Spine J.*, **16** (6), 771–776.

15 Helgason, T., Gargiulo, P., Ingvarsson, P., and Yngvason, S. (2007) Using mimics to monitor changes in bone mineral density of femur during electrical stimulation therapy of denervated degenerated thigh muscles. Annual International Conference on Computer Guided Implantology and Advanced 3D Medical Image Processing, Washington, June 1–3, 2007.

16 Gargiulo, P., Vatnsdal, B., Ingvarsson, P., Knútsdóttir, S., Gudmundsdottir, V., Yngvason, S., and Helgason, T. (2009) Density distribution of denervated degenerated rectus femoris muscle in electrical stimulation treatment. *IFMBE Proc.*, **25** (IX), 399–402.

17 Kern, H., Stramare, R., Martino, L., Zanato, R., Gargiulo, P., and Carraro, U. (2010) Permanent LMN denervation of human skeletal muscle and recovery by h-b FES: management and monitoring. *Eur. J. Trans. Myol.*, **20**, 91–104.

18 Boncompagni, S., Kern, H., Rossini, K. et al. (2007) Structural differentiation of skeletal muscle fibers in the absence of innervation in humans. *Proc. Natl. Acad. Sci. USA*, **104**, 19339–19344.

19 Squecco, R., Carraro, U., Kern, H., Pond, A., Adami, N., Biral, D., Vindigni, V., Boncompagni, S., Pietrangelo, T., Bosco, G., Fanò, G., Marini, M., Abruzzo, PM., Germinarlo, E., Danieli-Betto, D., Protasi, F., Francini, F., and Zampieri, S. (2009) Despite lost contractility, a sub-population of rat muscle fibers maintains an assessable excitation–contraction coupling mechanism after long-standing denervation. *J. Neuropathol. Exp. Neurol.*, **68** (2009), 1256–1268.

20 Kern, H. and Carraro, U. (2008) Translational myology focus on clinical challenges of functional electrical stimulation of denervated muscle. *Basic Appl. Myol.*, **18**, 37–100.

21 Zanato, R. (2009) Ecomiografia funzionale del muscolo denervato: Risultati preliminari. MD thesis. University of Padova, Italy, pp. 1–44.

22 Zanato, R., Martino, L., Carraro, U., Kern, H., Rossato, E., Masiero, S., and Stramare, R. (2010) Functional echomyography: thickness, ecogenicity, contraction and perfusion of the LMN denervated human muscle before and during h-bFES. *Eur. J. Trans. Myol.*, **20**, 33–40.

11
CAD-CAM Construction of a Provisional Nasal Prosthesis After Ablative Tumour Surgery of the Nose: A Pilot Case Report

Clinical note

CAD-CAM construction of a provisional nasal prosthesis after ablative tumour surgery of the nose: a pilot case report

L. CIOCCA, DDS, PHD, ASSISTANT PROFESSOR, *Maxillo-Facial Prosthetics, Section of Prosthodontics, Department of Oral Science, Alma Mater Studiorum University of Bologna*, G. BACCI, LAB. TECHNICIAN, *SILAB Laboratory, Department of Architecture, Faculty of Engineering, Alma Mater Studiorum University of Bologna*, R. MINGUCCI, DOCTOR, DEAN, PROFESSOR, *SILAB Laboratory, Department of Architecture, Faculty of Engineering, Alma Mater Studiorum University of Bologna*, & R. SCOTTI, DMD, DDS, PROFESSOR, DEAN, *Oral and Maxillo-Facial Rehabilitation, Section of Prosthodontics, Department of Oral Science, Alma Mater Studiorum University of Bologna, Bologna, Italy*

CIOCCA L., BACCI G., MINGUCCI R. & SCOTTI R. (2009) *European Journal of Cancer Care* **19**, 97–101
CAD-CAM construction of a provisional nasal prosthesis after ablative tumour surgery of the nose: a pilot case report

The computer-aided design of a nasal prosthesis based on pre-operative virtual laser scanning of the affected site was virtually adapted to the post-operative laser-scanned surface. The designed volume of the nose was rapidly prototyped and used to fabricate a provisional prosthesis and a computed tomography diagnostic template to check the available premaxilla bone for implants. The mould for the nasal prosthesis was prototyped using a computer-aided design and manufacturing (CAD-CAM) procedure. In addition, the mesiostructure of an eyeglasses-supported provisional prosthesis was also designed and prototyped using CAD-CAM procedures.

Keywords: maxillofacial prosthesis, nasal prosthesis, CAD-CAM, rapid prototyping.

INTRODUCTION

New technologies of computer-aided design and manufacturing (CAD-CAM) for facial prostheses have increased rapidly in the last decade. Although microvascularized free flaps or rotated frontal flaps can be used to restore a defect surgically, with good aesthetic results, sometimes plastic surgery cannot restore the entire volume of the nose (Harrison 1982; McGuirt & Thompson 1984; DiLeo

Correspondence address: Dr Leonardo Ciocca, Via S. Vitale 59, 40125 Bologna, Italy (e-mail: leonardo.ciocca@unibo.it).

The English in this document has been checked by at least two professional editors, both native speakers of English. For a certificate, see: http://www.textcheck.com/cgi-bin/certificate.cgi?id=nzigQZ

Accepted 13 July 2008
DOI: 10.1111/j.1365-2354.2008.01013.x

European Journal of Cancer Care, 2009, **18**, 97–101

© 2008 The Authors
Journal compilation © 2008 Blackwell Publishing Ltd
Computer Aided Biomanufacturing, Edited by Roger Narayan and Paul Calvert
© 2011 WILEY-VCH Verlag GmbH & Co. KGaA. Published 2011 by WILEY-VCH Verlag GmbH & Co. KGaA.

et al. 1996; Fornelli *et al.* 2000; Hecker *et al.* 2002). In such patients, a facial prosthesis provides aesthetics and respiratory function (Javid 1971; Ugadama & King 1983; Dumbrigue & Flyer 1997; Nabadalung 2003). Many attempts at reducing the number of manual steps during ear prosthesis construction have been made (Lemon *et al.* 1996; Choi *et al.* 2002; Jiao *et al.* 2004; Mardini *et al.* 2005; Coward *et al.* 2006; Ciocca *et al.* 2007). Other reports have focused on nasal prostheses, with or without implant support (Flood & Russell 1998; Ciocca *et al.* 2007). Even if a protocol was presented by the authors concerning the CAD-CAM procedures for the virtual design and rapid prototyping of the mould for an ear prosthesis, a CAD-CAM system has never been used for this specific application (Ciocca *et al.* 2007). This article describes the CAD-CAM construction of an eyeglasses-supported provisional nasal prosthesis. It also describes

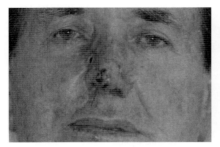

Figure 1. Squamous cell carcinoma of the nose.

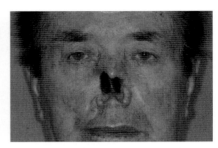

Figure 2. Aesthetic disfiguration after tumour removal.

the CAD-CAM construction of diagnostic templates for the computed tomography (CT) examination, for positioning implants for retaining the nasal prosthesis.

CLINICAL REPORT

Before surgery

Using a new laser scanner (NextEngine Desktop 3D Scanner, NextEngine, Santa Monica, CA, USA) connected to a Notebook computer (Vajo, Sony, Corp, Tokyo, Japan) to acquire the 3-dimensional (3D) spatial coordinates of the pre-surgical nasal surface, using Scanstudio Core software (NextEngine, Santa Monica, CA, USA), the first measurement was made after positioning the patient (Fig. 1) in front of the laser scanner. Three coloured balls (Ballpin, Buffetti, Milan, Italy) (diameter 2.5 mm) were positioned randomly around the site using a skin adhesive (Bloom-Singer Brush-on Silicone Skin Adhesive, In-health Technologies, Hansa Medical Products, Carpentaria, CA, USA). In situations where the scheduling of the surgery does not allow a laser scan, instead of laser scanning the patient, a stone cast of his or her nose may be used. In such a case, an alginate impression is made and a stone cast of the pre-surgical anatomy is made using conventional techniques. The cast is positioned on a platform with coloured pins (Ballpin, Buffetti, Milan, Italy) (diameter 2.5 mm) positioned around it randomly, as described by Ciocca and Scotti (2004), for laser scanning.

After tumour surgery

After surgery for tumour removal, the patient is placed in three random positions to obtain three laser measurements of the defect from different angles to detect all undercuts. A skin adhesive (Bloom-Singer Brush-on Silicone Skin Adhesive, Pomona, CA, USA) was used to attach three small balls to the skin around the defect (Fig. 2). These patterns were recorded using the laser scanner. The scanned surface was represented by four clouds (the entire number of 3D points representing a volume surface) of 50 000 points each, in 3D point coordinates. These digitalized surfaces were elaborated using Inus Rapidform 2006 CAD ver. 2006 (INUS Technology, Seoul, Korea), to recombine, align and blend the different surfaces into a single virtual model, eliminating any surface abnormalities, while remeshing the organization of the triangulated mesh of points and filling any surface gaps that remained after data elaboration. To merge the 3D point clouds, the same 3D points in each digital image were located and the centre of each coloured sphere was overlapped with the corresponding sphere in the other angled image scans, and all measurements were integrated. The resin substructure was developed using a CAD-CAM design to be included in the volume of the silicone prosthesis for connecting the prosthesis to the eyeglasses. To elaborate the final stereolithographic (STL) file of the prosthesis, the pre- and post-operative 3D images were superimposed and the correct position of the nose in relation to the patient's face was determined (Fig. 3). Once the STL file of the nose was made, it was represented as a negative volume and this pattern was transformed into a new STL file for rapid mould prototyping. For the provisional prosthesis, the substructure was projected and positioned in relation to the external volume of the prosthesis straight in the mould (Fig. 4). The resin substructure was prototyped alone; it was not connected to the base of the mould and was positioned in the mould before silicone processing using two landmark holes in the base on the side of the defect. The STL file was processed using a computer system (Z Printer 310, Z Corporation, Burlington, MA, USA) to manufacture the mould in a single step, developing the entire volume of the mould through layer-by-layer apposition of 3D-printer materials (resin and powder). After allowing 60 min for the acrylic resin to polymerize, the mould was extracted from the powder and then the surfaces of the cast were coated with epoxy resin (Renlam M-1, Fuchs, Milan, Italy) to further harden the prototyped material. Using conventional silicone (VST 50F, Factor II, Lakeside, AZ, USA) processing procedures, the definitive prosthesis was manufactured, as for conventional stone mould processing. A spectrophotometer was used to determine the intrinsic colour of the silicone (SpectroShade™ Office, MHT, Verona, Italy). Extrinsic colours (Extrinsic; Factor II) were applied and a silicone adhesive (A-564; Factor II) was applied as a coating. Finally, matting dispersion liquid (MD564; Factor II) mixed with silicone dispersion liquid (TS564; Factor II) was used to give the prosthesis a matt appearance (Fig. 6).

DISCUSSION

The mould used for silicone processing was rapid prototyped entirely using CAD-CAM procedures. The mesiostructure was also projected virtually, designed and prototyped. A retention system with holes in the mould was constructed to retain it during silicone polymerization. An eyeglasses-supported provisional prosthesis was manufactured, with the resin mesiostructure connected to the eyeglasses using a screw in the bridge of the eyeglasses. The patient did not have to use a skin adhesive. The same volume designed for the prosthesis was used to construct an acrylic rapid-prototyped diagnostic template (Fig. 5). The best position for the implants for retaining the definitive prosthesis was determined using three spherical gutta-percha markers inside the base of the template, corresponding to the premaxillar region below crista-galli bone lamina. Time and costs of the CAD-CAM procedure are presented in Table 1. The clinical timing of the protocol for the provisional prosthesis is presented in Table 2, even if the timing for the definitive nasal prosthesis is longer than this. After the delivery of the provisional, the implants for the retention of the definitive nasal prosthesis have to be inserted as soon as possible (6–8 weeks after the tumour surgery) and, after a further 6 months healing period, the bar for the retention and the definitive nasal prosthesis may be delivered to the patient.

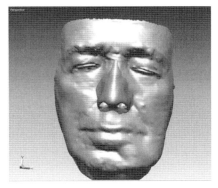

Figure 3. Superimposition of the pre-surgical anatomy on the residual defect after tumour removal.

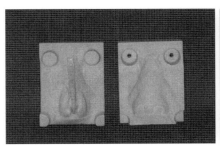 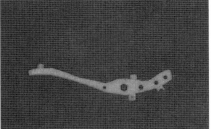

Figure 4. Rapid prototyping of the mould and substructure.

CIOCCA *et al.*

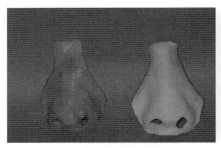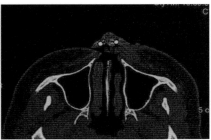

Figure 5. Developing the diagnostic template with two gutta-percha landmarks, and the CT result. CT, computed tomography.

Table 1. Time and cost of the procedure

	CAD time (h)	ABS model material (cm³)	Support material (cm³)	Build time (min)	Cost of material (€)
Pre-operative nose CAD	2	46.75	23.81	2 h 31	16.98
Post-operative nose CAD-CAM	2	40.68	15.84	3 h 27	13.71
Nasal prosthesis for try-in/diagnostic template	–	7.33	4.42	2 h 14	3.67
Mould	3	6.03	3.12	1 h 1	3.07
Total	5	100.79	47.19	8 h 33	37.43

CAD-CAM, computer-aided design and manufacturing.

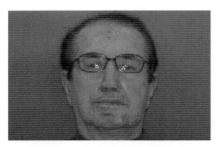

Figure 6. Final eyeglasses-supported provisional prosthesis.

Table 2. Timing of the procedure of the provisional prosthesis

Step	After surgery (weeks)
Pre-operative laser scanning	–
Post-operative laser scanning	4
Try-in	5
Delivery	6

The CAD-CAM procedure presented here reduced the number of manual steps needed to construct a provisional nasal prosthesis. The main advantages of this technique are:

- All corrections may be made straight onto the PC screen: if you use the pre-surgical anatomy of the nose, where the tumour is present, all the morphological alterations to the external volume due to the tumour will be replicated in the final prosthesis. This protocol allows to correct the anatomy taking into account a perfect symmetry with respect to the face.
- It is a good option for producing both a provisional prosthesis supported by eyeglasses, and a CT diagnostic template.
- The design may also be used for an immediate provisional adhesive prosthesis that can be delivered to the patient in a few days after surgical resection, to restore an acceptable aesthetic appearance.

Further improvements to our protocol may include using a metal bar for retention on the eyeglasses instead of an acrylic resin one, and using a nose model from a virtual library instead of the pre-surgical anatomy, which may have been altered by tumour involvement in this area.

REFERENCES

Choi J.Y., Choi J.H., Kim N.K., Kim Y., Lee J.K., Kim M.K., Lee J.H. & Kim M.J. (2002) Analysis of errors in medical rapid prototyping models. *International Journal of Oral and Maxillofacial Surgery* **31**, 23–32.

Ciocca L. & Scotti R. (2004) CAD-CAM generated ear cast by means of a laser scanner and rapid prototyping machine. *The Journal of Prosthetic Dentistry* **92**, 591–595.

Ciocca L., Maremonti P., Bianchi B. & Scotti R. (2007) Maxillofacial rehabilitation after rhinectomy using two different treatment options: clinical reports. *Journal of Oral Rehabilitation* **34**, 311–315.

Ciocca L., Mingucci R., Gassino G. & Scotti R. (2007) CAD/CAM ear model and virtual construction of the mold. *The Journal of Prosthetic Dentistry* **98**, 339–343.

Coward T.J., Scott B.J.J., Watson R.M. & Richards R. (2006) A comparison between computerized tomography, magnetic resonance imaging, and laser scanning for capturing 3-dimensional data from a natural ear to aid rehabilitation. *The International Journal of Prosthodontics* **19**, 92–100.

DiLeo M.D., Miller R.H., Rice J.C. & Butcher R.B. (1996) Nasal septal squamous cell carcinoma: a chart review and a meta-analysis. *Laryngoscope* **106**, 1218–22.

Dumbrigue H.B. & Flyer A. (1997) Minimizing prosthesis movement in a midfacial defect: a clinical report. *The Journal of Prosthetic Dentistry* **78**, 341–345.

Flood T.R. & Russell K. (1998) Reconstruction of nasal defects with implant retained nasal prosthesis. *The British Journal of Oral and Maxillofacial Surgery* **36**, 341–345.

Fornelli R.A., Fedock F.G., Wilson E.P. & Rodman S.M. (2000) Squamous cell carcinoma of the anterior nasal cavity: a dual institution review. *Otolaryngology and Head and Neck Surgery* **123**, 207–210.

Harrison D.F. (1982) Total rhinectomy-a worthwhile operation? *The Journal of Laryngology and Otology* **96**, 1113–23.

Hecker D.M., Wiens J.P., Cowper T.R. & Eckert S.E. (2002) Can we assess quality of life in patients with head and neck cancer? A preliminary report from the American Academy of Maxillofacial Prosthetics. *The Journal of Prosthetic Dentistry* **88**, 344–51.

Javid N. (1971) The use of magnets in a maxillofacial prosthesis. *The Journal of Prosthetic Dentistry* **25**, 334–341.

Jiao T., Zhang F., Huang X. & Wang C. (2004) Design and fabrication of auricular prostheses by CAD/CAM system. *The International Journal of Prosthodontics* **17**, 460–463.

Lemon J.C., Chambers M.S., Wesley P.J. & Martin J.W. (1996) Technique for fabricating a mirror-image prosthetic ear. *The Journal of Prosthetic Dentistry* **75**, 292–293.

Mardini M.A., Ercoli C. & Graser G.N. (2005) A technique to produce a mirror-image wax pattern of an ear using rapid prototyping technology. *The Journal of Prosthetic Dentistry* **94**, 195–198.

McGuirt W.F. & Thompson J.N. (1984) Surgical approaches to malignant tumors of the nasal septum. *Laryngoscope* **94**, 1045–1049.

NaBadalung D.P. (2003) Prosthetic rehabilitation of a total rhinectomy patient resulting from squamous cell carcinoma of the nasal septum: a clinical report. *The Journal of Prosthetic Dentistry* **89**, 234–8.

Ugadama A. & King G.E. (1983) Mechanically retained facial prostheses: helpful or harmful? *The Journal of Prosthetic Dentistry* **49**, 85–86.

Update

CAD–CAM Construction of Nasal Prostheses

Leonardo Ciocca, Massimiliano Fantini, Francesca De Crescenzio, and Roberto Scotti

1
Provisional Nasal Prostheses: An Update

A 58-year-old man lost his entire nose in a self-inflicted gunshot injury and was scheduled for a definitive nasal prosthesis anchored to osseointegrated craniofacial implants. His general medical condition did not allow surgical reconstruction. To enable the patient to recover socially, an immediate temporary solution in the form of an eyeglass-supported provisional prosthesis was constructed.

A three-dimensional (3D) laser scan was taken of the patient's facial defect and of the surrounding anatomical structures. Scanning included both ears as they would be used for positioning the digital model of the eyeglasses. A digital model of the entire face was constructed using a laser scanner (NextEngine Desktop 3D Scanner; NextEngine, Santa Monica, CA). Although the class 1M laser beam is classified as enabling eye-safe scanning, the patient's eyes were protected by a protective anti-ultraviolet (UV) mask. Five different perspectives (left, right, frontal, upper, and lower) were used in scanning the patient's face to detect all undercuts. The patient was asked to keep his head firmly positioned in the headrest without moving, to refrain from smiling, and to keep his maxillary arches closed in the maximum intercuspal position. It is important to avoid any movement or alteration in the external profile of the face, caused by smiling or contracting muscles, in order to get good results and achieve good alignment of the different scans during the post-processing operations.

The patient had previously selected a pair of eyeglass frames that were then digitized using a Konica Minolta VI-9i laser scanner (Konica Minolta Sensing, Tokyo, Japan). The temple arms of the eyeglasses were opened and then the eyeglasses were coated with talc powder so as to avoid scanning problems due to the transparency of the lens and the highly reflective nature of the frame. As is usual for reverse engineering postprocessing, the data sets for both the patient's face and the eyeglasses were carefully aligned and merged to obtain the final digital models in a solid-to-layer

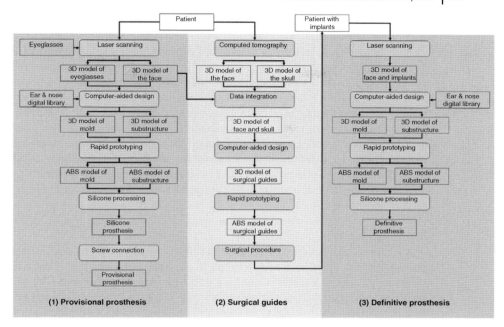

Figure 1 The flowchart of the process updates.

(STL) format. Any surface abnormalities were eliminated during further finishing operations, followed by remeshing and smoothing of the two triangular meshes using Rapidform XOS software (INUS Technology, Seoul, Korea).

The customized prosthesis was then designed using an "ear and nose digital library." This is used when no contralateral healthy side of the patient's face is available for prosthesis development using the mirroring-based approach, as would be the case, for example, with an ear prosthesis. Beginning with the 3D model of the patient's face, a digital anatomic nose was selected as a reference model from the digital library using preinjury photographs of the patient in addition to his facial dimensions. The digital model nose was superimposed on the defect and positioned in a correct anatomic location ensuring that the entire defect was covered. The margin of the prosthesis was adjusted to fit the patient's skin and holes were designed for the nostrils. Once the volume of the prosthesis was designed, the thickness was selected, aiming to reduce as much as possible the mass while giving a minimum 6 mm backward offset to the prosthesis. Due to the need to reduce the weight of the prosthesis to enable it to be supported by the eyeglasses, the prosthesis does not fill the entire volume of the defect; moreover, a thinner prosthesis has the advantage that it is more easily adaptable to the patient's defect, thanks to silicone's elastic properties.

Next, the digital model of the eyeglasses was superimposed on the 3D model of the patient's face using the previously scanned existing anatomical structures as reference points in addition to the designed nasal epithesis. Specifically, the lens rims were centered on the eyes, the temple arms placed over the ears, and the bridge of the eyeglass frame was positioned relative to the upper part of the nasal prosthesis. Once the digital models of the nasal prosthesis and eyeglasses were both in position on the 3D image of the patient's face, the relative connecting substructure was designed, taking into account the volume constraints. The substructure must be entirely contained within the silicone nasal prosthesis with the exception of the upper part, which is connected to the frame of the eyeglasses. This part allows the technician to correctly position the eyeglasses with respect to the substructure and is removed after the silicone is processed. By subtracting the volume of the bridge of the eyeglasses from the upper part of the substructure, the seat for the connection was obtained in a single computer-aided (CAD) environment (Boolean volume difference). In this way, the substructure can be positioned accurately and unambiguously and then attached to the eyeglasses. In addition, three rectangular holes were made in the main body of the substructure to guarantee a firm mechanical fixing within the silicone prosthesis.

Finally, the nasal prosthesis was represented as a negative volume and divided into two sections to create a two-part mold for subsequent conventional silicone processing. A reference seat was designed in the upper part of the mold to fix the substructure in place during silicone processing. When the silicone polymerized, the upper part of the substructure was removed, thereby making it invisible behind the interocular connector of the eyeglasses.

The substructure and the two-part mold were manufactured directly using rapid prototyping techniques. The physical models in acrylonitrile butadiene styrene (ABS) were made using a Stratasys Dimension soluble support technology (SST) 3D printer (Stratasys, Eden Prairie, MN) based on fused deposition modeling (FDM). The working principle of this system is based on a layer-by-layer deposition with a 0.254 mm layer thickness of fused ABS and soluble support material to sustain the overhanging parts of the component being constructed. Once the building process is complete, the model is placed in a bath of hot soapy water and agitated in order to remove the support material.

Before continuing with the silicone molding procedure, the ABS substructure was positioned on the eyeglasses to check that there was no ambiguity with the planned connection and its ease of determination. Next, a hole was drilled in both the eyeglasses and in the connecting region of the substructure at the level of the eyeglasses. An implant abutment (Multi Unit abutment, external connection; NP, Nobel Biocare, Kloten, Switzerland) was fixed to the eyeglasses using epoxy resin, and an implant replica (NP, Nobel Biocare) was inserted into the corresponding part of the substructure. A rigid connection to retain the nasal prosthesis was ensured by a bolt.

The substructure was disconnected from the eyeglasses during the conventional silicone processing procedure and positioned in the mold using the reference hole that had been made in the upper section to facilitate the simple repositioning of the substructure in the mold. The silicone (VST-50F; Factor II, Lakeside, AZ) was processed to obtain the provisional nasal prosthesis using a conventional stone mold processing method, injecting the silicone with a syringe to ensure that it was deposited all around the substructure. The excess silicone was trimmed at the margins to refine the prosthesis.

The intrinsic color of the prosthesis was determined using a spectrometer (SpectroShade Office; MHT, Verona, Italy). The coloring (Extrinsic, Factor II) was applied, a silicone adhesive (A-564, Factor II) was used as a sealant, and a matting dispersion liquid (TS-564, Factor II) was added to give a matte finish to the final prosthesis. Finally, the provisional prosthesis was fixed to the eyeglasses with the bolt and delivered to the patient.

2
Radiological and Surgical Templates for Guiding Craniofacial Implant Insertion: An Update

2.1
Computed Tomography Elaboration Using NobelGuide

The computed tomography (CT) data were uploaded into the NobelGuide software (Nobel Biocare, Kloten, Switzerland) and elaborated to plan the implant surgery in the nasal region, where sufficient bone was available. Two implants (RP, Nobel Biocare, Kloten, Switzerland) were positioned in the premaxillary area, one in the nasal floor and the other in the glabellar region. The implants were 11.5 mm long with a diameter of 3.75 mm. Once the implants were positioned, frontal, lateral, and upper orthographic views (including and excluding the skeletal region of interest) were collected as JPG images.

2.2
CT and Laser Scanner Integration

The CT data were uploaded into Amira 3.1.1 software (Mercury Computer Systems, Chelmsford, MA) and elaborated to reconstruct a 3D model of the skull surface by setting the same threshold value as is used with NobelGuide (276 HU). A 3D digital model of the patient's skin was also obtained by selecting a suitable threshold value. Both models were achieved semiautomatically using threshold-based segmentation, contour extraction, and surface reconstruction, which is a particularly useful process for distinguishing between skeletal structures and soft tissues.

Laser scanner data had been previously collected for the design and manufacture of an eyeglass-supported provisional nasal prosthesis using a laser scanner (NextEngine Desktop 3D Scanner; NextEngine, Santa Monica, CA) to acquire the facial skin surfaces from five different perspectives (right, left, frontal, upper, and lower). The five scans were aligned very carefully, as is usual in reverse engineering postprocessing and merged to obtain the final digital model of the patient's entire face.

The skin surfaces acquired by both CT and laser scanner data were imported into Rapidform XOS2 (INUS Technology, Seoul, Korea). A registration process was used to integrate the data into a single coordinate system. Three pairs of corresponding reference points were chosen on both the laser scanner and the CT skin surfaces to give a rough initial alignment. During this operation, the first shell selected (the skin surface from the laser scanning) was transferred to the second shell selected (the skin surface from the CT data). Iterative closest points (ICP)-based registration was used to semiautomatically refine the alignment.

The surface deviation between the CT and the laser scanner data was analyzed in order to evaluate the accuracy of the registration process. A mean distance of less than 1 mm was found.

Once the registration process is completed, it is simple to use the skin surface acquired from the laser scanner to replace the skin surface reconstructed from the CT after data integration between the skull surface obtained using CT and the skin surface using the laser scanner.

2.3
Virtual Planning Transfer

The frontal, lateral, and upper images (excluding the skeletal region of interest) that were collected using NobelGuide were imported into Rhino 3.0 (Robert McNeel & Associates, Seattle, WA) as background bitmaps in the corresponding views (scaled to match one another and aligned in space). In each of the three views, all construction lines representing the axis of each of the three implants were traced over using background bitmaps as a guide. The *Crv2View* command (curves from two views) was used to create the axis of each implant within the 3D space by choosing the corresponding construction lines in two views. The implants were modeled as cylinders (diameter 3.75 mm and height 11.5 mm) and placed in the 3D space as determined by the relative axis and background bitmaps. Only two views are necessary for this kind of construction, although three views avoid eventual problems caused by overlapping of the reference features in the images.

Digital models of the skull surface obtained using CT and of the skin surface obtained with the laser scanner were also imported in 3D space for referencing. Once the skeletal region of interest, collected using NobelGuide, had been substituted for the background bitmaps with the images, both digital models were moved so as to overlap the skull surface with respect to the new background in each view.

2.4
Designing the Template

Once the transfer into Rhino 3.0 was completed, a three-part template with surgical guides for implant placement was designed. This was composed of a main template for referencing on the patient's head and two interchangeable overhanging surgical guides.

The main template was designed as a customized helmet with a 5 mm offset of the frontal–upper part of the 3D digital model of the scanned face to ensure a correct match with the patient's head. A dovetail joint was added in the front to connect the two surgical guides, both of which were provided with guide cylinders.

The first surgical guide was designed just to mark the skin corresponding to the implant axis before the soft tissues are surgically cut, and the second one guides the drilling of the bone for implant placement.

2.5
Rapid Prototyping the Template

The helmet template and the two interchangeable overhanging surgical guides were manufactured directly using a 3D soluble support technology rapid prototyping system (Stratasys, Eden Prairie, MN). The working principle is based on fused deposition modeling using an ABS P400 and soluble support material that supports the prototype while under construction. With this process, the prototypes are built up in layers (thickness 0.254 mm) with a choice of two available filling options: solid and sparse. In the former, each section of the model is completely filled with ABS material. In the latter, the interior of the model is replaced with a honeycomb structure. Solid fills are stronger and heavier, whereas sparse fills are weaker and lighter, requiring less material and speeding up the building process. This allowed the digital models to be exported in STL format and prototyped directly in a single work session by choosing the sparse fill option for the helmet template and the solid fill option for the overhanging guides so as to obtain stronger elements. The process was finished by removing all the support material by washing the models in an agitation system with a hot soapy water bath for a hands-free models completion.

3
Implant-Supported Definitive Nasal Prostheses: An Update

A 67-year-old man was referred to the Maxillofacial Prosthesis section of the Department of Oral Sciences at the University of Bologna for a nasal prosthesis following ablative surgery of the nose for a squamous cell carcinoma and failure of reconstructive plastic surgery. On examination, the nasal floor appeared suitable for implants insertion. The available bone was evaluated using computed tomography before placing two oral implants (MKIII Ti Unite RP 8.5 Nobel Biocare, Kloten, Switzerland) in the nasal floor.

After 4 months, a second surgical exposure was made. First, a transfer impression (Permadyne Garant 2:1, 3M ESPE, Seefeld, Germany) of the implants was made. Then, a cross-shaped metal bar (Cendres & Métaux SA, Biel/Bienne, Switzerland) was manufactured for retention of the bar clip (Cendres & Métaux) that was connected to the implants. A laser scan (NextEngine Desktop 3D Scanner; NextEngine, Santa Monica, CA) of the patient's facial defect was obtained while the patient's eyes were covered with a protective anti-UV mask. Taking the defect as the ideal center of a hexagon, the defect was scanned from six different angles around the patient's head to detect all undercuts. These meshes were saved as STL files using NextEngine ScanStudio software. The digitalized surfaces were elaborated using Rapidform 2006 software (INUS Technology, Seoul, Korea) to align and merge the different meshes into a single virtual model. All surface abnormalities were eliminated, the organization of the triangulated mesh of points was remeshed, and the surface holes that remained after data elaboration were filled in. A digitalized anatomic nose of correct anatomy was selected from an "ear and nose library" for the patient. This volume was superimposed on the defect, taking into consideration the correct modeling of the emerging profile in the marginal zones of the prosthesis and the design of the holes for the nostrils.

Once the STL file of the nose was developed, the substructure was designed within this space and was rapid prototyped with a Stratasys Dimension soluble support technology 3D printer (Stratasys, Eden Prairie, MN). This rapid prototyping system is based on fused deposition modeling and produces physical models in ABS P400 plastic. The nose was represented as a negative volume and was transformed into a new STL file for the two-part mold design. The upper and lower parts of the mold were processed using the same procedure as used for the substructure. The ABS substructure was positioned in the mold before silicone processing using the scanned bar on the implants as a reference. Conventional silicone (VST-50F; Factor II, Lakeside, AZ) processing procedures were performed in order to obtain the definitive prosthesis [1].

References

1 Beumer, J., Curtis, T.A., and Marunick, M.T. (1996) *Maxillofacial Rehabilitation:* *Prosthetic and Surgical Consideration*, Elsevier, St. Louis, MO, pp. 377–453.

12
Individually Prefabricated Prosthesis for Maxilla Reconstruction

CLINICAL REPORT

Individually Prefabricated Prosthesis for Maxilla Reconstruction

Sekou Singare, PhD,[1] Yaxiong Liu, PhD,[2] Dichen Li, PhD,[2] Bingheng Lu, PhD,[2] Jue Wang, PhD,[4] & Sanhu He[3]

[1] Mechanical Engineering School, Dongguan University of Technology, Guangdong, China University, Xi'an, China
[2] State Key Lab for Manufacturing Systems Engineering, Xi'an Jiaotong University, Xi'an, China
[3] Department of Maxillofacial Surgery, School of Stomatology, Xi'an Jiaotong University, Xi'an, China
[4] Key Laboratory of Biomedical Information Engineering of the Ministry of Education, and Institute of Biomedical Engineering, Xi'an Jiaotong

Keywords
Individual template; designed prosthesis; computer-aided reconstruction; rapid prototyping; rapid tooling.

Correspondence
Sekou Singare, The Key Laboratory of Biomedical Information Engineering of Ministry of Education and Institute of Biomedical Engineering, Xi'an Jiaotong University, Xi'an, 710049, China. E-mail: sekou2d@yahoo.com, sekousingare@hotmail.com

Accepted 18 September 2006

doi: 10.1111/j.1532-849X.2007.00266.x

Abstract

The reconstruction of maxillofacial bone defects by the intraoperative modeling of implants may reduce the predictability of the esthetic result, leading to more invasive surgery and increased surgical time. To improve the maxillofacial surgery outcome, modern manufacturing methods such as rapid prototyping (RP) technology and methods based on reverse engineering (RE) and medical imaging data are applicable to the manufacture of custom-made maxillary prostheses. After acquisition of data, an individual computer-based 3D model of the bony defect is generated. These data are transferred into RE software to create the prosthesis using a computer-aided design (CAD) model, which is directed into the RP machine for the production of the physical model. The precise fit of the prosthesis is evaluated using the prosthesis and skull models. The prosthesis is then directly used in investment casting such as "Quick Cast" pattern to produce the titanium model. In the clinical reports presented here, reconstructions of two patients with large maxillary bone defects were performed using this new method. The custom prostheses perfectly fit the defects during the operations, and surgery time was reduced. These cases show that the prefabrication of a prosthesis using modern manufacturing technology is an effective method for maxillofacial defect reconstruction.

Conventionally, reconstructions of maxillary defects have been achieved with autografts[1-3] or prosthetic maxillary obturators.[4] Bone grafts have become the common method used in maxillofacial surgery; however, use of a bone graft increases length of surgery, blood loss, and donor site morbidity, and risks failure of the graft due to bone resorption.[5] A prosthetic maxillary obturator is an alternative for maxillary defect reconstruction. Although acceptable results can eventually be achieved in many cases, patients may become dissatisfied, because the removable prosthesis lacks sufficient retentiveness for adequate speech, swallowing, and acceptable esthetic appearance. Poor retention because of denture bulkiness and poor residual dentition can result in leakage and oronasal regurgitation. Patients must maintain adequate hygiene at the surgical site and around the prosthesis.[2] Due to these limitations, a bridging titanium implant can be used as an alternative for functional maxillary reconstruction. Reconstruction of the defect by means of bridging titanium implants avoids the need for bone grafting and the problems associated with resorption of grafted bone, and requires only a minor surgical procedure for implant insertion.

Conventional CT and MRI scans are standardized and are important diagnostic tools for assessing the extent of tumor resection.[6,7] The reconstructed 3D data from the CT can be transferred in the operating room to accurately determine the resection margins of the tumor, simplifying the surgical procedure;[8] however, tumor resection or defect reconstruction based on 3D imaging modalities presents difficulties in defining the resection plane with sufficient accuracy. On the other hand, stereolithographic models are more concrete, allowing the surgeon to actually simulate the surgical procedure or even to generate patient-specific templates that can be used in the surgery.

In the field of maxillofacial surgery, implants are often manufactured on life-size stereolithographic models.[9] Because of the manual sculpting necessary for anatomically-shaped implant geometry, this technique does not allow an accurate geometrical modeling approach as does computer-aided design (CAD)-based implant modeling. As the result of the development of modern design and manufacturing technology, a customized medical implant and surgical resection template that matches skeletal anatomy can now be accurately designed

Individually Prefabricated Prosthesis for Maxilla Reconstruction

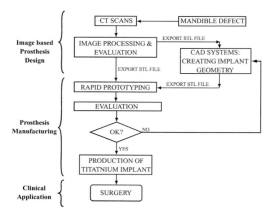

Figure 1 Computer-aided geometric modeling for the production of custom implants.

using a CAD technique.[10-12] The physical model of the individual implant, template, or skull replica can be produced through rapid prototyping (RP), rapid tooling (RT), and computer aided manufacturing/computer numerical control (CAM/CNC) processes.[13-24] The RP model facilitates surgical simulation and planning.[9,25-28]

This report describes a new method of constructing a prefabricated implant based on modern CAD and RP techniques. The method provides a long-term, stable, precisely-fitting replacement prosthesis for large maxillary bone defects. The CAD model prosthesis is designed using reverse engineering (RE) software and is directly fabricated using a stereolithography machine. This direct fabrication avoids the necessity for indirect manual modeling on full-size models. Two patients have received maxillary reconstruction with this type of implant with satisfactory results.

The proposed approach as shown in Figure 1 includes an image-based prosthesis design process, manufacture, and clinical application.

Image-based prosthesis design

The skull of the patient is scanned using CT, and the 2D image slices from the CT scans are imported into commercial Materialise Interactive Medical Image Control System (MIMICS) software (Materialise NV, Leuven, Belgium). The CT data are then segmented to generate a 3D volumetric image of the patient's skull anatomy. Once the 3D volumetric has been generated, contours are calculated and exported as follows:

1. As Initial Graphics Exchange Specification (IGES) format, which is directly imported into Geomagics Studio 6.0 (Raindrop Geomagic, Inc., Research Triangle Park, NC) as a point cloud for implant CAD design.

2. As binary data such as standard tessellation language (stereolithography)(STL) format, which is directly imported into stereolithography for the production of a life-size skull model.

After 3D reconstruction in MIMICS, the next step is to reconstruct the CAD model of the implant from the point cloud. The imported point cloud first must be processed in RE software (Geomagic Studio 6, Raindrop Geomagic, Inc.) to reduce the file size. The points are then denoised and wrapped as polygonal surfaces. Certain defects, such as holes in the surface, must be removed to obtain close manifolds (Figs 2A and 3A).

Prosthesis geometry modeling before tumor resection

The prosthesis for repairing the maxilla can actually be designed before resection of the tumor. First, the approximate area occupied by the tumor is identified on the initial CT diagnostic images. Using the information acquired from imaging diagnostics, the location of the exact tumor borders are identified, traced (Fig 2B), and cut out to isolate the tumor image. The cut out tumor image serves as the design template for the tumor resection. The prosthesis geometrical design includes: the segment to be resected, the margin from the border of the segment to be resected, and microplates for fixation (Fig 2C). Three individual microplates with bone-adherent surfaces for fixation are constructed to blend well with the outer contours of the segment to be resected to allow prosthesis fixation; these bone adherent surfaces are derived directly from the data of the maxilla contour, and the resection border planes are used for the margins of the prosthesis body. The nonuniform rational B-spline (NURBS) surfaces are then fitted into these geometrical contours to generate the individual prosthesis CAD model and tumor resection template. Basically, the resection template

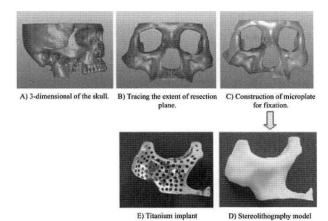

Figure 2 CAD implant construction before tumor resection.

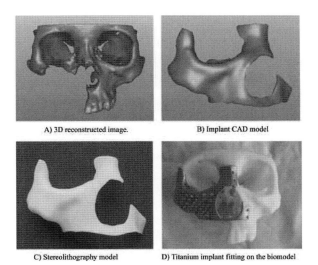

Figure 3 CAD implant construction after tumor resection.

geometry can be used as a surgical aid for tumor resection, with the prosthesis used to bridge the maxillary defect after tumor removal.

Prosthesis geometrical modeling after tumor resection

For a unilateral bone defect, such as the one shown in Figure 3A, the missing tissue is reconstructed by using mirror imaging techniques. First, the mirror plane is created (reference system), and the nondefect side (healthy maxilla) is mirrored to the defect side. The overall implant shape is obtained by applying a Boolean subtraction of the damaged portion of the maxilla with the skull. Individual microplates for fixation are derived directly from the maxilla contour data, and the prosthesis margins are derived from the border of the defect. Next, NURBS patches are used to fit across these geometrical contours to generate the prosthesis CAD surface model, and the surface is thickened to generate the solid model (Fig 3B).

Manufacturing

The CAD data for the prosthesis with corresponding resection templates are translated into an STL file format and imported into the RP machine to fabricate the physical object (Figs 2D and 3C). During surgery, the individual SLA template will be placed in its predefined position, and the optimal position of the resection plane can be found easily. Alternatively, the SLA model prosthesis can be fitted on the skull biomodel to evaluate symmetry, accuracy of surface fitting, etc. In addition, the surgery can be simulated on the biomodel (Fig 3D).

Finally, the stereolithography apparatus (SLA) prosthesis pattern is directly used in investment casting such as Quick-Cast for production of the titanium prosthesis (Figs 2E and 3D). Holes are inserted in the implant body after completion of the CAD/CAM process for better soft-tissue integration.

Clinical application

Case 1

As shown in Figure 4B, a 64-year-old patient, who had been diagnosed with gingival carcinoma of the right upper jaw, underwent maxillary reconstruction. Using the information acquired from imaging diagnostics, a resection template was CAD/CAM fabricated with the titanium implant to provide one-step reconstruction. During surgery, the tumor was exposed, and the resection template was fitted to the surface of the affected bone in order to mark the resection margin. Then the segment of the affected bone inside the marked area was resected based on the contour of the individual resection template SLA model to ensure adequate tumor clearance. The upper jaw was then immediately reconstructed with the custom-made titanium prosthesis as shown in Figure 4A. In this case, the information acquired from 3D-CT reconstructed data have contributed to

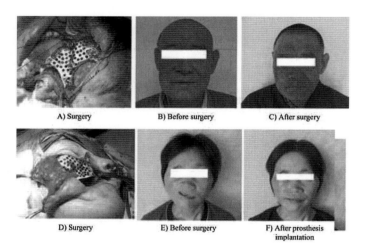

Figure 4 Maxilla reconstruction.

the assessment of tumor extension, as well as its location in the patient's anatomy, and also were helpful in the determination of adequate limits of tumor resection. As a result, resection and reconstruction were thus highly precise, safe, and fast. There were no difficulties during reconstruction, because the individual titanium implant is prefabricated with a geometry fitting to that of the template. As a consequence, the implant closes the bone defect perfectly and so the contour is reconstructed precisely. No complications or tumor recurrences were seen in a 1-year follow-up period, and the patient was satisfied with the result.

Case 2

As shown in Figure 4E, a 34-year-old female patient presented at the hospital reporting pain in her right upper teeth for the past 2 months and nasal blood secretions for the past 20 days. Clinical examination revealed swelling of her right maxilla sinus with middling density and uneven quality, extending into the middle nasal meatus. The inner wall of the maxillary sinus had broken into the nasal septum. Adenocarcinoma of the maxilla was diagnosed.

The patient underwent maxillary bone resection for the first surgery; her wound healed well with no recurrence of the tumor, but with 1/3 facial deformation and severe diplopia. She returned to the hospital for deformation correction and repair. The customized titanium maxillary prosthesis was fabricated as shown in Figure 3 and implanted successfully at the correct position during surgery (Fig 4D).

Clinical outcome

Three-dimensional CT images and stereolithographically-produced models were helpful for the determination of the extent of the necessary resection area and defect reconstruction.

The customized prefabricated prostheses fit the maxillary defects well in both patients, and no adjustments were needed during the surgery. As a result, briefer surgical time was required. Rigid fixation of both implants was achieved using screws. The reconstructed maxillary contour and facial symmetry were judged to be good in both patients, as shown in Figures 4C and 4F. (Post-surgical swelling is obvious in Fig 4C, but this swelling was eventually relieved.) Complications were not observed during the follow-up period.

Discussion

The maxillary skeleton serves as the functional and esthetic keystones of the midface. Defects in the palatomaxillary complex can lead to devastating functional and cosmetic consequences.[29] Multiple reconstructive techniques, such as autologous tissue transfers and alloplastic materials, have been available for many years, but reconstruction of extensive defects with autologous bone is limited by the amount of available donor bone, difficulty with 3D contouring, and poor tissue tolerance and acceptance.[30] The use of alloplastic materials, such as reconstruction plates, has several risks, including plate exposure, plate and screw fracture, screw loosening, infection, and limited esthetic and functional restoration.[31] On the other hand, some studies have recommended a bridging plate for advanced oral cancer with a poor prognosis or poor performance status rather than vascularized free bone.[32,33]

Until now most implants have been manually shaped intraoperatively on the surgical site. Intraoperative adaptation of the implant is a difficult task, however, due to lack of visualization of the facial anatomy, with the result that an undesirable shape can be obtained when use of complex 3D contouring is required.[28] Furthermore, intraoperative modeling is time-consuming and reduces accuracy, often leading to more invasive surgery, and impairing esthetic results. The use of a CAD/CAM system is an adequate method for the design and manufacture of very complex 3D prosthesis shapes that are difficult, if not impossible, to create with conventional techniques. Intraoperative adaptation can be avoided when using prefabricated individual titanium implants. On the other hand, the use of CAD-based prosthesis modeling can avoid indirect manual fabrication on a life-size stereolithography model, which always increases cost, decreases precision, and does not use the advantages of geometric design in CAD/CAM.[18]

As the majority of tumor-related maxilla deformities are unilateral, CAD using RP technologies is an effective technique for generating a precise prosthesis shape for reestablishing maxilla symmetry and an individual template for tumor resection. Compared with intraoperative navigation systems for tumor resection, the use of an individual resection template eliminates the need for complex equipment and time-consuming work under radiographic control or registration procedures in the operating room.[34]

Creating the 3D model of bone structures extracted from CT image data allows not only for prosthesis design, but also provides very good visualization of the defect for preoperative surgical evaluation and planning. The preoperative preparation, symmetry, and precise fit implant evaluation can be performed much more easily on the physical model generated by RP. As a consequence, the operating time is reduced, and potential intraoperative errors can be modified preoperatively and thus avoided during the actual surgery.

The cases presented demonstrate the efficacy and accuracy of using combined technologies of 3D-CT data and a stereolithography-produced model for tumor resection guidance and defect reconstruction. One drawback of this approach is that it depends on preoperative CT imaging and, therefore exposes the patient to high radiation exposure. On the other hand, the solid modeling of implant and surgical template in a CAD system is time-consuming, which makes it unsuitable for emergency cases.

We can conclude that CT imaging, RP, and computer modeling have improved the surgical planning and the manufacture of customized implants and have also achieved efficient immediate reconstruction. In such clinical cases, a computer-generated model allows the fabrication of a custom prosthesis that very accurately represents the anatomic defect. The use of these techniques leads to reduced operating time, fewer surgical errors, more precise fit, and high stability after screw fixation. Other advantages include simplification of the surgical procedure; the method also permits testing implant fit before the actual surgery, and determination of accurate positioning of the implant. As result, the actual surgery consists only of defining the defect and placement and fixation of the implant.

Acknowledgments

The authors express their deepest gratitude and thanks to the National Natural Science Foundation of China (No. 50235020, No. 50575170) and DongGuan Research Development Special Foundation (No. 2006D015) for their assistance with the rapid prototyping activities presented in this paper.

References

1. Ostric SA, Martin WJ, Stock C, et al: The model graft: reconstruction of the maxilla using a fibular bone graft template. J Craniofac Surg 2006;17:145-147
2. Peng X, Mao C, Yu GY, et al: Maxillary reconstruction with the free fibula flap. Plast Reconstr Surg 2005;115: 1562-1569
3. Pryor SG, Moore EJ, Kasperbauer JL: Orbital exenteration reconstruction with rectus abdominis microvascular free flap. Laryngoscope 2005;115:1912-1916
4. Uckan S, Oguz Y, Uyar Y, et al: Reconstruction of a total maxillectomy defect with a zygomatic implant-retained obturator. J Craniofac Surg 2005;16:485-489
5. Okura M, Isomura ET, Iida S, et al: Long-term outcome and factors influencing bridging plates for mandibular reconstruction. Oral Oncol 2005;41:791-798
6. Gagliardi G, Bayar S, Smith R, et al: Preoperative staging of rectal cancer using magnetic resonance imaging with external phase-arrayed coils. Arch Surg 2002;137:447-451
7. Kahler DM, Zura RD, Mallik K: Computer guided placement of iliosacral screws compared to standard fluoroscopic technique. 5th Symposium on CAOS Computer Assisted Orthopaedic Surgery. 2002, Davos, Switzerland
8. Bettega G, Dessenne V, Cinquin P, et al: Computer assisted mandibular condyle positioning in orthognatic surgery. J Oral Maxillofac Surg 1996;54:553-558
9. Bill JS, Reuther JF, Dittmann W, et al: Stereolithography in oral and maxillofacial operation planning. Int J Oral Maxillofac Surg 1995;24:98-103
10. Dean D, Min KJ, Bond A: Computer aided design of large-format prefabricated cranial plates. J Craniofac Surg 2003;14:819-832
11. Singare S, Dichen L, Bingheng L, et al: Design and fabrication of custom mandible titanium tray based on rapid prototyping. Med Eng Phys 2004;26:671-676
12. Singare S, Dichen L, Bingheng L, et al: Customized design and manufacturing of chin implant based on rapid prototyping. Rapid Prototyping J 2005;11:113-118
13. Barker TM, Earwaker WJ, Frost N, et al: Integration of 3-D medical imaging and rapid prototyping to create stereolithographic models. Aust Phys Eng Sci Med 1993;16: 79-85
14. Bouyssie JF, Bouyssie S, Sharrock P, et al: Stereolithographic models derived from x-ray computed tomography. Reproduction accuracy. Surg Radiol Anat 1997;19:193-199
15. D'Urso PS, Barker TM, Earwaker WJ, et al: Stereolithographic biomodelling in cranio-maxillofacial surgery: a prospective trial. J Craniomaxillofac Surg 1999;27:30-37
16. Ellis DS, Toth BA, Stewart WB: Three dimensional imaging and computer-designed prostheses in the evaluation and management of orbitocranial deformities. Adv Ophthalmic Plast Reconstr Surg 1992;9:261-272
17. Eufinger H, Wehmoller M, Machtens E, et al: Reconstruction of craniofacial bone defects with individual alloplastic implants based on CAD/CAM-manipulated CT-data. J Craniomaxillofac Surg 1995;23:175-181
18. Eufinger H, Wehmöller M: Individual prefabricated titanium implants in reconstructive craniofacial surgery: Clinical and technical aspects of the first 22 cases. Plast Reconstr Surg 1998;102:300-308
19. Goh JC, Ho NC, Bose K: Principles and applications of computer-aided design and computer-aided manufacturing (CAD/CAM) technology in orthopaedics. Ann Acad Med Singapore 1990;19:706-713
20. Heissler E, Fischer FS, Bolouri S, et al: Custom-made cast titanium implants produced with CAD/CAM for the reconstruction of cranium defects. Int J Oral Maxillofac Surg 1998;27:334-338
21. Hieu LC, Bohez E, Vander Sloten J, et al: Design for medical rapid prototyping of cranioplasty implants. Rapid Prototyping J 2003;9:175-186
22. Warnke PH, Springer IN, Wiltfang J, et al: Growth and transplantation of a custom vascularised bone graft in a man. Lancet 2004;364:766-770
23. Winder J, Cooke RS, Gray J, et al: Medical rapid prototyping and 3D CT in the manufacture of custom made cranial titanium plates. J Med Eng Technol 1999;23:26-28
24. Winder J, Bibb R: Medical rapid prototyping technologies: state of the art and current limitations for application in oral and maxillofacial surgery. J Oral Maxillofac Surg 2005;63:1006-1015
25. Abe M, Tabuchi K, Goto M, et al: Model-based surgical planning and simulation of cranial base surgery. Neurol Med Chir (Tokyo) 1998;38:746-751
26. Anderl H, Zur Nedden D, Muhlbauer W, et al: CT-guided stereolithography as a new tool in craniofacial surgery. Br J Plast Surg 1994;47:60-64
27. Sailer HF, Haers PE, Zollikofer CP, et al: The value of stereolithographic models for preoperative diagnosis of craniofacial deformities and planning of surgical corrections. Int J Oral Maxillofac Surg 1998;27:327-333
28. Muller A, Krishnan KG, Uhl E, et al: The application of rapid prototyping techniques in cranial reconstruction and preoperative planning in neurosurgery. J Craniofac Surg 2003;14:899-914
29. Genden EM, Wallace D, Buchbinder D, et al: Iliac crest internal oblique osteomusculocutaneous free flap reconstruction of the postablative palatomaxillary defect. Arch Otolaryngol Head Neck Surg 2001;127:854-861
30. Blake GB, MacFarlane MR, Hinton JW: Titanium in reconstructive surgery of the skull and face. Br J Plast Surg 1990;43:528-535
31. Doty JM, Pienkowski D, Goltz M, et al: Biomechanical evaluation of fixation techniques for bridging segmental mandibular defects. Arch Otolaryngol Head Neck Surg 2004;130:1388-1392
32. Head C, Alam D, Sercarz JA, et al: Microvascular flap reconstruction of the mandible: a comparison of bone grafts and bridging plates for restoration of mandibular continuity. Otolaryngol Head Neck Surg 2003;129:48-54
33. Poli T, Ferrari S, Bianchi B, et al: Primary oromandibular reconstruction using free flaps and thorp plates in cancer patients: a 5-year experience. Head Neck 2003;25:15-23
34. Birnbaum K, Schkommodau E, Decker N, et al: Computer-assisted orthopedic surgery with individual templates and comparison to conventional operation method. Spine 2001;26:365-370

Update

Individually Prefabricated Prosthesis for Maxilla Reconstruction

Sekou Singare, Yaxiong Liu, Dichen Li, Bingheng Lu, Jue Wang, and Sanhu He

At present, most of the maxilla/mandible restoration implants are fabricated by hand-forming technique. The method involves prebending the reconstruction plate on the stereolithography model to cover the defect. The precision of fit and durability of implant mainly rely on the abilities of the technicians.

Requirements for developing a mandible reconstruction implant from CAD/CAM are durability, precision of fit, and cost. To fulfill these requirements, an approach was developed that integrated computer-aided design (CAD) and rapid prototyping (RP) systems with medical imaging systems and rapid tooling technology to fabricate the maxilla reconstruction implant. The advantage of this method is that a 3D hard copy of the patient maxilla can be generated for use in surgical rehearsal, surgical planning, and custom implant design and prostheses production so that the patient satisfaction can be achieved.

In general, an image-based bio-CAD modeling process involves the following three major steps: (1) noninvasive image acquisition such as a stack of computed tomography (CT) cross-sectional images; (2) imaging process and three-dimensional reconstruction of the region of interest (ROI) to form voxels that describe the 3D shape of the model to be used for further modeling, analysis, or prototyping; and (3) prosthesis design.

1
Data Acquisition

Data acquisition for 3Dmodeling was performed using a helical tomography (CT) imaging. CT scanning was performed with a Picker MX8000 with the following parameter: 120 kV and 150 mA, 512 × 512 matrix, and 1.3 mm slice thickness. The data were transferred to a CD-ROM and loaded into the Mimics software (Materialise, Belgium) to segment CT data so as to expose the anatomy of interest.

Computer Aided Biomanufacturing, Edited by Roger Narayan and Paul Calvert
© 2011 WILEY-VCH Verlag GmbH & Co. KGaA. Published 2011 by WILEY-VCH Verlag GmbH & Co. KGaA.

2
Image Processing and 3D Geometry Extraction

Materialise's Interactive Medical Image Control System (Mimics) is an interactive tool for visualization and segmentation of CT images. Mimics can be used for diagnostic, operation planning, or rehearsal purposes. Mimics can also be used either to export the medical data to CAD software to design the custom-made prosthesis or to transfer the segmentation directly to rapid prototyping systems for building the segmentation objects (physical 3D model). The 3D image processing is described in the following sections.

2.1
Thresholding

In thresholding technique, one can select a region of interest such as soft tissue or bone by defining a range of threshold value. In order to select as much bone tissue as possible without selecting any soft tissue, a threshold value of 1441 HU (Hounsfield units) was chosen to identify the bony region.

2.2
Region Growing: Separation of Different Tissues

The region growing was used to isolate only the bony structure from the overall CT image.

2.3
3D Calculations

By applying 3D calculation feature, Mimics automatically calculates a 3D model of the region of interest.

2.4
3D Displays

Mimics can display the 3D model in any of the windows with visualization functions that include real-time rotation, pan, zoom, and so on.

When segmentation and visualization is complete, the data can be translated into instructions for designing the implant using reverse engineering and manufacture of parts often by rapid prototyping.

The International Graphics Exchange Standard (IGES) format or the Standard for Exchange of Product (STEP) model can be used for models to be exported to CAD and the STL format used to import models from CAD to the rapid prototyping system interface.

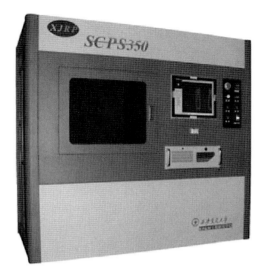

Figure 1 RP systems.

3
Rapid Prototyping Medical Model Production

Finally, 3D virtual model in STL format should be inputted into the RP software for production of 3D physical model (see Figure 1). In this study, the prosthesis and the skull model were manufactured using the stereolithography system of the SCPS laser RP machine type. SCPS laser RP machines use a solid freeform fabrication method to build a physical model through a layer-by-layer building process.

To build the part, the solid model was converted to STL file format. STL is a facet-based representation that approximates surface and solid entities only. It is a triangulated file containing the information about vertices of the triangles and the normal vector directions. The STL file was loaded into the data-processing software (RP-Data were developed in our institute) to check for the closeness at all surfaces and edges. RP-Data allow the file to be checked and repaired if the conversion software has made any omission. The optimal orientation for part building was selected and the CAD model was sliced into 0.1 mm layer thickness and the support was created. The data was imported into the RP machine to fabricate the physical object.

SCPS laser RP machines directly control UV light through CAD data to scan the resin and produce a prototype layer by layer.

4
Technical Parameters

Scanning speed: 0.1–0.25 m/s
Light spot diameter: <0.4 mm

Building volume: 350 × 350 × 350 mm^3
Power consumption: 3 kW

5
Prosthesis Casting

The RP model was embedded in a high-temperature-resistant phosphate investment material. After successive drying and dipping, the entire RP part was placed in an oven to burn out the resin at 300–600 °C. This led to a casting mold. Then, the molten pure titanium was protected in an inert atmosphere and poured into the mold. After the solidification of the metal, the mold was broken down to take out the titanium prosthesis; and the gating system was cut off. The titanium prosthesis was then subjected to postprocessing including, among others, trimming, sandblasting, and drilling.

6
Discussion

The maxillary skeleton serves as the functional and aesthetic keystone of the midface. Defects in the palatomaxillary complex can lead to devastating functional and cosmetic consequences [1]. Multiple reconstructive techniques, such as autologous tissue transfers and alloplastic materials, have been available for many years, but reconstruction of extensive defects with autologous bone is limited by the amount of available donor bone, difficulty with 3D contouring, and poor tissue tolerance and acceptance [2]. The use of alloplastic materials, such as reconstruction plates, has several risks, including plate exposure, plate and screw fracture, screw loosening, infection, and limited esthetic and functional restoration [3]. On the other hand, some studies have recommended a bridging plate for advanced oral cancer with a poor prognosis or poor performance status rather than vascularized free bone [4, 5].

Until now most implants have been manually shaped intraoperatively on the surgical site. Intraoperative adaptation of the implant is a difficult task, however, due to lack of visualization of the facial anatomy, with the result that an undesirable shape can be obtained when the use of complex 3D contouring is required [6]. Furthermore, intraoperative modeling is time consuming and reduces accuracy, often leading to more invasive surgery and impairing aesthetic results. Hieu *et al.* [7], Gopakumar [8], and Lohfeld *et al.* [9] after studying the designing cranial and maxillofacial implant claim that there is a reduction of time in implementing the integrated approach of medical imaging, CAD, FEA, and LM for fabricating personalized medical implants.

The development and advancement of three-dimensional CT imaging has been very helpful in evaluating skull deformities and surgical planning. Medical imaging provides important data on various body structures for diagnostic purposes. These data can be used to obtain geometrical information of the body structures for three-dimensional modeling. Once the acquisition process of the CT scan is complete, the CT images are processed, segmented, and three-dimensionally reconstructed. Solid models can then be generated for use in CAD systems to design the custom implants, and the export of data to a RP machine for the manufacture of the solid models. The use of a CAD and RP system is an adequate method for the design and manufacture of very complex 3D prosthesis shapes that are difficult, if not impossible, to create with conventional techniques. Intraoperative adaptation can be avoided when using prefabricated individual titanium implants. On the other hand, the use of CAD-based prosthesis modeling can avoid indirect manual fabrication on a life-size stereolithography model, which always increases cost, decreases precision, and does not use the advantages of geometric design in CAD/CAM [10].

As the majority of tumor-related maxilla deformities are unilateral, CAD using RP technologies is an effective technique for generating a precise prosthesis shape for reestablishing maxilla symmetry and an individual template for tumor resection. Compared to intraoperative navigation systems for tumor resection, the use of an individual resection template eliminates the need for complex equipment and time-consuming work under radiographic control or registration procedures in the operating room [11].

Creating the 3D model of bone structures extracted from CT image data not only allows for prosthesis design but also provides very good visualization of the defect for preoperative surgical evaluation and planning [12]. The preoperative preparation, symmetry, and precise fit implant evaluation can be performed much more easily on the physical model generated by RP. As a consequence, the operating time is reduced, and potential intraoperative errors can be modified preoperatively and thus avoided during the actual surgery. The cases presented demonstrate the efficacy and accuracy of using combined technologies of CT 3D data and a stereolithography-produced model for tumor resection guidance and defect reconstruction. One drawback of this approach is that it depends on preoperative CT imaging and, therefore, exposes the patient to high radiation. On the other hand, the solid modeling of implant and surgical template in a CAD system is time consuming, making it unsuitable for emergency cases.

We can conclude that CT imaging, RP, and computer modeling have improved the surgical planning and the manufacture of customized implants and have also achieved efficient immediate reconstruction. In such clinical cases, a computer-generated model allows the fabrication of a custom prosthesis that very accurately represents the anatomic defect. The use of these techniques leads to reduced operating time, fewer surgical errors, more precise fit, and high stability after screw fixation. Other advantages include simplification of the surgical procedure; the method also permits testing implant fit before the actual surgery and determination of accurate positioning of the implant. As a result, the actual surgery consists only of defining the defect and placement and fixation of the implant.

Acknowledgments

The authors acknowledge the support provided by Dongguan Science and Technology Project (2007108101007) and DongGuan Research Development Special Foundation (No. 2006D015) in this study.

References

1 Genden, E.M., Wallace, D., Buchbinder, D. et al. (2001) Iliac crest internal oblique osteomusculocutaneous free flap reconstruction of the postablative palatomaxillary defect. *Arch. Otolaryngol. Head Neck Surg.*, **127**, 854–861.

2 Blake, G.B., MacFarlane, M.R., and Hinton, J.W. (1990) Titanium in reconstructive surgery of the skull and face. *Br. J. Plast. Surg.*, **43**, 528–535.

3 Doty, J.M., Pienkowski, D., Goltz, M. et al. (2004) Biomechanical evaluation of fixation techniques for bridging segmental mandibular defects. *Arch. Otolaryngol. Head Neck Surg.*, **130**, 1388–1392.

4 Head, C., Alam, D., Sercarz, J.A. et al. (2003) Microvascular flap reconstruction of the mandible: a comparison of bone grafts and bridging plates for restoration of mandibular continuity. *Otolaryngol. Head Neck Surg.*, **129**, 48–54.

5 Poli, T., Ferrari, S., Bianchi, B. et al. (2003) Primary oromandibular reconstruction using free flaps and thorp plates in cancer patients: a 5-year experience. *Head Neck*, **25**, 15–23.

6 Muller, A., Krishnan, K.G., Uhl, E., and Mast, G. (2003) The application of rapid prototyping techniques in cranial reconstruction and preoperative planning in neurosurgery. *J. Craniofac. Surg.*, **14**, 899–914.

7 Hieu, L.C., Bohez, E., Vander Sloten, J. et al. (2003) Design for medical rapid prototyping of cranioplasty implants. *J. Rapid Prototyping*, **9**, 175–186.

8 Gopakumar, S. (2004) RP in medicine: a case study in cranial reconstructive surgery. *Rapid Prototyping J.*, **10** 207–211.

9 Lohfeld, S., McHugh, P., Serban, D., Boyle, D., O'Donnnell, G., and Peckitt, N. (2007) Engineering assisted surgery: a route for digital design and manufacturing of customised maxillofacial implants. *J. Mater. Process. Technol.*, **183**, 333–338.

10 Eufinger, H. and Wehmöller, M. (1998) Individual prefabricated titanium implants in reconstructive craniofacial surgery: clinical and technical aspects of the first 22 cases. *Plast. Reconstr. Surg.*, **102**, 300–308.

11 Birnbaum, K., Schkommodau, E., Decker, N. et al. (2001) Computer-assisted orthopedic surgery with individual templates and comparison to conventional operation method. *Spine*, **26**, 365–370.

12 Singare, S. et al. (2009) Rapid prototyping assisted surgery planning and custom implant design. *Rapid Prototyping J.*, **15/1**, 19–23.

13
The Use of Rapid Prototyping Didactic Models in the Study of Fetal Malformations

Letters to the Editor

The use of rapid prototyping didactic models in the study of fetal malformations

The importance of rapid prototyping (RP) in the biomedical sector has been increasing steadily during the past decade. Different uses of RP models have been reported widely in the medical scientific literature[1,2]. In our eight studied cases, of which the final models of two are presented, RP was performed after magnetic resonance imaging (MRI) (Figure 1) or computed tomography (CT) (Figure 2) of fetuses at gestational ages greater than 26 weeks. The indications for MRI were central nervous system, thoracic, gastrointestinal or genitourinary malformations, and skeletal malformations for CT. All cases were examined first by ultrasound imaging. MRI examinations were performed using a 1.5-T scanner (Siemens, Erlangen, Germany). The protocol consisted of: T2-weighted sequence in the three planes of the fetal body (HASTE; repetition time, shortest; echo time, 140 ms; field of view, 300–200 mm; 256 × 256 matrix; slice thickness, 4 mm; acquisition time, 17 s; 40 slices). The entire examination time did not exceed 30 min[3]. CT was performed using a multislice 64 scanner (Philips, Solingen, Germany) with the following parameters: 40 mA, 120 kV, 64 slices per rotation, pitch 0.75 and slice thickness 0.75 mm. This corresponds to a mean radiation dose to the fetus of 3.12 mGy (CT dose index weighted). The acquisition lasted around 20 s and was performed during maternal apnea[4].

In order to construct physical models from the medical examinations (MRI and CT) of the cases described, with the aim of didactic use, the first step was the production of three-dimensional (3D) virtual models. These models are made by the use of medical segmentation software (ScanIP version 2.0, Simpleware Ltd., Exeter, UK) to select the contours, allied to design and engineering software (Dassault Systèmes, SolidWorks Corp., and Autodesk Maya) that is used when connections are necessary between parts, and also for surface smoothing and adjustments. When the 3D virtual model is ready, the next step is its physical materialization using RP technology, which works by the principle of overlapping of layers of materials (selected according to the RP technology)[5].

In the first case, to build the model presented (Figure 1), the technology adopted was fused deposition modeling. The material used was thermoplastic acrylonitrile butadiene styrene and the total machine time for the RP construction was 32 h. The model required a supporting water-soluble material, which was removed after the construction process through immersion in an ultrasound bath in a liquid release agent. The final production cost of this model was US$280.

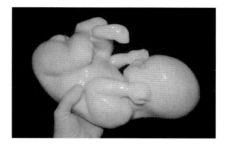

Figure 1 Rapid prototyping model of a fetus created using fused deposition modeling after magnetic resonance imaging at 34 weeks.

The second model presented was made using the 3D Systems Viper Stereolithography process (Figure 2), in which a laser is used to 'draw' successive cross-sectional layers in a photosensitive resin. The building process was followed by a postprocessing stage, in which the support was removed and the piece cleaned by removing polymer residues that did not harden during the building process. The model was then totally hardened under ultraviolet light. The RP machine time was 26 h, with a final production cost of US$240.

Through the associated use of MRI and CT with RP technologies, we believe that physical models will help, in a didactic, tactile and interactive manner, the study of complex malformations by a multidisciplinary staff.

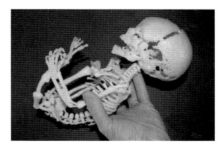

Figure 2 Rapid prototyping model of the skeleton of a fetus created using stereolithography after computed tomography at 35 weeks.

H. Werner*†, J. R. Lopes dos Santos‡§, R. Fontes‡,
E. L. Gasparetto†¶, P. A. Daltro†, Y. Kuroki†
and R. C. Domingues†
†*Clínica de Diagnóstico por Imagem,*
‡*Instituto Nacional de Tecnologia and*
¶*Department of Radiology,*
Federal University of Rio de Janeiro School of Medicine,
Rio de Janeiro, Brazil, and
§*Royal College of Art, London, UK*
*Correspondence.
(e-mail: heron.werner@gmail.com)
DOI: 10.1002/uog.6253
Published online 13 November 2008

References

1. Armillotta A, Bonhoeffer P, Dubini G, Ferragina S, Migliavacca F, Sala G, Schievano S. Use of rapid prototyping models in the planning of percutaneous pulmonary valved stent implantation. *Proc Inst Mech Eng* 2007; **221**: 407–416.
2. Robinoy M, Salvo I, Costa F, Zerman N, Bazzocchi M, Toso F, Bandera C, Filippi S, Felice M, Politi M. Virtual reality surgical planning for maxillofacial distraction osteogenesis: the role of reverse engineering rapid prototyping and cooperative work. *J Oral Maxillofac Surg* 2007; **65**: 1198–1208.
3. Prayer D, Brugger PC, Prayer L. Fetal MRI: techniques and protocols. *Pediatr Radiol* 2004; **34**: 685–693.
4. Cassart M, Massez A, Cos T, Tecco L, Thomas D, Van Regemorter N, Avni F. Contribution of three-dimensional computed tomography in the assessment of fetal skeletal dysplasia. *Ultrasound Obstet Gynecol* 2007; **29**: 537–543.
5. Willis A, Speicher J, Cooper DB. Rapid prototyping 3D objects from scanned measurement data. *Image and Vision Computing* 2007; **25**: 1174–1184.

Cerebral blood flow in a case of fetal brain death syndrome

The clinical features of fetal brain death syndrome include fixing of fetal heart rate (FHR) without decelerations, and loss of fetal body, eye and breathing movements[1–11]. The etiological mechanism is thought to be chronic or acute hypoxia, resulting from a pathological state such as a temporary disruption of umbilical blood flow[1,4,5]. However, it is unknown when the fetal brain damage occurs and how it progresses in fetal brain death syndrome.

A 28-year-old woman, gravida 1 para 1, was admitted to our hospital owing to onset of labor at 36 weeks and 2 days of gestation. However, she had noticed an absence of fetal movement 2 days before this. The FHR on arrival showed a fixed pattern of 150 bpm without accelerations or decelerations, and it did not change during uterine contractions. Sonographic examination revealed normal amniotic fluid volume. A pale and floppy male infant was delivered vaginally. The umbilical cord was thin and attached to the margin of the placenta. The neonate weighed 2700 g and measured 46.0 cm in length, 31.0 cm in head circumference and 31.6 cm in chest circumference. Apgar scores were 1 and 3 at 1 and 5 min, respectively. After endotracheal intubation and resuscitation, the infant was admitted to the neonatal intensive care unit. Body temperature was 36.2°C, heart rate was 130 bpm and blood pressure was 60/26 mmHg. No spontaneous breathing or body movements, somatic or primitive reflexes, or pupillary light reflex were observed. There was no abdominal distension, edema, bleeding or external malformation. Limb tonus and joint contracture were absent.

A venous blood sample showed pH 7.145 and a partial pressure of carbon dioxide of 44.9 mmHg; base excess −13 and metabolic acidosis were noted. Also recorded were: white blood cell count 7700/mm^3, red blood cell count 372×10^4/mm^3, hemoglobin 14.2 g/dL, hematocrit 41.3% and platelet count 18.2×10^4/mm^3; these were all normal. The following protein and ion concentrations were found: C-reactive protein 0.3 mg/dL, sodium 140 mEq/L, potassium 3.9 mEq/L, aspartate transaminase 82 IU/L, alanine transaminase 21 IU/L, lactate dehydrogenase (LDH) 852 IU/L and creatine kinase (CK) 243 U/L. None of these levels was elevated. Neonates with hypoxic–ischemic encephalopathy show CK and LDH levels ranging from a few thousand to tens of thousands in blood tests during the first few days after brain injury. The values become normal after about a week[12,13]. The fact that this infant's CK and LDH levels were normal at birth suggests that the brain damage had occurred before the mother noticed the absence of fetal movement.

Cerebral ultrasound examination was performed on the day of delivery. We measured peak systolic and end-diastolic velocity in the middle cerebral artery (MCA) using transtemporal sonography (SONOS 1000, Hewlett-Packard, Palo Alto, CA, USA), and a resistance index (RI) was calculated using the Pourcelot formula: RI = (peak systolic velocity − end-diastolic velocity)/peak systolic velocity[14]. The MCA showed a high diastolic blood flow velocity, the RI was at an extremely low level of 0.45 and luxury perfusion was noted, indicating a brain-sparing effect, as reported in cases of severe hypoxic–ischemic encephalopathy[15] (Figure 1a). A repeat ultrasound examination at 2 days of age showed that the RI was still low at 0.40 and luxury perfusion continued (Figure 1b). However, computed tomographic examination of the head at 4 days of age showed widespread ischemic changes of the brain parenchyma, but no ventricular dilatation, multicystic encephalomalacia or atrophy (Figure 2a). A further cerebral ultrasound examination at 15 days of age showed multicystic encephalomalacia, and that cerebral blood flow velocity was decreased (also suggesting a decrease in blood flow volume). The decrease in diastolic blood flow velocity was particularly marked. The RI had risen to 0.91 and the brain-sparing effect had disappeared (Figure 1c). Magnetic resonance imaging at 43 days of age documented almost no brain parenchyma and showed the presence of multicystic encephalomalacia; the brainstem and medulla oblongata

Update

The Use of Rapid Prototyping Didactic Models in the Study of Fetal Malformations

H. Werner, J.R. Lopes dos Santos, R. Fontes, E.L. Gasparetto, P.A. Daltro, Y. Kuroki, and R.C. Domingues

The importance of rapid prototyping (RP) technologies in the biomedical sector has been steadily increasing since the past decade. Different uses of RP models have been reported widely in the medical scientific literature [1, 2]. Of the 50 cases studied, 3 final models are presented. Some of the results achieved were used by the physicians to demonstrate and explain physical characteristics to parents and other medical specialists.

RP was performed after three-dimensional (3D) ultrasound (US), magnetic resonance imaging (MRI), or computed tomography (CT) of fetuses at different gestational ages. The indications for MRI were central nervous system, thoracic, gastrointestinal, or genitourinary malformations, and for CT, skeletal malformations after a period of 30 weeks. The ethical issues associated with this work were carefully considered.

All cases were examined first by ultrasound imaging. Three-dimensional US scans were performed transvaginally or transabdominally using a high-resolution ultrasound probe with harmonic imaging for all examinations (4–8 MHz transducer, Voluson 730 Pro/Expert system, General Electric, Kretztechnik, Zipf, Austria). MRI examinations were performed using a 1.5 T scanner (Siemens, Erlangen, Germany). The protocol consisted of T2-weighted sequence in the three planes of the fetal body (HASTE: repetition time, shortest; echo time, 140 ms; field of view, 300–200 mm; 256 × 256 matrix; slice thickness, 4 mm; acquisition time, 17 s; 40 slices and TRUFI: repetition time, 3.16 ms; echo time, 1.4 ms; field of view, 340 mm; slice thickness, 1.5 mm; acquisition time, 18 s; 96 slices). The entire examination time did not exceed 30 min [3]. CT was performed using a multislice 64 scanner (Philips, Solingen, Germany) with the following parameters: 40 mA, 120 kV, 64 slices per rotation, pitch 0.75, and slice thickness 0.75 mm. This corresponds to a mean radiation dose to the fetus of 3.12 mGy (CT dose index weighted). The acquisition lasted around 20 s and was performed during maternal apnea [4].

In order to construct physical models from the medical examinations (3D US, MRI, and CT), with the aim of didactic use, the first step was the production of three-dimensional virtual models. All 3D US, MRI, and CT images were exported to a workstation in Digital Imaging and Communications in Medicine (DICOM) format for manual, slice-by-slice segmentation by a single observer using a digital high-definition screen tablet (Cintiq Wacom 21 UX, Tokyo, Japan). The 3D structure of the fetus was reconstructed by generating skinning surfaces that joined the resulting profiles. Software that converts medical images into numerical models (Scan IP version 2.0, Simpleware Ltd., Exeter, UK and Mimics v. 12, Materialize, Leuven, Belgium) were used for 3D virtual model reconstruction, and the model was exported into a standard triangular language (STL) format and converted into an "OBJ" extension for adjustment using 3D modeling polygonal software (Autodesk Mudbox, San Francisco, CA). Using this software, the volumetric surface was smoothed, to be later compared and analyzed as a topographic construction. After this procedure, the 3D model was again converted and exported as an STL extension. The model file was again opened in Simpleware/Mimics software for correlating the contours of the 3D US, MR, or CT images with the generated 3D surface.

The physical modeling process was done using three different RP technologies that are classified by different authors [5] into three main categories, according to the physical state of the materials to be transformed: liquid-based systems (associated with photosensitive resins), powder-based systems (associated with sintering or agglutination of grain particles), and solid-based systems (associated with nonpowder formats, such as sheets or thermoplastic extruded filaments).

The experiments on 3D fetal modeling began by using CT files to build physical models of a fetal skeleton (Figure 1) [6]. This study generated a series of bone connection structures in a 3D virtual environment. In this case, we also used the design modeling software Autodesk Maya to keep the skeleton whole, preserving its shape and spatial coordinates and allowing the production of a physical model without losing accurate bond positioning. A liquid-based system (stereolithography system) [7] was selected and the process started by resolving the layers of a

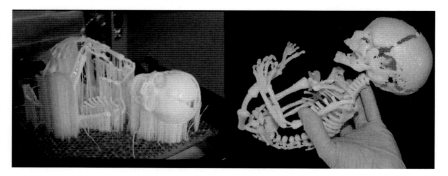

Figure 1 Rapid prototyping model of the skeleton of a fetus at 34 weeks created using stereolithography technology (3D Systems – VIPER si2) after computed tomography.

photocurable resin solidified with a laser beam. For generating the physical models, the data from each slice were used to direct the laser beam over the X and Y axes of the surface of a liquid photopolymer reservoir. The 3D geometry was achieved by hardening the photopolymer and gradually lowering the supporting structure. A necessary postprocessing was done through hardening the physical model in a special chamber under ultraviolet light.

The next challenge using the same CT file and RP technology was representing the body of the fetus as well as its external surface or skin, which was met by virtual separation of the CT slices. This interactive process visually detects the boundaries of the fetal body parts using a digital stylus pen that directly interacts with the computer screen. The resulting layers of the relevant fetal area were virtually overlapped, generating a 3D volumetric model.

Based on results from the CT files, MRI files were studied using alike manual segmentation techniques in which every slice was virtually contoured and separated according to medical interpretation by a radiologist who assigned actual thicknesses to the MR scan. The main difference in CT and MRI images was the quality of the contrast between the internal organs on the MRI images. The high gray scale contrast between internal regions allowed easier visual separation of the relevant areas using an LCD screen tablet. On CT scans, only the skeleton was easily identified. On MRI scans, the image quality is best in the final stages of pregnancy, since the fetus has little space to move, and image quality is better if fetus is immobile during the sweep [8].

The RP technology adopted in this case was the fused deposition modeling (solid-based system). The material used was thermoplastic acrylonitrile butadiene styrene (ABS), and the model required a supporting water-soluble material (Figure 2), which was removed after the construction process through immersion in an ultrasound bath in a liquid release agent.

The most substantial challenge in this study was the construction of models from 3D US. This examination modality allows a faster sweep of the fetus, and the image is automatically transformed into 3D virtual images on the screen [9]. Depending on the

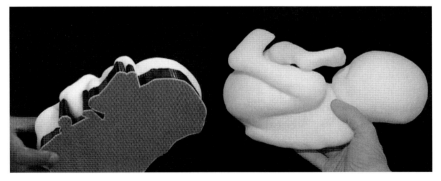

Figure 2 Rapid prototyping model of a fetus at 32 weeks created using fused deposition modeling technology (Stratasys – Vantage) after MRI imaging.

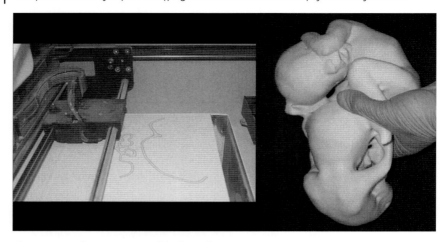

Figure 3 Rapid prototyping model of twin fetuses at 28 weeks created using Z Corporation technology (Z 510) after the combination of 3D US and MRI scan.

size of the fetus, this process can permit the visualization of the complete body in the first trimester or, from the second trimester, parts of the fetal body captured in separate sequences. We used the tomographic ultrasound imaging (TUI) function of the GE 4D View software to process the 3D US images and superimposed the results on MRI or CT files. The obtained images were exported to Mimics software for reconstruction of the 3D image, while maintaining accuracy and reliability. The protocols for the two preceding experiments were adopted for subsequent processing.

In the example of twins (Figure 3) combining 3D US and MRI, the choice was the use of a powder-based system (Z Corporation Technology, Burlington, MA). This procedure uses a printer head to deposit an agglutination liquid whose composition is similar to plaster as a top layer of the material. As the printer head elevator moves down, additional layers of material can be added and this is repeated until the model is completed. This process does not use a support structure, since the model is positioned inside the powder that sustains the prototype.

Using 3D US, images from the entire gestation period could be captured for potential use with MRI and CT, including adding and combining features from these techniques. Since all 3D US, MRI, and CT files were obtained on the same day, detailed characteristics of the body could be combined, for example, using 3D US images for the face, hands, or feet and MR images for the body (Figure 3), maintaining distances by obtaining several measures by both technologies. The segmentation and reconstruction techniques developed for fetal modeling can be applied to the construction of both virtual 3D models and physical models, using the same data.

By the time of this study, only two articles that use medical ultrasound scans and 3D models were found. Nelson and Bailey [10] converted 3D US data to a set of polygons representing an isosurface that could be transferred to RP equipment to create a solid 3D object. This is considered the first attempt to transform fetal 3D US data into RP physical models. The second project was developed by Blaas et al. [11], who calculated the volume of embryos and first trimester fetuses by transforming the area of the embryo into a 3D virtual model.

In this study, the main outcomes presented were the possibility to create 3D virtual models from 3D US, MRI, or CT, both separately and in various combinations. RP systems allow the conversion of a 3D virtual model to a physical model in a fast, easy, and dimensionally accurate process [6]. The construction process transfers a 3D data file that specifies surfaces and solid internal structures to RP equipment that builds physical models through the superimposition of thin layers of raw materials. This study introduced the use of RP models into fetal research, an area where studies on digital 3D modeling have been scarce. The results suggest a new possibility for interaction between parents and their unborn child during pregnancy, by physically recreating the interior of the womb during gestation, including physical appearance, actual size, and malformations in some cases.

References

1 Armillotta, A., Bonhoeffer, P., Dubini, G., Ferragina, S., Migliavacca, F., Sala, G., and Schievano, S. (2007) Use of rapid prototyping models in the planning of percutaneous pulmonary valved stent implantation. *Proc. Inst. Mech. Eng.*, **221**, 407–416.

2 Robinoy, M., Salvo, I., Costa, F., Zerman, N., Bazzocchi, M., Toso, F., Bandera, C., Filippi, S., Felice, M., and Politi, M. (2007) Virtual reality surgical planning for maxillofacial distraction osteogenesis: the role of reverse engineering rapid prototyping and cooperative work. *J. Oral Maxillofac. Surg.*, **65**, 1198–1208.

3 Prayer, D., Brugger, P.C., and Prayer, L. (2004) Fetal MRI: techniques and protocols. *Pediatr. Radiol.*, **34**, 685–693.

4 Cassart, M., Massez, A., Cos, T., Tecco, L., Thomas, D., Van Regemorter, N., and Avni, F. (2007) Contribution of three-dimensional computed tomography in the assessment of fetal skeletal dysplasia. *Ultrasound Obstet. Gynecol.*, **29**, 537–543.

5 Hopkinson, N., Hague, R., and Dickens, P. (2006) *Rapid Manufacturing: An Industrial Revolution for the Digital Age*, John Wiley & Sons, Inc., pp. 55–80.

6 Werner, H., dos Santos, J.R., Fontes, R., Gasparetto, E.L., Daltro, P.A., Kuroki, Y., and Domingues, R.C. (2008) The use of rapid prototyping didactic models in the study of fetal malformations. *Ultrasound Obstet. Gynecol.*, **32**, 955–956.

7 Willis, A., Speicher, J., and Cooper, D.B. (2007) Rapid prototyping 3D objects from scanned measurement data. *Image Vis. Comput.*, **25**, 1174–1184.

8 Prayer, D., Brugger, P.C., Kasprian, G., Witzani, L., Helmer, H., Dietrich, W., Eppel, W., and Langer, M. (2006) MRI of fetal acquired brain lesions. *Eur. J. Radiol.*, **57**, 233–249.

9 Campbell, S. (2007) 4D and prenatal bonding: still more questions than answers. *Ultrasound Obstet. Gynecol.*, **27**, 243–244.

10 Nelson, T.R. and Bailey, M.J. (2000) Solid object visualization of 3D ultrasound data. *Med. Imaging*, **3982**, 26–34.

11 Blaas, H.G., Taipale, P., Torp, H., and Eik-Nes, S.H. (2006) Three-dimensional ultrasound volume calculations of human embryos and young fetuses: a study of the volumetry of compound structures and its reproducibility. *Ultrasound Obstet. Gynecol.*, **27**, 640–646.

14
Non-invasive Archaeology of Skeletal Material by CT Scanning and Three-dimensional Reconstruction

SHORT REPORT

Non-invasive Archaeology of Skeletal Material by CT Scanning and Three-dimensional Reconstruction

NIELS LYNNERUP,[1†] **HENRIK HJALGRIM,**[2] **LENE RINDAL NIELSEN,**[3] **HENRIK GREGERSEN**[4] **AND INGOLF THUESEN**[5]

[1]*Laboratory of Biological Anthropology, Institute of Forensic Medicine, University of Copenhagen, Denmark;* [2]*Danish Epidemiology Science Centre, Statens Seruminstitut, Denmark;* [3]*Laboratory of Dental Anthropology, Dental School, University of Copenhagen, Denmark;* [4]*Department of Radiology, Aalborg University Hospital, Denmark and* [5]*The Carsten Niebuhr Institute, University of Copenhagen, Denmark*

ABSTRACT The remains of an ancient Sumerian skeleton, approximately 7000 years old, were investigated using the techniques of stereolithography. The very fragile and delicate skeletal material was recovered in a block, thus retaining it in the soil matrix. The excavated block was CT-scanned and the skeletal material was rendered in three dimensions. This formed the basis for a stereolithographic model of the mandible, which was used for physical and dental anthropological studies. Skeletal remains may thus be made available for research without having to remove them from the local matrix, which may be an advantage in an archaeological or palaeoanthropological setting.

Key words: three-dimensional imaging; stereolithography; bone; Sumeria.

Introduction

Stereolithographic modelling is a novel technique for rapid production of models of three-dimensional structures. Recently, stereolithographic models of anthropological specimens have been produced on the basis of digitized CT-scanning images.[1–3] This technique was applied here for the first time on archaeological skeletal material still embedded in the soil matrix.

The Danish Khabur Expedition has conducted archaeological excavations since 1990 at Tell Mashnaqa in north eastern Syria, an early Sumerian (Ubaid) settlement dating approximately to 5000 BC.[4,5] In the course of the excavations, 24 human burials were located. However, even though outlines of complete skeletons and bones could be discerned in the graves, the human remains were very delicate and fragmented, precluding the retrieval of intact skeletal material. Traditional techniques usually applied in such circumstances, e.g., application of liquid stabilizers, proved unsatisfactory, and this prompted us to attempt CT-scanning and stereolithographical modelling.

Material and methods

During the excavation of burial no. XV, soil was removed to a level where most larger skeletal elements were recognizable, so that the approximate location of the skull could be determined.

†Corresponding address: Niels Lynnerup, Laboratory of Biological Anthropology, The Panum Institute, Blegdamsvej 3, DK-2200 Copenhagen, Denmark.

CCC 1047–482X/97/010091–04
© 1997 by John Wiley & Sons, Ltd.

Received 14 May 1996
Accepted 18 June 1996

Computer Aided Biomanufacturing, Edited by Roger Narayan and Paul Calvert
© 2011 WILEY-VCH Verlag GmbH & Co. KGaA. Published 2011 by WILEY-VCH Verlag GmbH & Co. KGaA.

The skull, still embedded in the soil matrix, was then removed *en bloc* completely encapsulated in wool and plaster of Paris.

The block, measuring approximately 30 × 25 × 20 cm, was transported to Aalborg University Hospital, Denmark, where it was CT-scanned (Siemens Somatron; 181 images made at 1 mm intervals with a gantry angle of 0°, at 125 kV and 280 mA s^{-1} and a scanning time of 3 s). The CT-scanning data was transferred to an ordinary 486 PC equipped with image-processing software (MIMICS^{TM}). This software allowed separation of bone and soil by means of grey-scale thresholding and manual editing on the single CT-scan slices and subsequent rendering in three dimensions of selected structures. The three-dimensional image may be viewed from any angle specified by the user or segmented to show cut-throughs of the structures. The CT-scans showed the cranial vault and facial skeleton to be fragmented, but the mandible was reasonably intact (Figure 1). The rendering of the mandible produced formed the basis for a stereolithographic model (Figure 2) subsequently made at the Danish Institute of Technology. The model was made on a SLA-250 device (3D Systems, Valencia, California). Basically, a stereolithographic model is produced by guiding a laser beam into a vat with liquid photosensitive polymer resins. The laser causes the resin to polymerize and thus solidify.[2,3] The precision of the method is claimed to be as fine as 0.2 mm (3D Systems, Valencia, California), making the CT-scan data the limiting factor in the resolution, because it is presently not technically possible to lower the CT-scan slice interval below 1 mm.

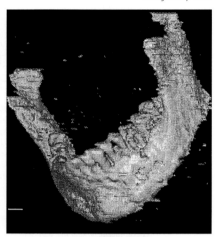

Figure 1. The mandible as rendered in three dimensions by the computer after CT-scanning. Horizontal white bar indicates 1 cm. The artefacts seen as white dots seen around the mandible are picture elements with the same grey-scale tone as the bone. These artefacts are eliminated automatically when the stereolithographical model is produced.

Results and discussion

It would have been possible theoretically to produce renderings and models of all the cranial bone fragments in the soil block and thus ultimately reconstruct the whole cranium. However, owing to the high degree of fragmentation of the cranial vault and facial skeleton this would have been very time consuming. Also, the stereolithographic technique is still rather expensive, especially due to the photosensitive resin (the mandibular model produced cost approximately £400). Therefore, we chose only the intact mandible for modelling.

The model clearly shows evidence of post-mortem diagenetic changes of the mandible, such as extremely brittle cortical bone tissue, especially at the rami, and fracture lines. It was possible to observe morphological characteristics, measure several standard physical anthropological variables (Table 1) and describes the gross (mandibular) dental status of the individual. This allowed for a tentative evaluation of sex (probably male) and age (adult, probably 25–50 years old). The crowns of the teeth were reproduced in less detail owing to occlusion (in the matrix) with the maxillar teeth. Although it is evident that there was no antemortem or post-mortem tooth loss, nor dental agensia, this lack of crown detail restricted the ability to evaluate dental wear

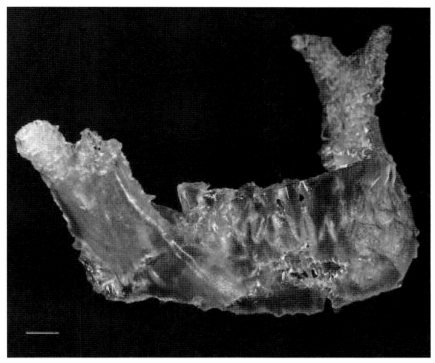

Figure 2. The stereolithographical model of the mandible. Horizontal white bar indicates 1 cm. The model is a 1:1 rendering of the real mandible (refer to Table 1 for dimensions).

(attrition and abrasion) and conditions such as enamel hypoplasia and calculus deposition. On the other hand, the dental root morphology could be assessed owing to the translucency of the model (Figure 2).

Table 1. Physical anthropological variables as measured on the model using a goniometer and a caliper.

Variable	mm
Maximum length	100
Maximum body length	70
Vertical height of ramus	50
Oblique height of ramus	55
Mental height	35

Until recently only a small number of institutions possessed the machines and facilities to produce stereolithographic models. However, there has been a great interest in this technique, both industrially and medicotechnically, as witnessed for example by the emergence of newsletters and workshops dealing specifically with medical applications of rapid prototyping and stereolithography.[6]

Partly damaged and fragmented skeletal remains embedded in soil may thus be made available for observation prior to actual removal and cleaning. We feel that this may be of use for palaeontologists and archaeologists dealing with extremely fragile skeletal remains. Indeed, archaeological field procedures of excavation of fragile materials may be improved, due to the non-invasive and non-destructive nature of the technique. Before attempting to remove the embedding matrix, stereolithographical models may be made, and these may then be used as a guide both during retrieval and preparation. If during these procedures the material is further damaged, they may serve as models for reconstruction. Finally, stereolithographical models may serve the role of accurate casts, and several models may (depending on their size) be produced simultaneously. In this case, models were made for study and exhibition purposes in Denmark and Syria.

Acknowledgements

We kindly thank the Directorate General of Antiquities, Syria, and the staff of the Danish Institute of Technology.

References

1. Zur Nedden, D., Knapp, R., Wicke, K., Judmaier, W., Murphy, W. A. Jr., Seidler, H. and Platzer, W. Skull of a 5,300-year-old mummy; reproduction and investigation with CT-guided stereolithography. *Radiology*, 1994; 193: 269–272.
2. Hjalgrim, H., Lynnerup, N., Liversage, M. and Rosenklint, A. Stereolithography: potential applications in anthropological studies. *American Journal of Physical Anthropology*, 1995; 97: 329–333.
3. Zollikofer, C. P. E., Ponce de León, M. S., Martin, R. D. and Stucki, P. Neanterthal computer skulls. *Nature*, 1995; 375: 283–285.
4. Thuesen, I. Tell Mashnaqa. *American Journal of Archeology*, 1991; 95: 691–692.
5. Thuesen, I. Tell Mashnaqa. *American Journal of Archeology*, 1994; 11: 111–112.
6. EARP. European Action on Rapid Prototyping, 1995; 5: 21 pp.

Update

Noninvasive Archeology of Skeletal Material by CT Scanning and Three-Dimensional Reconstruction

Niels Lynnerup

Stereolithography is one of a number of rapid prototyping protocols and methods. Basically, rapid prototyping (RP) means exactly that: the rapid production of a prototype. As all industrial design is carried out on CAD/CAM systems, this means that the designed objects exist as virtual 3D objects. RP machines simply convert such an element directly into a physical object [1, 2]. A typical example would be the design of a new cell phone. It is designed using CAD/CAM and by RP directly made into a 1 : 1 prototype. Although perhaps only the shell is produced, this is enough to allow user testing in terms of size, fit, and general handling, before starting up a real production of a working cell phone. Traditionally, such test models were manufactured in wood or sculpted.

The use of RP in the medical sciences came with the advent of CT scanning. CT scan images of specific bodily elements can be rendered as 3D objects on the CT scanner workstation. Essentially, one then has the same situation as mentioned above: an object rendered virtually in 3D. Usually, however, the CT scan images and visualizations need some degree of postprocessing with specialized software, in order to produce a file format that can then be read by RP machines.

As such, RP is now used to generate 1 : 1 models of various bodily structures, for example, to plan surgery [3–5]. We have used this whole process to look at human skeletal remains of a very old age.

Since our first stereolithographical productions, there has been a tremendous increase in the number of resins and materials used for the solid-state models. Various resins may offer different capabilities, for example, in terms of serving as positive forms for casting in other materials, either metals or silicone.

This publication was among the first that addressed the use of RP to study as yet not fully excavated human remains in an archeological context. Since this publication, we have worked extensively with the method, especially with a view to producing exact replicas of skulls. Skulls form the basis of facial reconstructions, and we [6] and other researchers have thus been able to perform facial reconstructions of Egyptian

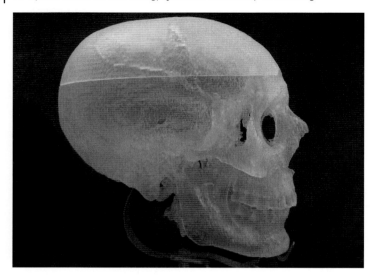

Figure 1

mummies, where the skull is encased in layers of soft tissue and embalming materials, or bog bodies, where the skull may be somewhat degraded due to taphonomic changes (Figure 1) [7, 8].

References

1 Peltola, S.M., Melchels, F.P.W., Grijpma, D.W., and Kellomäki, M. (2008) A review of rapid prototyping techniques for tissue engineering purposes. *Ann. Med.*, **40**, 268–280.

2 Sun, W., Darling, A., Starly, B., and Nam, J. (2004) Computer-aided tissue engineering: overview, scope and challenges. *Biotechnol. Appl. Biochem.*, **39**, 29–47.

3 Perez-Arjona, E., Dujovny, M., Park, H., Klyanov, D., Galaniuk, A., Agner, C., Michael, D., and Diaz, F.G. (2003) Stereolithography: neurosurgical and medical implications. *Neurol. Res.*, **25**, 227–235.

4 Sinn, D.P., Cillo, Jr., J.E., and Miles, B.A. (2006) Stereolithography for craniofacial surgery. *J. Craniofac. Surg.*, **17**, 869–875.

5 Hidalgo, H.M., Romo, G.W., and Estolano, R.T.R. (2009) Stereolithography: a method for planning the surgical correction of the hypertelorism. *J. Craniofac. Surg.*, **20**, 1473–1477.

6 Asingh, P. and Lynnerup, N. (2007) *Grauballe Man*, Århus University Press, Århus, p. 351.

7 Lynnerup, N. (2007) Mummies. *Yearb. Phys. Anthropol.*, **50**, 162–190.

8 Lynnerup, N. (2008) Computed tomography scanning and three-dimensional visualization of mummies and bog bodies, in *Advances in Human Paleopathology* (eds R. Pinhasi and S. Mays), John Wiley & Sons, Ltd, Chichester, pp. 101–120.

Index

a

acrylonitrile butadiene styrene (ABS)   181
adenocarcinoma of maxilla   167
adhesives
– cyanoacrylate adhesives   86, 87
– medical adhesives   89
– synthetic adhesives   83, 89
– use   83
alkaline phosphatase (ALP)   35, 43
– activity   118
allograft tissue   93
AMD processors   15
American Society for Testing and Materials (ASTM)   123
anthropological variables   186
Apgar scores   178
asymptotic analysis approach   18
atomic force microscopy (AFM)   85, 88, 89
autograft tissue, use   93

b

bacterial adhesion   55, 63
barrier materials
– microbial colorization   56
Beriplast® P   83
bioadhesives, inkjet printing   83
– conclusions   89
– materials and methods   84, 85
– results and discussion   85–89
bioceramic drug-release matrices
– bioactives during 3D powder printing, simultaneous immobilization   113, 114
– discussion   116
– polymer modification   116, 117
– printed drugs, biological activity   117, 118
– release profile and drug/polymer modification dependency   117

– results   114–116
bioceramic scaffold   113
biocompatible polymers   113
biodegradable scaffolds   33, 39
biomaterials   113
bioreactors   94
– spinner flask   36, 46
blood analysis techniques   104
bone   9, 26
– defect   167
– grafting   163
– grafts   163
– hierarchical biocomposite materials   26
– hierarchical structure   10, 11
– micro-architectural deterioration   9
– micro-scale structure   9
– – characterstics   11
– tissue, mechanical evaluation   15
bone mineral density (BMD)   9, 11, 26, 136
– assessment techniques   11
– testing limitations   12
bone tissue engineering applications
– hierarchical starch-based fibrous scaffold for   33, 34, 39
– – alkaline phosphatase quantification   43
– – cell adhesion, morphology, distribution, evaluation   35, 42
– – cell seeding and culture   34, 35, 42
– – cell viability assay   35, 43
– – DNA quantification   35, 43
– – dynamic mechanical analysis (DMA)   42
– – future perspectives   49
– – results and discussion   35–37, 44–49
– – scaffold fabrication   34, 41
– – scaffolds' structure characterization   34, 41
– – statistical analysis   35, 44
Bose EnduraTEC Systems Group   106

Computer Aided Biomanufacturing, Edited by Roger Narayan and Paul Calvert
© 2011 WILEY-VCH Verlag GmbH & Co. KGaA. Published 2011 by WILEY-VCH Verlag GmbH & Co. KGaA.

brain heart infusion (BHI) 57
brushite-based bioceramic implants
– multijet 3D printing strategy 114

c

cage fabrication
– selective laser melting process 123
calcium phosphate (CaP) matrix 114
calcium/sodium alginate scaffolds 57
calculas deposition 187
Candida albicans
– scanning electron micrographs 61
cell medium/cell suspensions
– characteristics 76
cell proliferation 35, 106
cell–prosthesis interactions 2
cell-seeded scaffolds 2
– development 1
CellTiter 99® aqueous one solution cell proliferation assay 43
cellular preference phenomenon 46
cell viability assay 35, 43
– box plot 47
cerebral blood flow 178
cerebral ultrasound 178
chemical vapor infiltration (CVI) process 122, 125
colony forming units (CFUs) 60
– determination 62
– number 58
compression test 125, 126
computational mechanics 14
computational method
– development 19
computed tomography (CT)
– analyser software 34
– scan data 116
– scanning 189
computer-aided biomanufacturing methods 1–6
– disadvantages 2
computer-aided design (CAD) model 1, 34, 40, 123, 169
– based implant modeling 163
– based prosthesis modeling 167
– CAD–CAM construction of nasal prostheses 149
– – aesthetic disfiguration after tumour removal 150
– – clinical reports after tumour surgery 150, 151
– – clinical reports before surgery 150
– – developing diagnostic template with gutta-percha 152

– – final eyeglass-supprted provisional prosthesis 152
– – rapid prototyping of moulds and substructure 151
– – squamous cell carcinoma of nose 150
– – time and cost of procedure 152
– – timing of procedure of provisional prosthesis 152
– CAD/CAM system 167, 189
– implant construction, after tumor resection 165
– implant construction, before tumor resection 165
– patterning 83
– program 106
– rapid prototyping techniques 84
– software 34, 41
computerized 3D virtual biopsy system
– 3D bone architecture 30
confocal laser scanning microscopy (CLSM) 59, 63
– use 60
congenital/acquired pathology 55
contact angle measurements 85
continuous multi-scale approach 16
contractile proteins in muscle 135
conventional bioreactors 94
conventional machining-based processes 5
conventional manual-based fabrication technique 61
cranial vault 186
C-reactive protein 178
cross-linking 105
customized titanium maxillary prosthesis 167

d

Danish Khabur expedition 185
data acquisition for 3D modeling 169
data transmission scheme 20
2D bone micro-structures
– finite element analysis, phases 19
3D calculation 170
3D-CT reconstructed data 166
degeneration time 136
degrees of freedom (DOFs) 13, 15
dehydrogenase enzymes 35
– NADH production 43
dental root morphology 187
dental wear 186
denture bulkiness 163
digital imaging and communications in medicine (DICOM) format 180
digital magnifying glass 27

digital zoom camera   85
3,4-dihydroxyphenyl-L-alanine (DOPA)   84
3D image processing   170
3-(4,5-dimethylthiazol-2-yl)2,5-diphenyl
  tetrazohum bromide (MTT) assay   105, 106
direct computer-aided biomanufacturing
  methods   1
3D mesh model   12, 15
3D micro-scale scanning methods
– development   12
– μCT and μMRI   26
DMP 2800 piezoelectric inkjet printer   84
2D multiscale finite element analysis   30
DNA quantification   35
domain decomposition (DD) methods   18, 28
– data transmission scheme   20
– for 2D micro-structures   20, 21
– drawback   21
– important aspects   20
– micro-structures, finite element tearing and
  interconnecting (FETI) method   21
– ratio of total strain energy   21
– stages in   28, 29
3D printing (3DP)   36
3D-ribotyping technology   63
dropcast mussel adhesive proteins (Mefp)
  materials   88
dual-energy X-ray absorptiometery
  (DEXA)   11, 12
dual photon absorptiometery (DPA)   11
Dulbecco's modified Eagle's medium
  (DMEM)   34, 42
dynamic mechanical analysis (DMA)   42, 44

e

Eagle's minimum essential medium   95
Earle's balanced salt solution   95
early Sumerian skeletons   185
electrical stimulation
– monitoring muscles growth and tissue
  changes induced by
– – data analysis   132, 133
– – spatial CT of RISE study   132
– – stereolithographic 3D modeling
  132, 133
– – tissue differentiation, display and   133
– of the muscle fibers   136
– muscles growth and tissue changes induced
  by   131
electric field driven jetting   73
– benefit of   73
– discussion   79, 80
– materials and methods   74–76
– results   76–78

electrohydrodynamic jetting (EHDJ)
  equipment   74, 79, 80
– experimental set-up   76
– schematic representation   75
electrospinning (ES)   34, 35
electrospun fibres   33, 40
– nanofiber matrices   49
endotracheal intubation   178
Enterococcus faecalis
– confocal laser scanning micrographs   62
ethylene oxide (EtO)   34, 41
European Collection of Cell Cultures
  (ECACC)   34, 42
extracellular matrix (ECM)   33, 38, 40, 94, 95

f

fabricated titanium alloy optimal-structure
  (OS) cage
– microstructural features   124
fabrication time   106
facial reconstructions of Egyptian   189
fetal brain death syndrome   178
fetal heart rate   178
fibrin matrix   37, 47
finite element (FE) mechanical analysis   10,
  27, 122
finite element tearing and interconnecting
  (FETI) method   21
– advantages   22
Fourier transform infrared spectroscopy
  (FTIR)   83, 85
– absorption spectra   86
Fourier transforming lens   76
fragile skeletal remains   188
Fraunhofer scattering model   76
fused deposition modelling (FDM)   37, 47

g

generative manufacturing
  processes   123
genitourinary malformations   179
gingival carcinoma   166
gold standard   93
– joining technique   83
goniometer   187
growing neural gas (GNG) method   13

h

heat-sensitive proteins, rhBMP-2   117
heparin   113, 115
– anti-coagulation activity   118
– biological activities   116, 117
hepatitis B transmission   93
hierarchical fibrous scaffolds   35

– application 49
– production 34
– SEM micrographs 37
hierarchical geometric multi-resolution model 18
HIV-1 antigen test 84
home-based functional electrotherapy (h-bFES) 137
homogenization based topology optimization 122
homogenization technique 10
Hondsfield values (Hu) 135
human epidermal keratinocytes 107
– light micrograph 109
– MTT viability 109
human osteoblast-like cells 36, 37, 39, 47, 56
– box plot of cell viability results 37
– cell viability and metabolic activity 46
– roy plot of DNA content 37
hydroxypropylmethylcellulose (HPMC) 113, 117
hypermesh software, remeshing tool 12
hypodermic needles, use 104
hypoplasia 187
hypoxic-ischemic encephalopathy 178

i

image-based bio-CAD modeling 169
image-based finite element analysis 123–125
image-based prosthesis design process 164
inkjet printed materials
– X-ray photoelectron peaks 88
inkjetted mussel adhesive protein solution 87
– Fourier transform infrared (FTIR) spectra 86
– topography-iattened atomic force micrograph 88
instron floor model testing system 123
interbody fusion cages, use 121
International Graphics Exchange Standard (IGES) format 170
inverse material model 29

j

jet-based processes 73
Jurkat cells 74, 76, 77, 79

k

keratinocyte growth medium-2 (KGM-2) 107
Korsemeyer-Peppas model 114
– fitting parameters of experimental data 115
Kruskal-Wallis test 35

l

lactate dehydrogenase 178
Langmuir-Blodgett (L-B) coatings 94
laser microfabrication
– hydroxyapatite and zirconia, MAPLE DW transfer
– – experimental procedure 95
– – results and discussion 96–99
– of hydroxyapatite-osteoblast-like cell composites 93–95
– matrix assisted pulsed laser evaporation direct write 95
– MG 63-hydroxyapatite composites, MAPLE DW transfer
– – results and discussion 100, 101
– MG 63 osteoblast-like cells, MAPLE DW transfer 95, 96
– – experimental procedure 95, 96
– – results and discussion 99, 100
laser spectroscopy 76, 77
laser system 75
liquid-based techniques 5
live-dead stained MG 63 osteoblast-like cells
– fluorescence image 98
– optical micrograph 98
lower motor neuron (LMN) lesion 135

m

macro-scale bone analysis 11, 12
mandible 186
Mann–Whitney U test 44, 47, 48
marine mussel adhesive protein materials 86
material compliance matrix 18
material properties analysis 23
matrix assisted pulsed laser evaporation direct write (MAPLE DW) process 94, 95
– hydroxyapatite and zirconia
– – experimental procedure 95
– – results and discussion 96–99
– laser microfabrication 95
– – MG 63-hydroxyapatite composites, results and discussion 100, 101
– – MG 63 osteoblast-like cells 95, 96, 99, 100
– optical micrographs 96, 97
– protocols used for 96
– scanning electron micrographs 97, 98
– schematic diagram 94
– X-ray diffraction 97
maxilla/mandible restoration implants 169
maxillar teeth 186
maxillary defects 163, 164, 167
maxillary skeleton 172
medical imaging technology 10, 17
medulla oblongata 178

meshing growing neural gas neural network (MGNG) method   13
mesh quality numerical analysis   13
metabolic acidosis   178
metabolic bone diseases   26
metallic biocompatible materials   127
metallic cage devices, stiffness   121
MG 63-hydroxyapatite composite matrix assisted pulsed laser evaporation direct write (MAPLE DW) process
– optical micrograph   99, 100
MG 63 osteoblast-like cells
– growth profiles   101
micro-computed tomography/micro magnetic resonance imaging (μCT/μMRI)   10, 15, 34, 39, 41
– 3D models, reconstruction   12–14
micro FE analysis   14, 15
– disadvantages   15
microhardness test   123
micro-nano fibre polymeric scaffolds   34
– architecture   36
micro-nanofibrous structures   49
micro-nano scaffold architecture   36
microneedles   104, 107
– array, load *vs.* displacement data   108
– computer-aided design diagrams   107
microplate reader   43
microstructures
– diagnosis   26
– homogenization for   23
microsyringe-based systems   2
middle cerebral artery (MCA)   178
monitoring human tissue *in vivo*   135
MS-130 high resolution Micro-CT Scanner   123
MTS Alliance RT30 electromechanical test frame   123
MTS assay   36, 46
multicolor 3D-powder printing system   118
multicystic encephalomalacia   178
multi-resolution geometrical model   24
– development   18
multiscale computational method   28
– challenge   28
multiscale computerized bone diagnostic system   9
– 2D microscale finite element analysis   9, 26, 27
– domain-based multiscale material properties   28–30
– multiscale finite element approach   27, 28
– – advantage   27
– summary and future work   30

multi-scale finite element (FE) analysis   9, 15–19, 18
– block diagram   17
– components   28
– domain decomposition (DD) using parallel computing   18–19
– geometric modeling   18
– limitations in   16
– material compliance matrix   18
– μCT/μMRI images, acquisition   17, 18
– post-processing   19
– pre-processing   18
multiscale material compliance matrix   28
multi-scale methods
– binary scales   16
– network structure   33
– strengths and weaknesses   16
muscle atrophy   131
muscle degeneration   137
muscle force   131
mussel adhesive proteins   84
– contact angle image   85
– contact angle measurements   85
– optical micrographs   85, 86
– three-dimensional representation   88
– X-ray photoelectron spectra   87
Mytilus edulis   89

n

nanofibre meshes (NFM)   34, 39, 40
natural graft therapies
– limitations   93
Nd:YAG-solid state laser system   123
neural network (NN)-based method   12
nonuniform rational B-spline (NURBS) surfaces   164
– patches   166

o

optical microscopy   77
optimal-structure (OS) cage   125, 127
– fabrication   125
oral microorganisms
– overview   57
Ormocer® material   105, 108, 109
– light-curable dental composites   105
oronasal regurgitation   163
osteoblast-like cells   42
– DNA content, box plot   48

p

palatomaxillary complex   167
parallel-aligned rapid prototyped microfibers
– 3D structure   44

phosphate-buffered saline (PBS)   42, 57
photolithography   73
photosensitive polymers   5
physical anthropological variables   187
physical/chemical stresses   116
PicoGreen dsDNA Assay Kit   35
piezoelectric crystals   74
piezoelectric inkjet printers   84
plaster of Paris   186
p-nitrophenyl phosphate (pNPP)   118
polycaprolactone (PCL)   34
– nanomotif   40, 49
polygons   1
poly(lactide-co-glycolic acid) (PLGA)   56, 62, 63
– application   62
– chemical constitution   63
polymer-ceramic hybrid materials
– materials and methods   105–107
– results and discussions   107–109
– two photon polymerization, for transdermal drug delivery   103–105
polymer-processing technique   34
polymer swelling   117
polytetrafluoroethylene surfaces   108
polyurethane   56
poly vinyl alcohol (PVA)   56
Pourcelot formula   178
powder-based computer-aided biomanufacturing techniques   5
printing liquid bioactives   116
prosthesis casting   172
prosthesis geometrical modeling
– after tumor resection   166
– before tumor resection   164
prosthetic maxillary obturators   163
prototyping didactic models for fetal malformations   177
pure marine mussel extracts
– adhesion characteristics   89

q

quantitative computerized tomography (QCT)   11, 12
QuantiT™ PicoGreen dsDNA assay kit   43

r

rapid prototyped microfibers   39
– combination   39
rapid prototyping (RP) model   40, 113, 189
– medical model production   171
– of skeleton of fetus at 34 weeks   180
– of twin fetuses at 28 weeks   182

rapid prototyping (RP) scaffolds   33–35
– adhesion of microorganisms on   66
– bacterial and *Candida albicans* adhesion on   55
– – biomaterials   56, 57
– – conforal laser scanning microscopy   59
– – inoculation and colonization   57
– – results   59, 60
– – scanning electron microscopy   57, 58
– – statistical analysis   59
– microbial adhesion and infection, monitoring   66, 68, 69
– perspective   66, 67
– SEM micrographs   37, 47
rapid prototyping (RP) technologies   56, 169, 171, 179
– comparison   3, 4
recombinant bone morphogenic protein 2 (rhBMP-2)   113
rectus femoris   136
remeshed meshes   14
representative volume element (RVE) homogenization approach   18, 28
resuscitation   178
reticulated vitreous carbon (RVC) skeleton   122
reverse engineering (RE)   164
RISE project   131, 136

s

scanning electron microscopy (SEM)   34, 39, 41, 57, 58, 123
– micrographs   125
– of scaffolds prior to microbial colonization   59
SCPS laser RP machines   171
seeding process   46
selective laser melting (SLM) process   122
– discussion   126–128
– image-based finite element analysis   123–125
– integrated topology optimization design, overview   122
– mechanical testing   123
– radiographic and imaging characterizations   123
– results   125, 126
– schematic process   123
– selective laser melting process for cage fabrication   123
– topology optimized titanium interbody fusion cage   121
selective laser sintering (SLS)   2, 5
Shapiro–Wilk test   44

Simpleware/mimics software   180
skeletal malformations   177
solid-based computer-aided biomanufacturing techniques   5
solvent-based direct writing techniques   94
solvent-based processes   94
spastic paraplegia   131
spine segments   128
squamous cell carcinoma of nose   150
Standard for Exchange of Product (STEP) model   170
standard triangular language (STL) format   180
starch and polycaprolactone (SPCL) polymer   34, 39, 41
– micromotif   40, 49
starch-based rapid prototyped
– SEM and μ-CT micrographs   45
starch-based scaffolds   46
– fibrous scaffold   34, 36, 38
state-of-the-art micro-FE methods   15
stereolithographic models   163
stereolithographic modelss   185
– 3D modeling   132
stereolithography   189
stereolithography apparatus (SLA)   2, 166
– model prosthesis   166
stereolithography format (STL)   123
storage modulus   44
– variation   45
Streptococcus sanguis   60
– scanning electron microscopy (SEM)   60
stress-strain curves   127
synthetic extracellular matrix   2

t

taphonomic changes   190
Tell Mashnaqa   185
tessellation process   1
thermal purging proces   118

three-dimensional (3D) fibrous structures, application   34
thresholding technique   170
titanium alloy   127
tomographic ultrasound imaging (TUI)   182
topological optimization methods   19
topology optimization algorithms   122
– designed microstructures   124
total muscle growth   131
tricalcium phosphate powder (TCP)   56, 62, 113, 117
T-score   26
tumor-related maxilla deformities   167, 173
two photon absorption process   105
two photon polymerization (2PP)   104, 107

u

ultrasound   11
umbilical blood flow   178
UV sensitive hybrid material   105
UV/vis spectrometer   118

v

vancomycin   114
– cumulative release   115
– deposition   115
Vetbond® Tissue Adhesive   84
Vickers hardness   126
volume of interest (VOI)   27

w

World Health Organization (WHO)   9

x

X-ray diffraction   105
X-ray photoelectron spectra   89
– peak deconvolution   87

y

Young's moduli   23, 30